Pediatric Telephone Triage Guidelines

Infant-Child (Birth to 6 Years)

A 5-Tier Approach
to Triaging Symptom Urgency

Sheila Wheeler

TeleTriage Systems Publishers

NOTICE TO THE READER

The authors and publisher have made every effort to provide accurate information. However, they are not responsible for errors, omissions, or for any outcomes related to the use of the contents of this book and take no responsibility for the use of the products and procedures described.

To the best of our knowledge, the dispositions in this book reflect safe practice; nevertheless, they cannot be considered absolute and universal recommendations. The authors and publisher disclaim any responsibility for any adverse effects resulting from any suggested home treatment, or from any undetected errors related to readers' misunderstanding of the text.

TeleTriage Systems Publishers
44 Madrone Avenue
San Anselmo, CA 94960
415.453.8382
teletriage@gmail. com

Printed in the United States of America

Library of Congress Cataloging in Publication Data

Wheeler, Sheila Q.

Pediatric Telephone Triage Guidelines - Infant-Child (Birth to 6 Years)
Includes bibliographical references and index

ISBN 0-9883212-1-1 ISBN 978-0-9883212-1-2

1. Pediatric emergencies 2. Triage (Medicine) 3. Telephone in medicine 4. Medical protocols.
(DNLM: 1. Triage-nurse's instruction 2. Triage- handbook 3. Pediatric Nursing-methods- handbooks. 4. Telemedicine. 5 Telephone. 6 Clinical protocols for Infants and Children

Dedicated to telenurses throughout the world and to the future of telephone triage and telehealth.

ACKNOWLEDGMENTS

To my friends and family for their belief in me, their moral support,
sense of humor, perspective and words of wisdom.

My deepest gratitude goes to my husband Richard, and my children, Joe and Kate
for their love, patience and encouragement
as I worked incessantly on this project.

A special thanks to Jeff Clawson, MD, and Vimla Patel, PhD,
for pioneering work that influenced this manual.

And many thanks to all Task Force members—
expert nurse reviewers and physicians-
who took pains to make this an excellent product.

Finally, a special thanks to Elsa Tsutaoka, MD
for her excellent and painstaking work as contributing author,
and to Cindy Lamendola, RN, NP,
for her invaluable contributions as expert reviewer.

Introduction to New Edition

The 2017 edition includes new research that supports the ongoing use of checklists (Gawande, 2009; Wachter 2015), prevention of root causes of error (Joint Commission), using a systems approach (Institute of Medicine), AAACN Practice Standards and Position Papers by the American College of Emergency Physicians and the Emergency Nurses Association.

New content includes: 5-Tier Triage Flow Chart for Telephone Triage, Standard Guideline, QA Audit, Standards and research on safety, root causes of error, and Five-Tier Triage. (IOM, 2011, IOM, Joint Commission, 2011, Donabedian, 2003, Patel, 1996, AAACN, 2012, ACEP & ENA, 2015).

Please note: This book was produced by scanning an earlier version. Imperfections in the format generated by the scanning process may be apparent. Also note: while the approach we have used since 1995 is bolstered by current research, symptom descriptions and supplemental home treatment information was last revised in 2009 and 2005 for the Adult and Pediatric versions respectively. Always have the medical director review any guidelines prior to implementation.

Customize this manual by placing pages in a binder with tabs for use as a base set. Add your facilities' preferences on colored sheets at the end of each guideline. "Growing your own" paper guidelines from scratch may take years to accomplish, may be more expensive than expected, and may not produce high quality results. Paper-based guidelines are economical; electronic algorithms can be extremely costly.

Structure and Process the guideline design is grounded in Medical Traditions of pattern recognition and is further supported by new safety trends, research and professional standards. This edition builds and expands upon previous editions in the following areas:

1. Nursing Process
2. Checklist (Gawande, 2009)
3. Avoidance of Root causes of error (Joint Commission)
4. 5-Tier Triage (ACEP & ENA (2015), Manchester Triage Group (2015))
5. AAACN Standards *(2011)*
6. QA Audit (2017)

NEW CONTENT 2017

"Triage represents a grey area between medicine and nursing, where medical diagnoses are not essential in order to make a decision about the appropriate interventions, and where the dimension of *urgency* become the primary focus of the reasoning process."(Lephrohon, Patel, 1995)

Like the Merck Manual, these guidelines are a reference. They have been "field tested" without incidence of errors, omissions or lawsuits since publication in 1995. In this edition, the five-tier triage approach has been refined and updated per standards set forth by the Manchester Triage Group, ACEP and ENA with improved Nomenclature (descriptions, definitions, examples) for clarity. Revisions to these guidelines include updated and enhanced design elements listed below:

- *Introduction & Afterword*
    - *Telephone Triage Flow Chart*
    - *Adult and Pediatric Master Guideline with Standards*
    - *QA Audit of Performance Standards based on AAACN standards*
    - Telephone Triage Position Papers: ACEP & ENA
    - *Call Center and Performance Standards*

PLEASE NOTE:

- Before using, please review carefully three major sections: Users Guide, Individual Guidelines and Appendices.
- *Due to the limitations in the production of the revised guidelines, we were unable to add page numbers.*
- Please refer to the Table of Contents to locate a given Guideline – listed alphabetically.
- The Appendices follow the Vomiting/Nausea Guideline and contains useful resources: i.e.Patient Brochure, QA Audit, 14-page Director of Hotlines and Websites for Support Groups. Please read the Afterword and CE course information as well.
- There will be occasional guideline formatting variability, due to changes in formats from the original design.
- Directory of Hotlines and Websites for Support Groups has not been revised, but it is a useful resource for web searches on a wide range of topics.
- *Clinical content* was revised per list below:
    i. *Adult: 2009*
    ii. *School-Age: 2005*
    iii. *Infant-Child: 2003*

Guideline Uses

These age-based guidelines integrate telephone triage Structure and Process for safe, timely telephone triage (appropriate outcomes) useable in several ways:

- *Multi-purpose* -- suitable for *both* telephone- *and* face-to-face on-site triage (in office, ED, health center or clinic settings)
- *Paper References* as a standalone reference or adjunct to electronic guidelines.

The Master Guideline contains general descriptions of a range of conditions with 5-Tier Triage time frames and access sites for timely dispositions. It can serve as a:

- Contingency policy or *"Fall Back"* for the "out of protocol experience" -- when no guideline seems to fit the patient symptoms.
- Pre-emptive policy or *"Go-to"* guideline *before* selecting a specific guideline
- The Master Guideline may be also viewed as an orientation tool for new practitioners to review current Policies and Procedures of your facility.

Please note: **Design and methodology** described in the Afterword section at the end of the manual. Please read this section, and the User's Guide before using the guidelines.

Customize the guidelines, by placing them in a binder with Alphabetical Tabs (45). Add your own facilities' policies, procedures and additional guidelines on colored paper after each tab.

Resources

- **For Telehealth Update CE Course**, please see the last pages of this manual
- **Preceptor Workbook with Answer key** (200-page) please see last pages of this manual

FOREWORD

More than 20 years ago, I earned a certificate as a nurse practitioner in adult medicine and began to practice in a staff-model HMO. There were several nurse practitioners working there, and one day a week each of us took a turn doing telephone triage. Telephone triage was a newly coined phrase at that time, and we understood it to mean assessing patients' needs for health care over the telephone. Generally, these were patients with immediate health problems who were calling the HMO for same-day care. We nurse practitioners would assess their symptoms and either bring them in for appointments or provide home-care treatment advice. We had some written standing orders for treating minor infectious conditions, but otherwise we relied upon our experience as registered nurses and training as nurse practitioners to assess the patients and provide appropriate advice.

Since that time, I have worked in other managed care group practice settings and have set up and administered several triage systems. Telephone triage has evolved into telephone nursing practice, and many large organizations now have very sophisticated call centers staffed by registered nurses equipped with telephone headsets and the latest computer technology. Health care in almost all settings—acute care, home health, outpatient clinics, and physicians' offices—is enhanced by the telephone. Patients call to seek advice or urgent care appointments, and as more care is delivered in outpatient settings, nurses and other health care providers call patients to follow up on procedures and treatment plans.

However, there is a significant problem with this scenario. Nurses and other providers do not automatically have the knowledge and skills to effectively assess and provide advice to patients on the other end of a telephone. Our education and experience primarily prepare us to assess patients by using several senses, including hearing, seeing, and touching. In telephone practice we can only listen to a patient's verbal description of what is going on. We cannot even fully use our sense of hearing to measure a blood pressure or detect an abnormal lung sound. Instead we must rely upon what a patient says and how it is said. What the patient says is in large part dependent upon the questions we ask and how we ask them. Professional nurses and other providers may possess the judgment skills to accurately assess the information provided by a patient over the telephone, but do we know what questions to ask to obtain the essential information? And other than "Come in and see the doctor this afternoon," do we know what advice to provide the patient in managing the problem?

For the past 12 years, Sheila Quilter Wheeler has devoted her professional career to telephone practice. She has developed highly acclaimed workshops in telephone practice, and in 1993 she published the classic text *Telephone Triage: Theory, Practice, and Protocol Development* (Delmar Publishers). This book contains detailed information about the methods of high quality telephone practice, linking these to the nursing process framework which is fundamental to all of nursing practice. Also, there is extensive direction provided in how to design and develop written protocols to guide the practitioner. I was very impressed with the excellent information in this initial publication, and I wished Ms. Wheeler had gone further to provide her students and readers with the actual protocols.

My wish has now been granted! These three volumes entitled *Telephone Triage Protocols for Pediatric and Adult Populations* surpass all my expectations. These volumes contain extensive, clearly written protocols for all commonly encountered health problems for infants, children, and adults. These protocols are brief, yet detailed enough to guide the health care professional through specific pathways to accurately assess the problem and provide appropriate advice. Essential supplementary pages are provided for many of the protocols, providing highly useful information for patient teaching. The protocols and teaching guidelines are all written in layman's language at the fifth- to eighth-grade levels to help ensure effective communication between the patient and the health care professional.

Other excellent features of these volumes include Ms. Wheeler's superb instructions about the telephone triage process and how to use the protocols. The books are well-organized, and formatted to allow the user to write in specific treatments or patient instructions, and yearly updates from the publisher can easily be inserted. The appendixes are particularly useful, including additional information about certain illnesses and problems, as well as instructions about working with caregivers and patients with special needs.

These days nurses and other health care professionals increasingly need expert knowledge and skills to provide high-quality patient care. Most of us feel we cannot work any harder, and we're looking rather desperately for ways to "work smarter." Using the telephone to assess patients' health care needs and guide them to the appropriate avenue of care, whether that be a visit to a health care provider, or self-care delivered at home or work, is an essential element of today's cost-effective health care delivery system. These comprehensive volumes provide the health care professionals who provide services via the telephone with the support they need to deliver excellent care to their patients. The nursing and medical managers who work in settings where telephone practice is part of their care delivery can stop the incredibly labor-intensive process of developing and revising "home grown" telephone practice protocols. Sheila Wheeler and her team of experts have done the work for us, and through the Quality Improvement and Utilization Satisfaction sheets that are included in each volume, we can participate in improving and updating these protocols for the future.

As I mentioned earlier, telephone practice has come a long way in the past 20 years. The publication of these meticulous and beautifully designed protocols is another milestone in this arena. Sometimes in these days of rapid and tumultuous change, we health care professionals feel like the quality that results from attention to detail has been lost. I believe we have regained some of this with these volumes.

Jo Ann Appleyard, PhD, RN
President
American Academy of Ambulatory Care Nursing
Pitman, New Jersey

TASK FORCE MEMBERS

Laura Wachter Alexander, RN, BSN, IBCLC
Lactation Consultant and Prenatal Instructor
California Pacific Medical Center
San Francisco, California

Stacy Bischoff, RN, NP
Women's Health Care Nurse Practitioner
ATM A Group
San Rafael, California

Patricia A. Crane, MSN, RNC, NP
Forensic Nurse Consultant
Sexual Assault Nurse Examiner
San Jose, California

Ariadne Endress, RN, NP
OB/Gyn Nurse Practitioner
Marin County, California

Carmen Eribes, RN, MS
Department of Community Health, Mental Health, and Administrative Nursing
University of California, San Francisco
San Francisco, California

Jeff Howell, RN, CEN
Private Practitioner, Emergency Department
California Pacific Medical Center
San Francisco, California

Russ J. Kino, MD
Director, Emergency Services
Saint John's Hospital and Health Center
Santa Monica, California

Donna Kuester, RN C, BSN
Assistant Head Nurse, Eye and ENT Units
Santa Clara Valley Medical Center
San Jose, California

Joan Marks, BSN, NP
Private Practice
Greenbrae, California

Edna McCready, RN, BSN
Ambulatory Services Quality Improvement/Risk Management Department
Chaboya Medical Clinic
California

Jean Berg Meddaugh, RN
Manager
East Valley Clinic
Santa Clara Valley Medical Center
San Jose, California

Suellen Miller, RN, CNM, MIIA, PhD
University of California Berkeley School of Public Health
Berkeley, California

Robert H. Pantell, MD
Chief, General Pediatrics Division
Professor of Pediatrics
University of California, San Francisco
San Francisco, California

Susan A. Perlman, RN, BSN
San Francisco, California

Edwin Cary Pigman, MD
Assistant Professor of Emergency Medicine
George Washington University Medical Center
Washington, DC

Deborah Qiiilter
Author, Consultant
Beyond Ergonomics
New York, New York

Bertha A. Ruiz, DNSc, RN, GNP, CS
Gerontological Nurse Practitioner
San Francisco, California

Elizabeth San Luis, MSN, PNP
Ambulatory Care Center
University of California Medical Center
San Francisco, California

Mary Scheib, RN, BSN
San Francisco General Hospital
San Francisco, California

Sally Thresher, MSN, NP
Clinical Nurse Specialist
San Francisco Youth Guidance Center
San Francisco, California

Susan Valeriote, RN, CPNP, MS
Pediatric Nurse Practitioner
San Francisco, California

Amalia L. Velez, RN
Triage/Advice Nurse
Santa Clara Valley Medical Center, South Valley Medical Clinic
San Martin, California

Sheila Quilter Wheeler, RN, MS
President
TeleTriage Systems
San Anselmo, California

Catherine Zappel, RN
Urgent Care Department
Santa Clara Valley Medical Center
Santa Clara, California

PROTOCOL DIRECTORY

User's Guide & Operating Standards

Master Guideline

Abdomen Problem:

1. (Upper & Generalized): Pain w or w/o Trauma
2. (Lower): Pain w or w/o Trauma
   Abdomen Problem Supplemental Information

Abuse:

Abuse 1 (Sexual) Reporting Tree

Abuse 1 (Sexual) Supplemental Information

Abuse 2 (Physical) Supplemental Information

Back Problem (Upper & Lower): Pain w or w/o Trauma

Back Problem Supplemental Information

Behavioral Problem Supplemental Information (School-Age Children manual; Infants and Children manual)

Bites (Skin Problem 1):

1. (Human/Animal): Human; Cat; Dog; Bat; Horse; Squirrel; Skunk; Raccoon; Fox
2. Snake; Jellyfish; Sea Urchin; Stingray
3. Bee Stings, Yellow Jacket, Hornet, Wasp; Spiders, Scorpions; Fleas; Ticks
   Bites (Skin Problem 1) Supplemental Information

Bowel Problem:

1. Diarrhea (Severe/Moderate/Mild); Bloody Stool
2. Constipation; Stool Color Change
   Bowel Problem Supplemental Information

Breast Problem: (Adults manual; School-Age Children manual) • See Women's Health section

1. Female (Non Pregnant, Non Postpartum): Pain w or w/o Trauma; Discharge; Lump; Lesions
2. Male: Pain w or w/o Trauma; Discharge; Lump; Lesions
   Breast Problem (Male/Female) Supplemental Information

Breastfeeding Problem: Pain w or w/o Fever; Sore Nipples; Painful Breasts • See Women's Health section

Breastfeeding Initial Assessment Questions

Breastfeeding Problem Supplemental Information

Burn (Skin Problem 2):

1. Thermal; Chemical; Electrical
2. Radiation (Sunburn)
   Bum (Skin Problem 2) Supplemental Information

Chest Pain: Pain w or w/o Trauma

Chest Pain Supplemental Information

Cold Exposure: Hypothermia; Frostbite

Cold Exposure Supplemental Information

Confusion: Sudden; Chronic

Confusion Supplemental Information

Dizziness: W or w/o Trauma

Fainting

Dizziness; Fainting Supplemental Information

Ear:

1. Pain w Trauma; FB; Hearing Loss; Ringing; Earlobe Trauma
2. Pain w/o Trauma; Discharge; Congestion; Earlobe Swelling
   Ear Supplemental Information

Emotional Problem: (Adult manual; School-Age Children manual)

1. Suicide in Progress; Threat; Ideation
   Suicide Supplemental Information
2. Panic; Depression; Anxiety; Agitation; Aggression; Withdrawal; Hallucination
   Emotional Problem Supplemental Information

Extremities:

Upper: Pain w or w/o Trauma; Swelling; Lacerations; Fractures

Lower 1: Pain w Trauma; Swelling; Lacerations; Fractures

Lower 2: Pain w/o Trauma; Swelling; Weakness/Non Use; Limp

Extremities (Upper & Lower) Supplemental Information

Eye:

1. Pain w Trauma; Bum; FB; Vision Changes; Blood In
2. Pain w/o Trauma; Photophobia; Blood In; Discharge; Swelling; Vision Changes
   Eye Supplemental Information

Face/Jaw: Pain w or w/o Trauma; Swelling; Weakness

Face/Jaw Supplemental Information

Fever: Fever w Assoc. Symptoms

Fever Supplemental Information

Temperature Taking Instructions Supplemental Information

Head Problem:

1. Pain; Laceration; Level of Consciousness Change w Trauma

2. Pain; Level of Consciousness Change w/o Trauma
Head Problem Supplemental Information

Heat Exposure: Heat Stroke; Heat Exhaustion; Heat Cramps

Heat Exposure Supplemental Information

Joint Problem (Upper & Lower): Pain w or w/o Trauma; Swelling (Shoulder, Elbow, Wrist, Hip, Knee, Ankle); Limp (See also Extremities, Upper/Lower)

Joint Problem Supplemental Information

Lip/Mouth; Teeth/Gums; Tongue: Pain w or w/o Trauma; Swelling; Laceration; Lesions

Lip/Mouth; Teeth/Gums; Tongue Supplemental Information

Neck Problem: Pain w or w/o Trauma; Swelling; Lumps

Neck Problem Supplemental Information

Newborn Concerns Supplemental Information (Infants and Children manual)

Nose/Sinus Problem: Pain w or w/o Trauma; FB; Bleeding; Discharge; Congestion

Nose/Sinus Problem Supplemental Information

Penile/Scrotal/Testicle Problem: Trauma; FB; Pain; Discharge; Lumps; Lesions

Penile/Scrotal/Testicle Problem Supplemental Information

Penile Problem: STD Supplemental Information

Postpartum Problem (Adults manual; School-Age Children manual) • See Women's Health section: Leg Pain; Painful Urination; Incisional Pain; Fever; Bleeding; SOB; Diarrhea; N/V; Abd. Pain

Postpartum Concerns Supplemental Information

Postpartum Emotional Problem Supplemental Information

Pregnancy Problems: (Adults manual; School-Age Children manual) • See Women's Health section

High Risk Pregnancy Initial Assessment Questions

1. Labor; Abdominal Pain; Vaginal Discharge; Vaginal Bleeding
2. Trauma; Headache; Chest Pain; < Fetal Movement; N/V; Swelling; Burning on Urination; Itching
   Pregnancy Concerns Supplemental Information

Rectal Problem: Pain w or w/o Trauma; FB; Bleeding; Itching; Discharge; Lesion

Rectal Problem Supplemental Information

Respiratory Problem:

1. Breathing Problem/Cough: Respiratory Distress; Choking; SOB; Stridor: w or w/o Trauma
2. Throat: Choking; FB/Trauma; Pain; Bum: Chemical/Thermal
   Respiratory Problem Supplemental Information

Seizures: W or w/o Trauma

Shock: Distributive; Cardiogenic; Hypovolemic

Skin Problem:

Bites: See Bites (Skin Problem 1)

Bum: See Bum (Skin Problem 2)

3. Discoloration: Bruise; Yellow; All Color Changes
   Skin Problem 3 (Discoloration) Supplemental Information

4. Laceration/Wound: Amputations; Major & Minor Lacerations; Abrasions; Puncture Wounds
   Skin Problem 4 (Laceration/Wound) Supplemental Information

5. Lesion/Lump/Swelling: W or w/o Trauma
   Skin Problem 5 (Lesion/Lump/Swelling) Supplemental Information

6. Rashes; Childhood Rashes: W or w/o Itching
   Skin Problem 6 (Rashes; Childhood Rashes) Supplemental Information

Substance Abuse: (Adults manual; School-Age Children manual)

Substance Abuse Supplemental Information

Urinary Problem: Pain w or w/o Trauma; Frequency; Urgency; Discharge; Output/Color

Changes; Blood in

Urinary Problem Supplemental Information

Vaginal Bleeding (Non-Pregnant) • See Women's Health section: Abnormal Bleeding: Painful, Irregular, Excessive;

Absence of Menses

Vaginal Bleeding (Non-Pregnant) Supplemental Information

Vaginal Problem (Non-Pregnant) • See Women's Health section: FB; Trauma; Discharge; Pain; Lesion; Itching; STD

Exposure

OB/GYN Procedures

Vaginal Problem: STD Supplemental Information Vomiting/

Nausea: w or w/o Diarrhea; Headache; Abdominal Pain

Vomiting/Nausea Supplemental Information

Questions\

Women's Health

USER'S GUIDE AND OPERATING STANDARDS

Notice to the User

- Medical Approval: The protocols should be reviewed and approved by the Medical Director prior to implementation.
- User Qualifications: These guidelines were designed to be used by experienced RNs with formal training in telephone triage.
- Training Program: For optimal results and optimal risk management, Sheila Wheeler provides a comprehensive on-site or home study training program in Practice and Protocol Competency.

For more information about home study programs, conferences, consultation, content licensing, medical call center referral, medical-legal services, please visit: ~~www.teletriage.com~~.

About Telephone Triage

What Does Research Reveal about RN Decision Making?

Telephone triage—the safe, effective, appropriate disposition of health-related problems by RNs—always involves "decision making under conditions of uncertainty and urgency" (Lephrohon and Patel 1995). It involves "Uncertainty" because decisions are often made based on partial or inaccurate information; "urgency" because calls must be processed within a brief time frame—usually 6-10 min average. In new research, telephone triage has been compared to the work of air traffic controllers, EMDs, and firefighters—all high-stake activities. Vimla Patel, PhD, described how a group of RNs working in an emergency department setting made "real world" decisions in telephone triage. She discovered that these nurses used pattern recognition, rules of thumb, and context as major strategies to make decisions.

How Does This Research Relate to These Protocols?

The research on nurse decision making by Patel (Lephrohon and Patel 1995) and other experts has important implications for protocol design and for these Protocols in particular. The strategies of pat- tern recognition, rules of thumb, and context have been incorporated into all elements of this system— training, Protocols, and forms. The goal of this design is to mimic how the brain naturally solves problems in "real world" situations.

Because patients are complex and symptom presentations often ill-structured, novel, variable, and unique, one needs a system that is correspondingly complex yet flexible, attuned to symptoms' nuances and subtleties while at the same time providing firm support for decision making. Protocols based on a pattern-recognition approach have these qualities. Furthermore, because telephone triage is a high-stakes activity, a well-integrated *system* is needed to manage the uncertainty and urgency. That system (an inter- dependent group of items forming a whole and serving a common purpose) should be operated by a pro- fessional. Thus, the designers of these Protocols intend them to be used by RNs with decision-making experience.

If Protocols Are Well-Developed and Comprehensive, Why Must RNs Manage the Calls?

While Protocols are an important component of the telephone triage system, the bottom line is the experienced, well-trained RN. Current standards of practice stress the use of the RN. Protocols alone cannot guarantee safe practice.

Don't Protocols Take the Place of Training?

This is an area of confusion and controversy. Managers should be aware of the risks of relying on Pro- tocols to take the place of formal instruction. Overreliance on the tool can lead to mistriage. Training in the principles and skills of history taking, communications, assessment, disposition, and decision mak- ing is the foundation, followed by an orientation to the Protocols. Potential problems and misunder- standings can be averted through instruction in the correct and safe operation of the Protocols and documentation form. It will also address "protocol bias" that develops when RNs who have been using one type of protocol must become acquainted with a new one.

In order to determine the right disposition, the nurse must go through a decision-making process, the task being to create context or build a picture or pattern. Linked to this concept is that of "drilling down" to excavate the information. The process, then, is to ask *enough* of the *right questions,* in the *right way* to elicit *enough* of the *right data,* and to choose the *right Protocol(s)* and *right disposition.* This process will be outlined in detail in the pages that follow. The first step often begins with a cursory or global approach.

► Assessment Strategies

A Global Approach

How Many Questions Must I Ask?

How far the RN must "drill down" to finally reach a decision is uniquely determined by the acuity of symptoms and the patient presenting them. Some problems require more in-depth questioning and RNs will pursue data collection to different degrees—sometimes referred to as "skimming" or "sleuthing." There are times to do both. For example, in the case of chest pain, most nurses quickly elicit the large chunks of information "skimming" before making a decision. In other cases, such as vague abdominal pain, the RN may spend more time and gather larger quantities of detailed information—"sleuthing." Problems arise when some protocol designs (or professionals) treat problems superficially and fail to drill down far enough. These protocols are designed to enable the RN to drill down as far as the instance requires—yet allow for quick skimming as well. The four acronyms summarized below (SAVED, SCHOLAR, PAMPER, and ADL) are described in detail in *Telephone Triage: Theory, Practice and Protocol Development* (Wheeler 1993).

How Can I Quickly Assess and Prioritize Problems?

The telephone triage process usually begins with a broad, global assessment. Most nurses quickly build a picture through gathering information about the patient's age, gender, chief complaint, literacy or language level, emotional state (determined via the words, tone, pacing of voice), and sometimes previous medical history. This key contextual information can quickly identify high-risk patients or situations. This process, while appearing superficial, yields key chunks of information and may take as little as 60 sec.

Broad categories of high-risk patients and symptoms are signified by the acronym "SAVED" standing for: *severe, strange,* or *suspicious symptoms, age, veracity* problems, *emotional* distress, *debilitation,* and *distance.* These "red flags" are loaded with information. Identifying high-risk status aids in prioritizing and helps to "defend" dispositions, facilitating decisions regarding upgrading and disposition time frames. Red flags help all practitioners to function more effectively. Listed below are examples of each category:

Severe, Strange, or Suspicious Symptoms

Patel (Lephrohon and Patel 1995) notes that "it is easier to identify an emergency than to rule one out." Severe pain ("9 on a scale of 10"), severe bleeding (spurting, bright red), or severe trauma (falls from a height of over 15 ft) are conditions that the average layperson could identify as urgent.

Strange symptoms include ill-structured, vague, atypical, or unusual presentations, symptoms that only astute professionals might recognize as urgent. Falling into this category are sudden, unexpected, or new symptoms, recurrent symptoms, or a marked change in the patient's condition.

Suspicious symptoms include the "big six": head, abdomen, chest, respiratory, dizziness, and "flu." These symptoms always require thorough investigation by a professional, primarily because they are often associated with underdiagnosed conditions such as ectopic pregnancy, MI, or appendicitis—all serious diagnoses. Suspicious symptoms also apply to any situation where the nurse has a "gut feeling" or a "hunch about a problem." If the nurse is uncomfortable with the Protocol disposition, he or she may upgrade a problem or bring the patient in sooner. When red flags of suspicion are raised, nurses are encouraged to use their intuition.

Age

Age is one of the most important pieces of data obtained. The very young, the very old, and women of childbearing age are always considered high-risk patients. Premature infants and those under 3 mo are typically considered at highest risk. The "frail elderly"—anyone over 75 yr of age, suffering from multiple or chronic diseases, functional disability, or psychosocial problems—must always be treated with extreme care. The childbearing years, always a high-risk period, now extend from age 11 into the 60s! In regard to chest pain, the latest research demonstrates that women over age 50 have the same risks of cardiac disease as men over age 35.

Veracity

Veracity refers to the ability to reproduce the facts of the situation accurately. Obstacles to data-gathering arise whenever there are second-party calls, low-literacy callers, language barriers, extremely young or very inexperienced mothers, or a caretaker unfamiliar with the patient.

Emotional Status (Caretaker and/or Patient)

Nurses can pick up many cues through careful attention to the words as well as the tone and pacing of the caller's voice. There may be hysteria or denial or inappropriate affect in parent or caretaker with a history of psychiatric problems or substance abuse. Anxiety is always a red flag. Frequent calls in a short period of time can be an indicator of both caller anxiety and problem acuity.

Debilitation

In general, debilitation refers to chronic illness. Chronic illness may include but is not limited to the following:

- All Populations: AIDS, asthma, diabetes, sickle cell, low-income homeless
- Frail Elderly: Cardiac problems, COPD, dementia
- All Immunocompromised: Lack of adequate immunizations, chemotherapy, HIV, splenectomy, steroid therapy/chronic, transplants, nephrotic syndrome
- Pediatric Populations: Congenital heart disease, cystic fibrosis, spina bifida, hydrocephalus, prematurity with secondary complications

Distance

Distance can become an important factor when (1) the parent/caretaker is calling from a remote location several hours from hospital; (2) in an urgent situation, the patient is unable to arrive by car within 1 hr owing to traffic or lack of available car; and (3) the patient must take public transportation that is sporadic or nonexistent after certain hours at night. Ail of these situations heighten the need for reliable, prompt, safe transportation.

After performing a global assessment, the nurse may quickly discover an emergent situation, abbreviating the assessment process and necessitating paramedic transport. However, in most cases, the call requires more sleuthing.

History Taking: Assessing the Problem and Patient

What Is the Key Information to Elicit about the Chief Complaint?

To elicit key information about most symptoms (SCHOLAR), ask the following questions:

Symptoms and associated symptoms

Characteristics

History of complaint in past

Onset of symptoms

Location of symptoms

Aggravating factors

Relieving factors

What Is the Key Information to Elicit about the Patient?

Sometimes getting a brief patient history is helpful. This "snapshot" provides additional context, sometimes necessary to make the correct decision. The acronym "PAMPER" is summarized below:

- Pregnancy/breastfeeding
- Allergies
- Medications
- Previous chronic illness
- Emotional stress
- Recent injury, illness, ingestion

How Does One Assess Elderly or Poor Historians?

With, some elderly, and poor historians, it is difficult to get adequate information for two major reasons: (1) the patient is a poor historian and/or (2) the patient has vague or ill-structured symptoms. In both cases, the acronyms SCHOLAR and PAMPER may not be applicable. Use activities of daily living (ADL) to elicit and compare the client's current state with their baseline state. With children and the elderly especially, these indicators of current health or illness may help paint the clearest picture, when symptoms are often vague, ill-structured, or absent. *Marked changes* in any of these indicators can be a red flag:

- *INTAKE*
- Eating
- Drinking
- *OUTPUT*
- Elimination (urine, BM, emesis)
- *ACTIVITY*
- Work/play/daily routine
- Sleep pattern
- Appearance
- Skin color
- Mood

The above lists may be duplicated and hung on the wall by the phone for quick reference. Complete descriptions of each of the acronyms may be found in *Telephone Triage: Theory, Practice and Protocol Development* (Wheeler 1993) (available at www.teletriage.coml.

▶ Decision-Making Strategies

Rules of Thumb for Age-Based Populations

Rules of Thumb is another strategy that forms the foundation for managing calls from high-risk groups. These strategies are derived from years of experience and often operate at an intuitive level. Several of the rules of thumb below are based on ACEP policies as well. The examples below are divided into those that apply to all ages followed by age-based rules specific to adult, adolescent, and child populations.

AH Ages

All severe pain should be seen urgently.

Trauma: Always be alert to unwitnessed accidents and to mechanism of injury (major trauma: MV A, falls > 15 ft, blunt trauma). Assess and investigate completely. Caretakers' assessments may be faulty or they may focus on a problem that is minor (e.g., avulsed tooth) and miss a more serious one (e.g., head injury).

Several calls in a short period of time (several hours) without ability to describe seriousness of patient's symptoms may be an indicator of acuity.

Beware of the developing disease: what starts out as vague abdominal pain with low-grade fever may, over several hours or days, develop into appendicitis.

Self-limiting symptoms existing > 1 wk but not becoming markedly worse can be treated at home with optimal appointment in 24+ hr.

Age is a major factor in many Rules of Thumb. In fact, age alone (and especially extremes of age) can markedly influence the level of risk—owing to certain illnesses as well as greater vulnerability because of communication barriers or dependency on caretakers, as illustrated below:

Adolescent Populations

Assess all children with unexplained symptoms for possible unintentional or purposeful ingestion/exposure to toxins, inhalants, street or prescription drugs.

Teenagers are especially vulnerable to depression and suicide (and rarely, homicide) because of several factors: easy access to alcohol and drugs, increased sexual activity, complex societal demands, negative role models, and increased family disruptions. The precipitating factor is usually a loss—betrayal of a trust, romantic breakup, failure in school or sports, move to a new neighborhood, peer pressures, conflict regarding dependence and independence, poverty, unwanted pregnancy, sexual problems, peer- or media-emphasized suicide, treatment for mental illness, and/or any legal problems.

Elderly Populations

Symptoms in the elderly may be atypical, silent, or late (e.g., the patient may feel fatigue as only symptom of pneumonia).

Assess all elderly patients for dehydration status (as appropriate).

Elderly populations are at greater risk for hypothermia and hyperthermia.

Assess all elderly with unexplained symptoms for adverse drug reaction (ADRs), "chemical restraints," or possible ingestion—intentional or accidental. Exposures may be caused by toxins, alcohol, or overmedication with prescription or OTC medications.

The elderly are at risk for ADRs. The greater the number of drugs the patient uses, the greater the incidence of ADRs. As the number of daily doses increases, compliance decreases.

Elderly patients may be poor or forgetful historians. Err on the side of caution.

▶ Protocol Design Features

Design Philosophy

These protocols are unique in both organization and content. The authors included everything that advice nurses might want in a triage and advice tool, and tried to avoid too many "bells and whistles." If the nurse thoroughly understands the design, it will not only enhance his/her practice but also expedite calls. The goal is to create a tool that is neither overly simplistic nor treat problems superficially, and yet not so complicated that it proves too cumbersome to use. The Protocols are simple enough to be user-friendly and yet comprehensive enough to provide constant support for the decision maker.

Decision Support versus Decision Making

According to one definition, computer systems may be one of two types: decision making or decision support. *Decision-making* systems are expert systems that allow an unqualified person to "make a decision that is beyond his/her level of training and experience." On the other hand, *decision-support* systems are expert systems that remind an experienced decision maker of options or issues to consider that she/he once knew but may have forgotten. These protocols are based on a *decision-support* approach.

Quick Reference

In the style of *The Merck Manual,* these Protocols are designed to be a "quick reference." However, that is where the similarities end. This manual is a working tool—to be consulted constantly rather than infrequently. Unlike *The Merck Manual,* the disease descriptions contained herein are highly distilled, organized by acuity level, and contain disposition, home treatment, referral, and teaching sections.

Symptoms Patterns

Each Protocol presents an array of descriptions of commonly encountered conditions or diseases—"classic pictures." In order to be most useful to the user, these descriptions are comprehensive rather than minimalistic. They are often described as a progression, from beginning symptoms to "full-blown" condition.

The rationale for this is the rule of thumb to "beware the developing disease." This information can be passed on to patients when instructing them about symptoms to watch for as indicators of worsening conditions.

Concise but Complete

According to some experts, patients call with a limited number of problems. The authors found that about 50 protocols cover 95% of all callers' problems. Since each protocol includes about 20 possible diagnoses, the 45-50 Protocols in this manual address over 1000 possible conditions.

Anatomical Site-Based Titles

The Protocols match "real world" wording and presentation as much as possible; patients usually describe symptoms in relation to location or site on the body. For example, "I have—a *headache,"* "—a swollen *ankle,* " "—an *eye* discharge," "— an earache." In addition, the anatomical site-based approach is very visual. Starting with the location of the problem on the body (e.g., Eye Problem) is a major chunk of context and makes sense in a pattern-matching approach. The next step would be to narrow it down further (or flesh it out more) to the particulars (e.g., Eye Problem: trauma, discharge, blood in, vision difficulties, pain, etc.).

While an anatomical site-based approach might resemble a "systems approach" (Urinary to GU; Abdomen to GI; Chest to Cardiology), it is different. Rely on the caller's description of the site and symptoms at first.

With a strict symptom-based approach, difficulties arise when people (Protocol designers and/or nurse and patient) can't agree on the best words to use for symptoms (e.g., "ear ringing" or *"ringing* in ears"; "*belching*" or *"gas"; "hives" or "rash"; "stomach* ache," *"pain* in stomach," or "abdominal pain"). Using a variety of lay terms for symptoms, even when listed alphabetically, predictably results in confusing, time-consuming searches for the nurse.

Unique Features

Age-Based Protocols and Content

Protocols such as Breastfeeding, Bums, Bites, and others apply to all ages. Within all Protocols, you will also find certain age-specific information. Thus, age is listed when it has significant bearing on a certain disease or condition.

Women's Health Section

Women's Health Protocols are now in a separate section.

Key Assessment Tools

The Master Protocol and Pain Assessment provide unique support when no Protocol applies, and to elicit more detail about pain, respectively . They are meant to be consulted frequently . Pain is a common presenting symptom; monitoring and measuring pain—the fifth vital sign—is now a standard.

Community Alert

This is a new feature, designed to enhance RN sensitivity and awareness of the influence of community-based events (such as Super Bowl Sunday) and environmental factors (heat waves and cold snaps) that can increase the incidence of problems such as domestic violence and heat-and cold-related illness, respectively. Telephone triage nurses and call centers, often the first point of contact, have the capability to serve as "early warning systems," to notify providers and local EDs, when call volume related to these problems increases.

Content

Most Protocols are written in conversational, "cook-book" style, and in lay language at fifth- to eighth-grade level. This feature facilitates communication with all callers, especially low-literacy callers. The information is intended to be read to the patient as needed. This saves time by eliminating the extra step of translating symptom descriptions and instructions for home treatment, first aid, or self-assessment from college level to fifth-grade level language.

Protocol Length

The original goal was to develop the Protocols to one page in length. However, many Protocols are divided into two parts (e.g., Ear Problem 1, Ear Problem 2). As a general rule, Protocols with "1" in the title (e.g., Ear Problem 1) include trauma, whereas those with "2" in the title do not. If there is no number in the title, there is only one Protocol, and all symptoms, including trauma and nonacute, will be in that Protocol. Most Protocols have an accompanying Supplemental Information which must be consulted when using the Protocol. In some cases (as with Menopause) there is a Supplemental Information but no Protocol chart.

Initial Assessment Questions (IAQs)

Breastfeeding and Pregnancy Problems have Initial Assessment Questions. This section must be consulted prior to using the Protocol, in order to identify or rule out risk factors, as well as Toxicity or Dehydration in the infants of mothers calling with breastfeeding problems.

Flexible Disposition Time Frames

All Protocols have three standard disposition time frames (Emergent, Urgent, and Acute/Nonacute). These time frames overlap slightly and are intended as flexible limits within which the RN can operate. The site of the patient visit may vary according to what is accessible. For example, lack of access to office visits on weekends, holidays, and after hours means the patient who needs a same-day appointment must be seen in the ED or Urgent Care.

Format Variations: Atypical Format

Some Protocols do not follow the standard format and are atypical. The Abuse 1 (Sexual) Reporting Tree is atypical and the only example of its kind. Fainting, Seizures, and Shock Protocols include First Aid as well as causes and descriptions for RN reference.

Diagnosis "Lumping"

In an effort to be consistent in descriptions of medical problems, the Task Force tried to keep each complex of symptoms for a particular diagnosis separate. However, in many cases symptom complexes are so similar that the diagnoses are "lumped" together. In these cases, the disposition was usually upgraded to the higher level of acuity—to err on the side of caution.

Recurring Standard Topics

While there are specific Protocols for Abuse and Fever, these topics are also standard items found in nearly every Protocol. There is no specific Protocol for Ingestion, however. Ingestion may go undetected. Therefore, it too is found in Supplemental Information, in the section entitled "Drug Side Effect". Ingestion also appears on the Documentation Form under "Recent Ingestion" as reminder to explore unexplained symptoms in adults, adolescents or elderly clients.

"Problems" and "Concerns"

Throughout the Protocols, "Problems" and "Concerns" have been differentiated: Problems are defined as acute symptoms and are covered in the triage chart. Concerns are defined as nonacute symptoms or informational issues, covered in the Supplemental Information sections as in Birth Control and Menopause, Pregnancy and Postpartum Concerns.

Abuse 1: Sexual

The Abuse Reporting Tree is in an algorithmic format unlike any other Protocol. This algorithm or decision tree takes the place of the Protocol. Establish first if there is major trauma or if assailant is nearby. When major trauma is ruled out, the next priority is to preserve evidence. See Instructions for Preserving Evidence in the Supplemental Information section. Abuse 2: Physical covers adult and teen domestic violence, and elder abuse.

Bowel Problem

Bowel Problem is primarily concerned with symptoms related to bowel movements—diarrhea, constipation, etc.

Breastfeeding Problem

Breastfeeding Problem has IAQs. Please refer to IAQs prior to using the Protocol. Since there are *two* patients involved in the Breastfeeding Problem, assess *both* the mother and infant. (See also Postpartum Emotional Problem.)

Confusion

Confusion in adults and children is always a serious symptom. In the elderly especially, remain alert to the possibility of accidental or intentional overdose, overmedication (chemical restraints) or polypharmacy. With adolescents, suspect accidental ingestion as well as intentional ingestion (suicide attempt) in teen and young adult population.

Fever

Fever is atypical because in order to follow the standard format and to keep it a manageable length, it was necessary to "punt" to other Protocols.

Rectal Problem

Rectal problem only addresses problems of the rectum: Pain with or without trauma, foreign body, bleeding in very small amounts, itching, and lesions. Diarrhea/constipation are covered under Bowel Problem. An exception to the rule is the reference to "large amount of rectal bleeding," which is covered.

► A Tour of Protocol Elements

Detailed descriptions correspond to examples in the sample Protocol on the following pages.

Item	Description/Purpose
1. Title and Subtitle	Subtitles indicate key symptoms in Protocol left-hand column.
2. Key Symptoms Assessment	Symptoms presented by patient must match one of these words in order to move into center column questions (Acuity Level).
3. Symptom Pattems/Associated Symptoms	[Preceded by *plus* (+).] If patient describes one symptom (usually very severe) or more (several lesser symptoms) that match the symptom patterns move, to the disposition box in the right-hand column, and follow the instructions.
4. Considerations/Diagnoses	[Possible diagnoses in *parentheses* ()•] *The advice nurse must never document or verbalize to the caller the diagnosis found within the parentheses; they are for the RN's information and reference only.*
5. Disposition/Advice	The Disposition/Advice column is composed of two parts: the Disposition and the Protocol Advice; always advise the patient of the disposition—when and where to come for treatment; the site of care may vary depending upon the hour and day of the call. For some acute problems when care within 8-24 hr is not feasible, after hours, patients may need to be seen in the ED. Please see Disposition Options for details of how to use this section.
6. Cross-References	(If applicable, at the end of the Protocol, in the Assessment column). This section is designed to provide users with other possible Protocol choices; specific cross-references are also found throughout the Protocol in parentheses.
7. Arrows	The Disposition/Advice section may include other directives, First Aid instructions, or self-assessment to perform immediately; each of these items is linked to a specific complex of symptoms by an arrow; *arrows* indicate actions for the RN to take: directives for pt. self-assessment, First Aid directives, or referral to ED.
8. Self-Assessment (SA)	In Disposition/Advice section designated as *SA.*
9. First Aid Directives	(Designated as *First Aid* in Disposition/Advice section).
10. Specific Referrals	Specific referrals to Suicide Prevention, Poison Center, and instructions to *COME TO ED NOW!*
11. Supplemental Information (SI)	On a separate sheet, this section includes Home Treatment Instructions; Tutorial Information for the nurse as well as information and home treatment instructions for the patient.
12. Home Treatment References	*Always consult the Home Treatment* (Home lx SI, Appendix A) when directed by the Protocol. This section may be developed in-house; see Appendix A for examples. Home Treatment may be found in the specific Protocol or in Appendix A.

SAMPLE PROTOCOL: BURNS

Skin Problem: Burns 1

Electrical; Thermal; Chemical

ASSESSMENT	ACUITY LEVEL	DISPOSITION/ADVICE
Key Questions	**Emergent Symptom Patterns**	**EDOmin-1 hr**
All electrical burns	+ ± Chest pain, palpitations, > heart rate, fainting, Hx of lightning strike? (cardiac dysrhythmia) —	- - ▶ All electrical burns have potential for progressive injury; may be worse than it looks! Seconds count
All thermal burns	--	► See Burns SI, First Aid
Burn w decreased consciousness	/+ Weak, dizzy, cold/mottled/pale skin, blue lips/nail beds, rapid/shallow breathing, unresponsive, loss of consciousness? (shock) (See Shock)	Y SA: Estimate using one palm of *victim's* hand (not including fingers) = 1%
Burn w respiratory / symptoms	+ Hoarseness, cough, wheezing, SOB, singed/black nares, facial bum, smoke inhalation, black sputum? (inhalation injury)	
Burn (deep)	+ White, dark, charred appearance, loss of skin, regardless of size? (3rd degree)	
Burn (over 9%)	+ Red, mottled, blisters, extreme pain? (2nd degree, major)	
Burn of finger(s) (circumferential)	• Unable to remove rings? (> risk circ.)	
Facial/neck burn? (retinal, inhalation burn)		
All chemical burns (Including eyes)	....- -	► All chemical burns have potential for progressive injury; may be worse than it looks! Seconds count!

Key Questions	Urgent Symptom Patterns	ED/UCC/Office 1 -8 hr•
Burn (circumferential)	+ Face/neck/hands/feet/arms/legs/perineum/anyjoint? (circ. obstruction) --»—	See Burns SI, First Aid
Burn w blisters	+ Red, mottled, extreme pain, 5%-9%? (2nd degree) - -<	See Burns SI, First Aid

Key Questions	Acute/Nonacute Symptom Patterns	FA 8+ hr ± Home Tx ©
Burn Hx	+ Foul smelling, purulent discharge, > swelling, > streaks and pain, fever? (infection)------- — ------------→	Check tetanus status See Burns SI, First Aid
Burn (moderate)	+ Tetanus immunization > 10 yr? (> risk infection) + Red, blisters, pain 1%-5%? (2nd degree)	
Burn (minor)	+ Reddened, mild, swelling, moderate pain, no blisters? (1st degree) + Red, mottled, blisters, pain, < the size of one hand (1%)? (2nd degree)	

Cross-Reference ©
Abuse

SKIN PROBLEM: BURNS 2

Sunburn

ASSESSMENT	ACUITY LEVEL	DISPOSITION/ADVICE
Key Questions	**Emergent Symptom Patterns**	**ED 0 min-1 hr**
Sunburn w < consciousness	+ Fever (high), sev. fatigue, confusion, fainting, hot, dry red skin, rapid shallow breathing? (See Heat Exposure)	
Key Questions	**Urgent Symptom Patterns**	**ED/UCC/Office 1-8 hr**
Sunburn	+ Eye pain, photophobia, < vision? (retinal involvement) + Extensive, deep sunburn, fever, pain (sev. to mod.), dehydration Sx, generalized swelling of burned area? (sun poisoning)	
Red, mottled, blisters	+ > 5%, Extreme pain? (2nd degree)	
Sunburn Hx	+ Foul smelling, purulent discharge, worsening swelling or pain, streaks, fever? (infection)	
Key Questions	**Acute/Nonacute Symptoms Patterns**	**FA 8+ hr± Home Tx**
Sunburn w blisters	+ Red, mottled, tender, covering 5% of body? (> risk infection)	
Open blisters	± Discharge ± fever? (> risk infection)	
Sunburn	+ Pain/tenderness, deeply pigmented skin types? (1st degree) + Red, mild swelling, moderate pain, no blisters? (1st degree)	

Cross-References

Abuse | Heat Exposure

SKIN PROBLEM: BURNS
Supplemental Information

▶ First Aid

Thermal Burn

SA: Estimate using one palm of *victim's* hand (not including fingers) = 1%.

If clothing sticks to skin, do not remove clothing! Immerse burned area for no more than 3 min in cool tap water.

If clothing does not stick to skin, remove it.

- If > 5%, do not immerse. Cover with clean wet sheet + plastic wrap.
- If < 5%, immerse immediately in cool tap water x 10 min.

Do not put butter, oil, or creams on burn!

Do not put ice on burn: could lead to > skin damage, > shock.

- For transport: Wrap burn in clean plastic wrap to keep warm, clean, and reduce pain.

Chemical Burn

Contact poison center immediately and quickly do the following:

- Wet Chemicals: Rinse skin/eyes w cool tap water.
- Dry Chemicals: Brush off from skin/eyes.
- Bring substance to ED w you.

▶ Burn Assessment

Rule of Nines: A useful, quick method to estimate percentage of body surface areas that were burned.

Rules of Nines

Adult

Palm of victim's hand, not including fingers = 1%

Perineum = 1%

Head/Neck = 9%

Arm = 9%

Leg= 18%

Ant. trunk = 18%

Post, trunk = 18%

▶ Burn Care

Immediate Care

- Pain: Tylenol.
- Pain/Swelling: Cold compress Q1D. (See Home Tx)

- Remove rings, bracelets, etc., only if you can do so easily. If not, you need to come in to have the items removed.
- Pain/Swelling: Raise the bum area above heart level.
- Don't use "Caines" or Benadryl sprays for bum—may cause a reaction.
- Check tetanus status. If you have a clean bum and your last tetanus shot was > 10 yr ago, you need a tetanus shot within 72 hr.

► Blister Care

- Don't break blisters. They are like "nature's Band-Aids" and will protect your skin from infection.
- If they break, leave them alone. Do not peel off skin from broken blisters.
- Cover w clean, dry dressing. Change as needed.
- Watch for signs and symptoms of infection. (See Bum Care; review with caller.)

TeleTriage Systems
Workflow Process

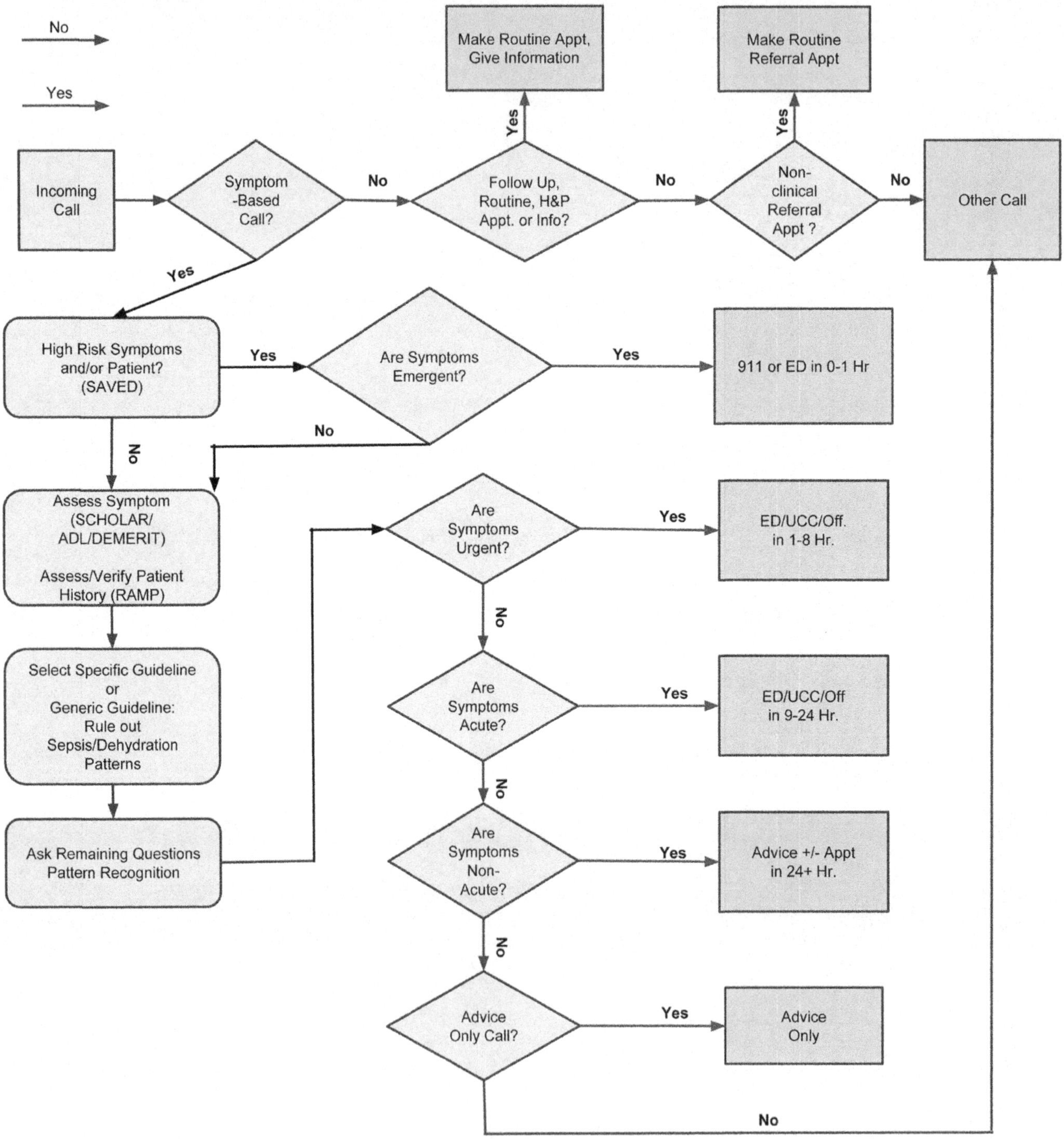

Disposition Options

FIVE-LEVEL TRIAGE APPROACH

The Five-level approach divides symptom patterns into five levels of Urgency, entitled as follows:

- Life Threatening
- Emergent
- Urgent
- Acute
- Non-Acute

Each level has a time frame and a range of sites to be further evaluated -- as appropriate and depending upon the time of day and day of the week. Each urgency level is intended as a flexible time frame within which the nurse must determine what is safe, timely and prudent. Nurses have a professional responsibility to use good judgment. A common rule of thumb to apply being "when in doubt, err on the side of caution, and bring patients in sooner rather than later".

Life threatening symptoms always require paramedic transport to ED within minutes. They must be kept NPO. Remain on the line with the caller. Whenever possible, institute a three-way conference call with both parties (patient and EMS services, Suicide Prevention, Rape Crisis or Poison center, for example) as directed by your policies.

Emergent level symptoms always require ED services. Some must be kept NPO. Some patients will require paramedic transport; some may be brought by car by a person who can safely bring them in within the appropriate time frame (0-1 hour). Always notify Labor and Delivery or Emergency Department of pending arrivals of any patient coming via car.

Urgent symptoms typically require evaluation within 1-8 hours (same-day appointment). Some may require evaluation within the hour and are instructed by guideline to "Come in now". Depending upon the time of day and day of the week, some patients may be directed, as appropriate, to Emergency Department, Urgent Care, or office settings for further evaluation.

Some patients in Urgent category may also require paramedic transport due to transportation problems. Some may require other reliable, timely transport as is practical, i.e. cabs, Uber, Lyft, etc. if there is no readily available car or if relatives are too anxious to drive them in. Always notify Labor and Delivery or Emergency Department of pending arrivals any patient arriving via car.

Acute Symptoms typically require evaluation within an 8-24 hour time frame, or a next day appointment. Depending upon the time of day and day of the week, some patients may be directed, as appropriate, to Emergency Department, Urgent Care, or office settings for further evaluation. Always notify Labor and Delivery or Emergency Department of pending arrivals of any patient arriving via car.

Non-Acute Symptoms may require evaluation within a 24+ time frame or future appointment or advice only. Depending upon the time of day and day of the week (available access), these patients may be directed to Emergency Department, Urgent Care, or office settings for further evaluation, as appropriate.

Continuity of Care

To prevent patients with emergent to acute symptoms from "falling through the cracks", policies should require nurses to notify managers in Labor and Delivery or Emergency Department *via phone call*, about pending arrivals of any patient who is arriving via car.

After Hours Lack of Access requires that provisions for safe, timely access be in place. Depending upon the time of day (After hours) and day of the week (Holiday or weekend), nurses should direct some patients as appropriate, to Emergency Department, Urgent Care, or office settings for further evaluation.

Informed Consent

According to Dan Tennenhouse, MD, JD, (1993) nurses must apprise patients of the urgency of their symptoms" ("the duty to terrify"), in order to motivate patients to comply with disposition instructions in a timely way. Thus, explicit directives define the time frame (when) and place (where) and the level of urgency (why) patients need further evaluation in clear, concise and understandable terms – thereby lessening the chance of delay in care.

PATTERN RECOGNITION & MATCHING

Patients rarely present with the "classic picture" of any condition. People are unique individuals, symptoms vary, and the advice nurse must deal with a myriad of variables. In truth, MI may present in various ways: with one key symptom (like chest pain); a few ill-structured or vague symptoms (nausea, vomiting, sweating without chest pain); or the "classic picture" of key and associated symptoms (crushing chest pain accompanied by shortness of breath, nausea, vomiting, dizziness, sweating, anxiety). The RN must use his/her best professional judgment to determine what constitutes a "match."

DOCUMENTATION STRATEGIES

Always start the assessment process using the above questions and the Documentation Form (below), rather than the Protocol. The rationale is to get a mental image of the problem, using the form and key questions, then fill in details using the Protocol.

Patients often present symptoms in erratic and disorganized ways, and may focus on one symptom to the exclusion of other, more important ones. Start with the Master Guideline and Documentation Form for the "first pass" to reduce the risk of premature selection of a Protocol that can lead to mistriage. The RN must be investigative, starting with a "clean slate" and performing a preliminary assessment before choosing a Protocol.

FORMING AN "IMPRESSION" OR "WORKING DIAGNOSIS"

In regard to the diagnosis, the most an advice nurse can hope for is a "working diagnosis" or "impression." Forming a working diagnosis is no great mystery. Use the patient's chief complaint in their own words—"headache," "nosebleed," "vaginal bleeding," "earache," etc. Then add modifiers or qualifiers (See Appendix for Approved Abbreviations) that will designate the level of acuity. For example:

> Abdominal pain, 9 on scale of 10, sudden onset
> Ankle pain, 4 on scale of 10, trauma history

Documenting high-risk patients and symptoms using SAVED may help "defend" dispositions. For example:

> Headache, non-English-speaking, yelling
> Abd. Pain, Prev. Hx, ectopic

The final steps, treatment, and evaluation are addressed in the Protocol. The treatment plan, formed from the Protocol's disposition and advice, is always a provisional one. Evaluation is carried out when the nurse provides patient teaching for self-evaluation through follow-up instruction from the Protocol.

The Documentation Form is based on the concept of charting by inclusion. Charting by inclusion requires that the RN chart normal negatives (pertinent negatives) as well as abnormal findings. Pertinent negatives are "findings that are normal and significant" (e.g., "no black or bloody stools," etc.). If you are charting by inclusion, pertinent negative findings should always be written.

PERTINENT NEGATIVES

In telephone triage, the issue of charting by inclusion or exclusion is best addressed by in-house counsel and formal policies. This guide proposes no directives about charting except to encourage charting by inclusion, where feasible.

The most conservative approach is to documenT pertinent negatives, especially with head, chest, respiratory, abdomen, dizziness, and flu symptoms. However, with other, less serious-sounding problems, if it is obvious that no emergent symptoms are present and all answers regarding urgent (or acute, Nona cute) symptoms are answered "no," the pertinent negatives may be noted as follows: "Denies all urgent symptoms." If, for example, the patient answers "yes" to certain urgent questions, one might write:

"Denies all urgent symptoms with exception of fever, shaking chills," or "Fever/chills"; denies all other urgent symptoms."

The Basic Assessment: Triage Form Key (See example next page)

1. All of the following demographic information is included here: Note vital statistics: Name, age, sex, and phone number, temperature, BP, weight, etc.
2. Immunization history: Elicit whether immunization is up to date and mark accordingly.
3. Chief complaint (CC).
4. "Key Questions": SCHOLAR, ADL are used to elicit detailed information about the chief complaint.
5. Note home care measures already tried.
6. Date of last normal menstrual period.
7. Note pregnancy status (circle one).
8. Note breastfeeding status (circle one).
9. Note allergies (circle one) and add if "Yes".
10. Note chronic illness (circle one) and describe.
11. Note emotional state.
12. Note medications (Rx, OTC, herbal, street, or recreational drugs).
13. Note recent injury or surgery and describe.
14. Note recent exposure to contagious illness.
15. Note recent possible ingestion of toxic substance.

Circle any/all emergent or urgent symptom patterns.

16. Note impression (working diagnosis), or circle one or more items in Emergent or urgent symptoms.
17. Note title of Protocol used, or note "Master Protocol."
18. Note any modifications to approved Protocol advice.
19. Mode of transport.
20. Note minutes or hour when patient to arrive at office, urgent care or ED.
21. Note date of appointment/time.
22. Note whether precaution was stated (circle one).
23. Note patient agreement to plan (circle one).
24. Signature/title.
25. Note time call ended.

NOTE: Boxes 5-15 relate to PAMPER.

TRIAGE/ADVICE FORM

1. Adult O Pediatric 0	Name	4
Age DOB M F	Date Time AM PM	SCHOLAR
Caller/Relation to Pt.		Sx
T. Oral AX Rec. BP	2. Immz Up to Date? Y N (N = Needs Appt.)	Char.
3. Chief Complaint:		Course
	4	Hx of Sx
		Onset
		Loc.
5. Home Tx Administered? Y N		Ag. Fac.
6. *IMP?* *7. Pregnant? YN*	*8. Breastfeeding?* Y *N*	Rcl. Fac.
9. Allergies? YN	*10. Chronic Illness? YN*	4
		ADL
	11. Emotional State?	Intake
12. Medications? YN	*13. Recent Injury? Y N*	Liquid
	14. Recent Illness? YN	Solid
		Output
	15. Recent Ingestion? YN	Urine
16. Impression:	SAVED	BM
EMERGENT SYMPTOMS	URGENT SYMPTOMS	Emesis
1. Extreme, unusual, new, sudden, suspicious, emergent or urgent sounding symptoms? 2. Trauma with suspicious history? 3. Unusual pain or symptoms • postoperative • postpartum • postprocedure	1. Infection symptoms; temp > 104? 2. Infection symptoms after 48 hours on antibiotic? 3. Moderate symptoms in patient with • Extreme Age/Childbearing Age • Communication Barrier • Chronic Illness • Severe emotional Distress (Pt. or Caretaker)	Sleep Activity Color
17. Protocol Advice/18. Modifications:		
19. Mode of Transport:	20. Advised to be here within Min. Hr.	
21.Appt. Date Time	22. Disclaimer Stated? Y N	
23. Client Agreement to Plan? Y N	24. RN Sig/Title 25. Time ended	

How Should I Chart?

Charting must be complete but cryptic, and include accurate, timely observations in patient's own words. Nurses must use approved abbreviations and terminology as well.

Please review the charting sample for examples to make charting more complete, accurate, and detailed.

1. Quantify where possible—avoid vague expressions.
2. Time frames (8,16,24,48 hr) as related to symptoms or treatment
3. "Working diagnosis" or "impression"
4. Advice per Protocol name
5. Protocol deviations/override/modifications

Must I Ask Questions in a Specific Order or According to the Order on the Form?

Elicit information in any order that seems appropriate to the caller and the situation. It is not necessary to let the form dictate the order of data collection. In real-world situations, people volunteer information when initially describing their chief complaint. To interrupt and begin mechanically asking questions is counterproductive, may lead the caller in the wrong direction, and may actually lengthen the call. Take notes in the appropriate spot on the form as the caller volunteers information. Then fill in the gaps with follow-up questions.

What about Documenting the Caller's Consent?

Always end your call with the precaution statement and document it. The precaution helps to ensure that the patient has given informed consent—in other words, they understand the problem definition and proposed treatment *with the following understanding:*

a. This is an "impression," *not* a medical diagnosis.
b. The treatment is based on the impression.
c. The final decision to follow advice rests with the patient.
d. If patients disagree with the impression, they may have an appointment.
e. If symptoms become markedly worse or fail to respond to the home treatment, the patient agrees to call back or come in.

Elicit and document what the caller plans to do at the end of the call. This will demonstrate that there was agreement to a certain plan of action.

What Calls Must Be Documented?

Again, this is an area for in-house counsel to address through formal policies. It is best to document all calls involving advice and calls involving same-day or later appointments. Calls for information or referral probably do not need to be documented, provided the caller has no symptoms.

How Important Is It to Document Medications?

Always chart medications, whether current prescriptions, OTC, recreational drugs, or herbal remedies. All medications have the potential to cause side effects or to interact with other medications, food, or chronic conditions. With women of childbearing age, always elicit pregnancy and breastfeeding status before advising any OTC or herbal remedy.

Should I Leave Blanks or Fill in All Spaces?

Don't leave any blank spaces. Such omissions may be interpreted as failure to chart completely. Write N/A if the question is not applicable (as in pregnancy status, if the caller is male) or "unknown" if patient does not know the answer (as in whether they have allergies or whether they are pregnant).

The acronyms SCHOLAR, PAMPER, and ADL are incorporated into the Documentation Form to serve as "triggers" to remind nurses what Key Questions to ask.

Once the nurse has elicited this information, she/he is ready to choose a Protocol. In some cases, the nurse will use the General Protocol, a "core protocol" that serves as "infrastructure" for all other Protocols. Understanding this Protocol is one of the best ways to understand and appreciate the overall design.

The Triage Process

The concepts of picture-building and "drilling down" underlie the telephone triage process. The instructions below incorporate these concepts as well as the strategies introduced on the preceding pages.

First Steps

Start with a global approach (SAVED) and the Documentation Form. Unless it is clearly an emergency, follow this quick assessment with Key Questions (SCHOLAR, PAMPER, ADL) as appropriate. Use open-ended questions where possible. Do *not* start with a Protocol, lest you fall prey to the "wrong track" syndrome. Clawson and Democoeur (1998) states that "if you get on the wrong track at the station, no matter how fast you travel, you still end up in the wrong place." Without the symptom and patient history, you may not know which Protocol to use or you may waste valuable time in the wrong Protocol and either delay treatment and/or mistriage.

How Do I Know Which Protocol to Use?

Once you have a general sense of the problem(s), turn to the Table of Contents or divider tab. Use the Protocol that best matches the site and/or symptoms of the patient's presenting problem(s). If patients present with multiple symptoms, use the Protocol that has the highest likelihood of leading to an appointment, or ask the patient which symptom is the most bothersome. If there is no Protocol that relates to the presenting symptom, use the General Protocol.

What Is the Purpose of the General Protocol?

Because of the variation in symptom presentation in unique individuals, it is not feasible to develop a set of Protocols to cover every condition. Not having a Protocol to cover a condition leads to what is commonly known as the "out of Protocol" experience. This is where the General Protocol is useful.

The General Protocol is especially useful in two instances: (1) when the nurse does not know which Protocol to use and (2) when responding to calls about elderly, and poor historians whose presenting symptoms are vague or ill-structured. In such cases, you may use the General Protocol alone.

The General Protocol (See Key Assessment Tools tab) acts as a safety net to keep patients from falling through the cracks by organizing problems in a very broad way. Each box contains general categories of problems that are emergent to nonacute (severe pain, major trauma, fever, acute infection, minor self-limiting symptoms, (etc.). Also included are general categories of high-risk patients because of age, veracity, emotional distress, debilitation, and distance. While it does not address symptoms or patients in a detailed way, the General Protocol provides general guidelines for the "out of Protocol" experience. However, there is always a need for more detailed Protocols that cover symptoms in depth. This is where site-specific Protocols come into play (e.g., Ear Problems, Urinary Problems, etc.).

How Do I Use the Protocol?

Generally speaking, each Protocol is divided into two sections—a triage "chart" and Supplemental Information (SI). For patients describing symptoms, start with the triage chart, reading from left to right and top to bottom. Reviewing the Bum Protocols, start with Key Questions first. For instance, if the patient responds "yes" to "electrical bums," question, go right to the middle column in "emergent symptom patterns." Continue asking more specific questions related to electrical bums. If the answer to *one or more* of these questions is "yes," shift to the right again for appropriate disposition and first aid. Many Protocols start with the key question of "Trauma." Thus, if the caller denies trauma (or pain, discharge, etc.), skip all questions related to it (to the right with pluses in front of them).

Always rule out emergent symptoms first, either by asking specific questions or from the patient history. Symptom patterns are listed in the middle column in descending order of acuity from emergent to nonacute. Corresponding Dispositions are listed in the right-hand column, also in descending order of acuity. Work your way down the list, ruling out emergent to nonacute symptoms. If the patient answers "no" to all key questions (left-hand column), consult the cross-reference section for other possibilities.

Some problems require immediate first aid or home treatment. First aid instructions are usually located in the "disposition" column (far right) or under Supplemental Information. Specific home treatment instructions are in the Supplemental Information (SI) section, and common home remedies are located under Flome Treatment Supplemental Information in Appendix A. The SI section provides information regarding particular conditions or treatments or for answering questions unrelated to symptoms or about conditions that have been previously medically diagnosed only.

► General Reminders

Remember, the most important task of telephone triage is to reduce uncertainty and urgency by asking *enough* of the *right questions,* in the *right way* to elicit *enough* of the *right data,* and to choose the *right Protocol(s)* and *right disposition.* Pattern recognition requires eliciting sufficient contextual information. The more preliminary information gathered, the more obvious the pattern.

General guide: *When in doubt, always err on the side of caution.* RNs must rely on their best professional judgment and use every means at their disposal to ensure that patients are treated in a timely manner. Time frames designated on the template are intended as a *general* guide. When in doubt, have the patient come in *sooner rather than later.* With the exception of emergent level dispositions, *time frames are intended to be flexible,* allowing for professional judgment. For example, when presented with a problem corresponding with a disposition time frame of 1-8 hr (essentially a same-day appointment), the RN may direct a caller to come in within 2 hr, if in his/her professional judgment it is more prudent or reasonable to do so.

Upgrading/downgrading: RNs may upgrade dispositions as appropriate (i.e., from urgent to emergent; nonacute to acute). However, never downgrade (i.e., urgent to nonacute) without a physician consultation. If a patient is noncompliant, always seek advice from the physician on call.

Ask questions in any order, or simply let the caller tell their story first.

Beware of the developing disease: What starts out as vague abdominal pain with low-grade fever may quickly develop into the classic picture of appendicitis. Follow-up calls should be mandatory for possible developing diseases, and especially for Abdominal Pain, Respiratory Problem, Diarrhea, N/V, Fever, or Marked Change in Activities of Daily Living.

► OTC Medications

Just because a medicine is over the counter does not mean it is harmless. Herbal remedies can have side effects, as can megadoses of vitamins. Prolonged use of any drug, over the counter or prescription, can produce unwanted or even dangerous side effects. Sometimes people become "functionally dependent," meaning that a body function has ceased to work naturally because it has been altered by the drug and must have it in order to continue to function. Remind patients that drugs should be taken in the smallest dose for the shortest time possible.

Currently many drugs that previously required a prescription are being approved for over-the-counter status. In order to avoid the possibility of delayed diagnosis, flawed triage, and possible complications, nurses must remain alert to possible side effects and cautions regarding all medications. There are three ways in which problems can arise with any drug, either over the counter or prescription. A few common examples are:

- Drug/drug interactions: Aspirin can interact with anticoagulants to increase the effect of anticoagulation. When combined with alcohol, long-term use of Tylenol may have a toxic effect on the liver.
- Drug/food interactions: Certain antidepressants (MAO inhibitors) can interact with foods that contain tyramine (Chianti wine, homemade bread, sour cream, avocado, aged game, liver, canned meats, eggplant, and many others) to cause a life-threatening rise in blood pressure.
- Drug/disease interactions: Salicylates are contraindicated in persons with bleeding disorders, ulcer, gout, asthma.

General Instructions

- Advise all patients using folk remedies of risk of two medications acting together; might cause harm.
- Most OTC brands come in numerous preparations, e.g., Robitussin, DM, AC, etc.

Some Final Words

If telephone triage is to continue to evolve into a formally recognized subspecialty, then standards, Protocols, and training must keep pace with developments in managed care and technology. Telephone triage nurses are being challenged by economic forces to prove themselves to be a viable component of this service. Telephone triage nurses can continue to uphold their unique traditional role as patient advocate and upgrade their profession and practice through ongoing training and standards development.

References

Clawson, J.J., and Democoeur, K.B. (1998). *Principles of Emergency Medical Dispatch.* (2nd ed.). Salt Lake City, UT: Priority Press.

Daugird, A.J., and Spencer, D.C. (1989). Characteristics of patients who highly utilize telephone medical care in a private practice. *The Journal of Family Practice, 27,* 420-421.

Fillit, H., and Capello, C. (1994). Making geriatric assessment an asset to your primary care practice. *Geriatrics, 49(*1), 27-30.

Finley, R. (1995). Telephone triage: Essentials for expert practice. *Polypharmacy and the Elderly.* Dublin, CA: Contemporary Forums.

► Pain Assessment Guidelines (ALL AGES)

"Pain is one of the most common reasons people seek medical attention" (JCAHO 2001).

Assessment Parameters/Descriptors

- Pain intensity
- Associated symptoms
- Characteristics (measure at present and at worst):
  —Quantity (8-10 on scale of 10; mild, moderate or extreme; worst or unbearable)
  —Quality (sharp, dull, throbbing, etc.)
- Onset/duration:
  —Sudden, gradual. How many hours, days, months?
- Location:
  —Local versus generalized (Have patient point to site and describe.)
- Aggravating factors:
  —What makes it worse? (Food, activity, position, etc.)
- Relieving factors:
  —What makes it better? (Meds, food, activity, position, etc.)
- Current Home Treatment
- Effects on daily life: Eating, sleeping, work, relationships, emotions, concentration

► Red Flags and Pain

"Red Flags" direct our attention to certain high-risk symptoms and populations (SAVED).

Severe

- Any severe, sudden or suspicious pain:
  —Awakens patient from sleep or keeps patient awake.
  —Described as "worst," "unexpected," "unusual," "sudden," "recurrent."
  —Any pain unrelieved by prescribed pain medication.
  —8-10 on scale of 10.
  —Sudden onset is considered to be more serious.
  —Localized pain is considered to be more serious.

Age Related

- Beware of pain symptoms in very young or very old.

Veracity

- Pain symptoms in non-English speaking children or poor historians

Emotional Distress

- Frequent calls about chronic, recurrent or unrelieved pain may signal emotional distress (Do not overlook physical problem, however.):
  —All ages with chronic pain have 40%-50% depression.
  —Untreated depression lowers ability to cope with pain.

Debilitation

- Pain in patients with history of chronic illness:
- Pain unrelieved by usual pain medication

- Pain in patients with recent surgical history
- Unusually bad postoperative pain

Rules of Thumb

- Localized pain *tends* to be more serious; diffuse pain tends to be less serious.
- Sudden onset of pain *tends* to be more serious; gradual onset, less serious.
- Recurrent episodes of pain may indicate high acuity.
- Take all patients' complaints of pain seriously.
- Severe pain is always treated as an emergency.
- Minority callers often fail to recognize acute symptoms, report fewer symptoms, or attribute them to other causes.
- Beware of any pain that awakens patient or keeps him or her awake at night.
- Ideally, preventive therapy starts the moment symptoms of pain appear.

Red Herrings

"Red Herrings" are common distractions (symptoms or situations) that lead the nurse astray, away from the main problem.

- Barriers to pain assessment:
  —Reluctance to discuss pain.
  —Denial of pain, when pain is likely to be present (postop, trauma, bums, cardiac emergencies).
- Remain vigilant to possible patient denial, minimization, and misinterpretation of symptoms.
- Regard with suspicion: all elderly callers and unusual sounding presentations, including pain that is new, sudden, or unexpectedly severe.
  —Patients who have been "seen recently" may still need to be seen today.
  —Don't be misled by concurrent complaints or patient self-explanation.
  —Symptom presentation may be early, late, silent, atypical, or novel.
  —Symptoms of two conditions may present concurrently, thereby causing confusion or misinterpretation.
  —Patients often misinterpret or stereotype their symptoms.

Pain Syndromes in the Elderly

In regard to pain management, the elderly are at risk for undertreatment and overtreatment. There is a common misperception that the elderly are less sensitive to pain. This is not true. While the elderly may be more accepting and resigned to pain, they have pain nonetheless. In regard to pain medications the elderly have a narrower range between therapeutic effect and drug toxicity, presenting the problems of polypharmacy.

The elderly have several conditions more likely to cause pain—cancer and shingles. The elderly comprise at least 80% of those with cancer and have significant pain with advanced cancer. Shingles affect about 40% of people over 70 yr of age; it is a major cause of suicide in the elderly. Cognitive impairment may create an obstacle to pain assessment. However, most elderly relate well to scales like "mild, moderate, or severe," or 1-10.

Pain Presentation in Comatose, Nonverbal Signs

- Comatose patients. The symptoms may be subtle: agitation, restlessness, irregular breathing, pupil dilation, and sweating (Todd 1998).
- Nonverbal signs of pain include grimacing, groaning, guarded posture, favoring a limb, isolation, irritability, or fatigue (Todd 1998).

► Chronic Pain

Chronic pain lasts longer than expected, may be continuous, repetitive, or intermittent. It may become a primary problem or lead to structural change in the nervous system. This can further lead to the "wind-up phenomenon" that can cause increased pain and lowered threshold for pain (Todd 1998).

► Pain as the Fifth Vital Sign

According to the American Pain Society, pain is the "Fifth Vital Sign." APS (1999-2001) and now JCAHO (2001) has set forth standards that promote routine evaluation of pain.

► JCAHO Standards*

Pain is assessed in all patients. (JCAHO 2001) Pain measurement standards mandate the consistent assessment of each patient complaint of pain through the use of pain measurement scales, number, picture, and/or verbal descriptions.

Patients are involved in making care decisions, including managing pain effectively. To this end, structures are developed, approved and maintained, such as a framework for addressing issues related to care at the end of life, providing for managing pain aggressively and effectively.

End of life pain issues. The health care organization addresses care at the end of life. Dying patients have unique needs for respectful, responsive care. All staff are sensitized to the needs of the patient at the end of life. Concern for the patient's comfort and dignity should guide all aspects of care during the final stages of life. The health care organization's frameworks for addressing issues related to care at the end of life provide for managing pain aggressively and effectively.

Patients have the right to appropriate assessment and management of pain. Pain that is unrelieved has adverse physical and psychological effects. The patient's right to pain management is respected and supported. The organization plans, supports, and coordinates activities and resources to ensure the pain of all individuals is recognized and addressed appropriately. This includes

- Initial assessment and regular reassessment of pain.
- Education of patients and families, when appropriate, regarding their roles in managing pain as well as the potential limitation and side effects of pain treatments. Taking into account personal, cultural, spiritual, and/or ethnic beliefs communicates to patients and families that pain management is an important part of their care.

Postprocedure: The patient is monitored continuously throughout the postprocedure period. The following specific items are monitored:

- Impairments and functional status.
- Pain intensity and quality (for example, pain character, frequency, location, education, and response to treatments).
- Unusual events or postoperative complications and their management. Results of monitoring trigger key decisions, such as change of care due to a precipitous change in vital signs.

Patients are educated about pain and managing pain as part of treatment, as appropriate. When appropriate, patient and families are instructed about understanding pain, the risk for pain, the importance of effective pain management, the pain assessment process and methods for pain management, when identified as part of treatments. Data that the organization considers for collection to monitor performance include the appropriateness and effectiveness of pain management.

- All patients are asked the following screening or general question about the presence of pain: "Do you have pain now?"

*Reprinted with permission from Joint Commission.(2002). *CAMH: 2002 Comprehensive Accreditation Manual for Hospitals.* Oakbrook Terrace, IL.: Joint Commission on Accreditation of Healthcare Organizations.

EMERGENCY MEDICINE ACUITY CATEGORIES

The *Master Guideline* is designed to serve as a "fall back" or "contingency "guideline in cases where no guideline seems to fit the problem. In the left-hand column are definitions of acuity from the Model of the Clinical Practice of Emergency Medicine. In the right-hand column are corresponding categories of acuity from the Wheeler design with examples of symptoms that fit each category.

Emergency Medicine Acuity Categories and Definitions	Wheeler Acuity Categories and Examples
CRITICAL	EMERGENT (0-1 Hr)
Signs or symptoms of a life-threatening illness/injury with a high risk of mortality if immediate intervention is not begun to prevent further airway, respiratory, hemodynamic, and/or neurologic instability	Loss of consciousness Major trauma Shock or impending shock OB crises, Impending birth Sudden confusion, disorientation Loss or threat of loss of vital functions: Respiratory, circulatory, or sensory organs Caretaker/patient presents danger to self or others *RN feels symptoms are emergent*
EMERGENT	URGENT (1-8 Hr)
Signs or symptoms of an illness/injury that may progress in severity or result in complications with a high probability for morbidity if treatment is not begun quickly	Trauma Severe pain Any severe symptom (See SAVED) Acute infection symptoms Any infection requiring antibiotics *RN feels symptoms are urgent*
LOWER ACUITY	ACUTE/NONACUTE (8+ Hr)
Signs or symptoms of illness/injury with low probability to worsen to a more serious disease or to develop complications	Moderate symptoms in high risk patient (See SAVED) Failure to improve on home treatment Minor trauma Self limiting Sx. not markedly worsening

"The Core Content Task Force It created and endorsed the 2001 Model of the Clinical Practice of Emergency Medicine (EM Model) as published in the June 2001 *Annals of Emergency Medicine* and *Academic Emergency Medicine.*

Emergency Medicine Model Review Task Force. (2007). Emergency model. *Annals of Emergency Medicine.* htto://wtvw.abem.orn/PUBLIC/Dortal/alias Rainbow/lanu en US/tablD 3590/DesktopDefault.aspx

MASTER GUIDELINE
Age Birth to 21 Years

	Acuity Level	Disposition
Key Symptom	**Emergent Symptom Patterns**	**911 or ED in 0-1 H**
■ Major Trauma?	Blunt/MVA/Fall > 15 FT	
■ Loss of Consciousness ?		
■ Shock or Impending Shock?		
■ OB Crisis or Impending Birth?		
■ Severe Respiratory Distress?		
■ Presents danger to sclf/othcrs? (Patient or caregiver)		
■ Disorientation, Confusion, Marked Behavior Change ?		
■ Damage or threat to Vital Functions?	Sensorium, Respiratory, Circulation, Excretion, Mobility or Sensory (Hearing, Sight) Organs?	
■ Suspected or Confirmed Infection and ANY:	■ Sudden change in mental state, confusion ■ Extremely Irritable, crying inconsolably, unable to comfort? ■ Extremely quiet, not moving, withdrawn, cannot engage? ■ Refusing breast, bottle, food? ■ Urine output: Markedly decreased ■ Bowel/Emesis Prolonger Vomiting/Diarrhea? ■ Color Pale, Blue or Red? *(Suspect Sepsis)*	
■ Severe Vomiting, Diarrhea or Extremely Low Intake and ANY:	*m* Extremely quict/inactivc/wcak ■ Very difficult to arouse, confused ■ Skin: cool/mottled/bluc, <Turgor/Tcnting ■ Mucous membranes: Extremely dry, parched lips/tonguc, difficult to swallow ■ Eyes: Sunken, absence of tears ■ Respirations: Mouth breathing - very fast ■ Intake: No fluids for 4-8 hr. ■ Output: Urine - No urine, or scanty amount *(Suspect Severe Dehydration)*	
■ Arc severe pain or suspicious or emergent symptoms ruled out?		

MASTER GUIDELINE
Age Birth to 21 Years

Key Symptom	Urgent Symptom Patterns	ED/UCC/Office 1-8 H First Aid or Home Tx
■ Trauma and ANY:	■ Suspicious History? (Possible Abuse)	COME TO ED NOW
■ Suspected or Confirmed Infection and ANY	■ History/Risk Factors: • *Immunodeficiency* • *Immunosuppression:* Chronic Disease (All), Cancer, Transplant • *Immunosuppressive* ***Med/Tx:*** Chemo/Corticosteroid/Radiation • *Implant, Invasive* Post-Op/Post-Partum, Post-Procedure/Trauma/Large Bum • *International Travel* • *Alcohol/Substance Abuse* • *Antibiotic therapy* (ongoing) • *(Suspect Sepsis)*	COME TO ED NOW
■ Pain or Unusual Symptoms and ANY:	*m* Post-Op, Post-Partum, or Post-Procedure? (Suspect Complications/Infection) ■ Recent Injury?	COME TO ED NOW
■ Symptoms of Infection and ANY:	■ Failure To Improve On Antibiotics X 48 Hr.? (Ineffective Rx)	
■ Decreased intake +/- moderate vomiting/diarrhea and ANY:	• Drowsy, Weak, Dizzy, Irritable? • Skin: Pale, Decreased Turgor? • Mucous Membranes: Very Dry Lips/Tongue? • Respirations: Moderately Fast? • Unable to retain small amt. fluids x 2-3 H • Urine - Dark yellow. Decreased *(Suspect Mod - Severe Dehydration)*	COME TO ED NOW
■ Possible Exposure: Inhalation, Ingestion, Eye/Skin Irritation or ANY:	Exposure to ANY Toxin, Adverse Drug Reaction, New Medication, Drug-Drug, Drug-Disease, Drug-Food Interactions, Intentional or Accidental Ingestion, Animal/Insect/Snake, Food or Mushroom Poisoning?	COME TO ED NOW Or CALL POISON CONTROL NOW
■ Fever +	> Infant < 3 Mo. Temp > 38 C or 100.4 F?	
■ ANY Condition -	With potential to result in ED/hospital admission within 24 hours (ACEP)	
■ Are urgent symptoms ruled out?		

MASTER GUIDELINE
Age Birth to 21 Years

Key Symptom	Acute Symptom Patterns	ED/UCC/Office 9 24 H +/First Aid or Home Tx
■ Moderate Symptoms and ANY:	■ High Risk Patient: - Extreme of Age: Newborn, < 3 mo. - Communication barrier - Emotional distress (Repeat phone calls) - Chronic illness History	Possible upgrade to Urgent?
■ Decreased Intake, Mild Diarrhea/Vomiting and ANY	■ Fatigue, low energy, irritable ■ Skin: Color - Normal, Turgor - WNL ■ Mucous membranes: Moist - si. dry ■ Respirations: WNL ■ Intake: Able to take small frequent amounts of fluid ■ Output: Urine slight decrease ■ BM: Infrequent, small, watery stools *(Suspect Mild Dehydration)*	
■ Moderate Symptoms and:	*m* Persistent or worsening? ■ Failure to improve on home treatment X 24-48 hr.	Possible upgrade to Urgent (> Risk)?
■ Are Acute symptoms ruled out?		
Key Symptom	**Non Acute Symptom Patterns**	**Future Appt in 24 + H First Aid or Home Tx**
■ Minor Symptoms and ANY:.	■ Self-Limiting, Existing > 1 Week, Not Becoming Markedly Worse? ■ Improving on home treatment	

Rule of Thumb: *Assess all sick children jor symptoms ofpossihle sepsis and dehydration.*

Dehydration

- May be the result of *the combined effect* of several conditions including: Extreme Weather Conditions (Heat, Humídity|, *Job Occupation or Exercise,* Fever or N/V, Diarrhea, Low or No Fluid Intake.
- Always consider patient history,such as Age, Degree and Duration of Fever, Past Medical Hx, Chronic Disease, Medication, etc.
- General descriptions of dehydration are based on alterations of Activities of Daily Living (ADL).

Acuity Definitions

- Emergent: S&S of life threatening illness/injury with *high risk of mortality* if immediate intervention is not begun to prevent further airway, respiratory, hemodynamic, and/or neurologic instability. ACEP
- Urgent: S&S of illness, injury that may progress in severity or result in complication with *high probability for morbidity* if treatment is not initiated quickly. *Any condition resulting in admission of the patient to a hospital within 24 hours* ACEP
- Acute: S&S of illness/injury with *some probability to worsen or develop complications.*
- Non-Acute: S&S of illness/injury with *low probability* to worsen or develop complications

Abdomen Problem

ABDOMEN PROBLEM (BIRTH-6)

PAIN W OR W/O TRAUMA; W OR W/O NAUSEA/VOMITING

ASSOC SX/SPECIFIC/CONSIDERATIONS	DISPOSITION/ADVICE
EMERGENT SYMPTOMS	**ED IN 0 MIN-1 HOUR**
• **PAIN W OR W/O TRAUMA (MAJOR): MVA, FALL, BLUNT TRAUMA** + ABD. RIGIDITY, N/V, WEAK, DIZZY, Cold/Mottled/or Pale Skin, Blue Lips/Nailbeds, Rapid/Shallow Breathing, Unresponsive, Loss of Consciousness? (Shock/Internal Hemorrhage) (See SHOCK)	• **ALL EMERGENT ABD. PAIN: KEEP NPO.**
• **PAIN ± SUDDEN ONSET OR SEVERE** + HX EXP. TO STREET DRUGS/Rx, Poisonous Plant or Inhalation/ Ingestion of Toxic Chemical/Lead/or Pesticide? (Toxic Exp.)------------------------- *-	• **CONTACT POISON CENTER.** BRING SUBSTANCE TO E.D. W YOU.
+ NEWBORN W INFECTED UMBILICAL STUMP, 'Toxic Child" (See Toxicity Assessment)? (Neonatal Tetanus)	
• Does RN feel Sx. are severe, extreme, emergent?	
URGENT SYMPTOMS	**ED/MD/APPT IN 1-8 HOURS**
• **PAIN W TRAUMA (MINOR-MOD.)**	• **ALL URGENT ABD. PAIN: KEEP NPO.**
+ SUSPICIOUS HX? (Possible Abuse) (See ABUSE) --→	• **BRING CHILD TO E.D. NOW.**
• **PAIN W NAUSEA/VOMITING** + +.CRAMPY ABD. PAIN; **WATERY STOOLS ± BLOOD/MUCOUS/PUS,** Alternating w Normal Stools, ± N/V, FEVER, Recent Immigration, Hx of Foreign Travel, Exp. to Contaminated Water, Undercooked Meat/ Seafood/Poultry/Improperly Stored Food? (Infectious Diarrhea, "Food Poisoning") --*-	• **BRING CHILD TO E.D. NOW.**
+ ± SEV.-MOD., **RADIATING FROM ABDVFLANK/BACK TO GROIN,** Colicky Then Constant & Severe, FEVER/Chills, N/V, Dysuria, ± Hematuria, Frequency/Urgency? (Pyelonephritis) ------------------------------------ ▶	• **BRING CHILD TO E.D. NOW.**
+ AGE < 2 YR: SUDDEN ONSET, RECURRENT, COLICKY, SHARP, **± BLOODY MUCUS STOOL (CURRANT JELLY STOOL),** ± Vomiting Thick, Bright Green Bitter Tasting Fluid, 'Toxic Child" (See Acuity Assessment), ± Severe Dehydration? (Intussusception) -------------------------------- ▶	• **BRING CHILD TO E.D. NOW.**
+ ± SUDDEN ONSET, CRAMPY, LOWER ABD., ± Vomiting Thick, Bright Green Bitter Tasting Fluid? (Volvulus) -- ▶	• **BRING CHILD TO E.D. NOW.**
+ ± SEVERE, SUDDEN OR GRADUAL ONSET, ± TRAUMA, Guarding, ± FEVER/Vomiting? (Acute Abdomen) --»	• **BRING CHILD TO E.D. NOW.**
+ **± LOCALIZED OR GENERALIZED TENDERNESS,** ± Vomiting, FEVER, Rigidity, Involuntary Guarding? (Peritonitis) -------------------------------------- ▶	• **BRING CHILD TO E.D. NOW.**
+ COLICKY, Abd. Distention, **HX OF MAJOR CHANGE IN BOWEL HABITS?** (Bowel Obstruction)--→	• **BRING CHILD TO E.D. NOW.**
+ ± VAGUE, POORLY DEFINED, CONSTANT, PROGRESSING FROM **PERIUMBILICAL TO RLQ,** Mild FEVER, ± Vomiting, ± Anorexia, ± Holds Abdomen, ± Walks Bent Over? (Appendicitis)------------------------------- ▶	• **BRING CHILD TO E.D. NOW.** + SA: Pain when hopping on right foot? (Yes = +)
+ W FIRMTENDER **BULGE AT GROIN/SCROTUM,** Groin Pain? (Incarcerated Hernia)---→	• **BRING CHILD TO E.D. NOW.**
• **PAIN W/O VOMITING** + (VAGUE), COUGH, FEVER, Shaking Chills, Substernal/Intercostal Retractions, Nasal Flaring, ± Wheezing, Rapid/Shallow Resp., Anorexia, Fatigue? (Pneumonia) --→	• **BRING CHILD TO E.D. NOW.**
+ "TOXIC" OR "VERY ILL CHILD" Severe-Mod. Dehydration Sx (See Toxicity/Dehydration Assessment)? --→	• **BRING CHILD TO E.D. NOW.**
+ (SEVERE), Hx of Sickle Cell Disease? (Sickle Cell Crisis)	
• **AGE < 3 MO + FEVER > 38°C or 100.4°F®? ---------------------------------------→**	• **BRING CHILD TO E.D. NOW.**
• FEVER >40°C or 104°F?	
• AGE < 3 MO + MOD. SX + RISK FX (AVED)?	
• FAILURE TO IMPROVE on Antibiotics X 24-48 Hr? (Ineffective Rx)	
• WORSENING SX After 24-48 Hr on Home Tx?	
• RECENT SURGERY or HOSPITALIZATION? (Poss. Complications)	
• Does RN feel Sx. are urgent?	

continues

ABDOMEN PROBLEM (BIRTH-6)

continued

ASSOC SX/SPECIFIC/CONSIDERATIONS	DISPOSITION/ADVICE
ACUTE SYMPTOMS	**ED/MD/APPT IN 8-24 HOURS**
• **PAIN** + FEVER, N/V, Anorexia, Yellow Skin, Yellow Sclera, Fatigue, Swollen Glands, Clay Colored Stools, Dark Urine, ± Exp. to Hepatitis? (Hepatitis) (See APPENDIX A) + Pain/Burning on Urination, Frequency, Urgency, ± Blood-Tinged Urine, ± Nocturia, ± Cloudy, Foul or Strong Smelling Urine, ± FEVER? (UTI) (See URINARY PROB) + (MOD.-MILD) ± Diarrhea, ± Constipation+ HxRx or OTC Med? (Drug Side Effect) (See BOWEL PROB INFO), Diarrhea w Antibiotic Use? (Drug Effect) + SICK CHILD (See Toxicity Assessment)? (Toxicity) + MILD DEHYDRATION (See Dehydration Assessment)? (Dehydration) • **PAIN W NAUSEA/VOMITING** + THROAT PAIN, Difficulty Swallowing, Headache, FEVER > 38.5°C or 101.3°F, Chills, Pus, Foul Taste, White Patches in Throat, ± Abd. Pain, Vomiting, Swollen Lymph Nodes, ± Hx Strep/Impetigo Exp.? (Strep Pharyngitis) (See RESPIRATORY PROBLEM 2: THROAT) • **LESION(S)** + NEWBORN: Umbilical Stump, Redness, Swelling, ± FEVER? (Omphalitis) • AGE 3 MO-6 YR + MOD. SX + (AVED) = POSS. UPGRADE? • Does RN feel Sx. are acute?	
NON-ACUTE SYMPTOMS	**HOME TREATMENT W OR W/O APPT IN 24+HOURS**
• **PAIN** + AGE 1-6 MO, Recurs Daily at Same Hr. Crying Inconsolably for 30 Min to 2-3 Hr, Then Sleeps? (Colic) (See NEWBORN CONCERNS) + (W BM), Hx of Constipation/Fissure, ± Blood Streaks on Stool &/or Toilet Paper, Large or Sm. Rabbit Stools? (Constipation) (See BOWEL PROBLEM) + Prolonged, After Milk Products? (Lactose Intolerance) (See BOWEL PROBLEM) + Crampy Abd. Pain, w/o Dehydration Sx: N/V, Diarrhea, ± FEVER, ± Headache? (Gastroenteritis) • **SWELUNG** + Painless, Easy to "Push Down," Near "Belly Button," > in Afro-American/Hispanic Population? (Umbilical Hernia) • MINOR SELF-LIMITING SX EXISTING > 1 WK, NOT BECOMING MARKEDLY WORSE? • HOME TX ITEMS OR PHONE NOT AVAILABLE = POSS. UPGRADE? • Does RN feel Sx. are non-acute?	

continues

ABDOMEN PROBLEM (BIRTH-6)

continued

ASSOC SX/SPECIFIC/CONSIDERATIONS	DISPOSITION/ADVICE
CROSS-REFERENCES	**STANDARD FOLLOW-UP INSTRUCTIONS**
• ABUSE • BACK PROBLEM • BOWEL PROBLEM 1; 2 • FEVER • HEPATITIS (APPENDIX A) • NEWBORN CONCERNS • RESPIRATORY PROBLEM 1; 2 • URINARY PROBLEM	PT TO CALL BACK: If symptoms become much worse or urgent or emergent symptoms arise (RN: review Protocol and advise caller). RN TO CALL BACK: If acute Sx in child AGE < 2 years. Routinely for Abdomen pain, Respiratory problems, Fever, Diarrhea, Marked change in ADL.

Abdomen Problem Supplemental Information (Birth-6 Yr)

QUICK REFERENCE: Abdominal Pain
Drug Side Effect (Abdominal Pain)

GENERAL AXIOMS

- Stomachache is a frequent complaint in young children, it may not be the actual source of the problem (e.g., stomachache is often a presenting Sx of pneumonia, strep throat, UTI, otitis).
- Age 3-6 yrs: Pain localized in one area is more suggestive of severe problem.
- Abdominal pain + fever ***w/o other associated Sx*** needs urgent appt.

ABDOMINAL PAIN

- Causes: Trauma, anxiety, obstruction, hernia, acute gastroenteritis, colic, UTIs, appendicitis, constipation, ingestion, pneumonia, viral syndrome, strep throat, otitis, sickle cell disease crises
- Abdominal Pain Tx Goal: Relieve abdominal discomfort.
  - Warm compress 20-30 min (see Home Tx Ref)
  - Lie down, rest
  - Prevent gas: Avoid spicy foods, gas-producing foods
  - Gas: Simethicone
  - Sips of fluid →"BRAT" -> soft -> reg. diet (see Home Tx Ref, Clear Liquids, "BRAT" Diet, Soft Diet)

DRUG SIDE EFFECTS—ABDOMINAL PAIN

(Possible explanation: Accidental ingestion)

The most common drugs and classes of drugs

- antibiotics (many) esp:
  tetracycline (Doxycycline)
  metronidazole (Flagyl)
- codeine
- erythromycin
- nonsteroidal anti-inflammatory drugs
  Aleve
  Advil
  Ibuprofen
  Midol 200
  Motrin
  Nuprin

Abuse
(Physical, Sexual, Emotional, Financial)

ABUSE 1 (SEXUAL) REPORTING TREE (AGE 18+)

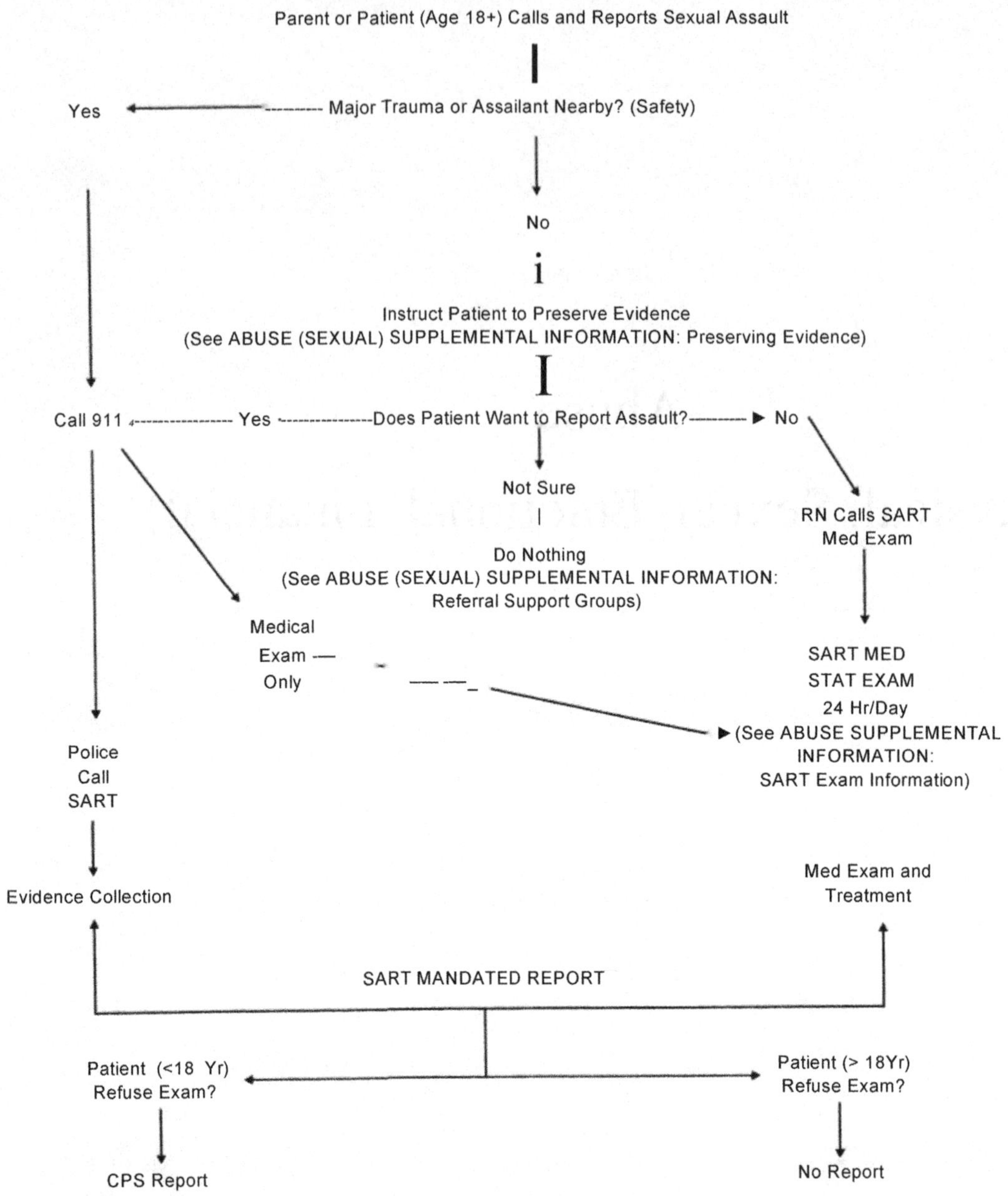

ABUSE 1 (SEXUAL) REPORTING TREE (AGE 6-18)

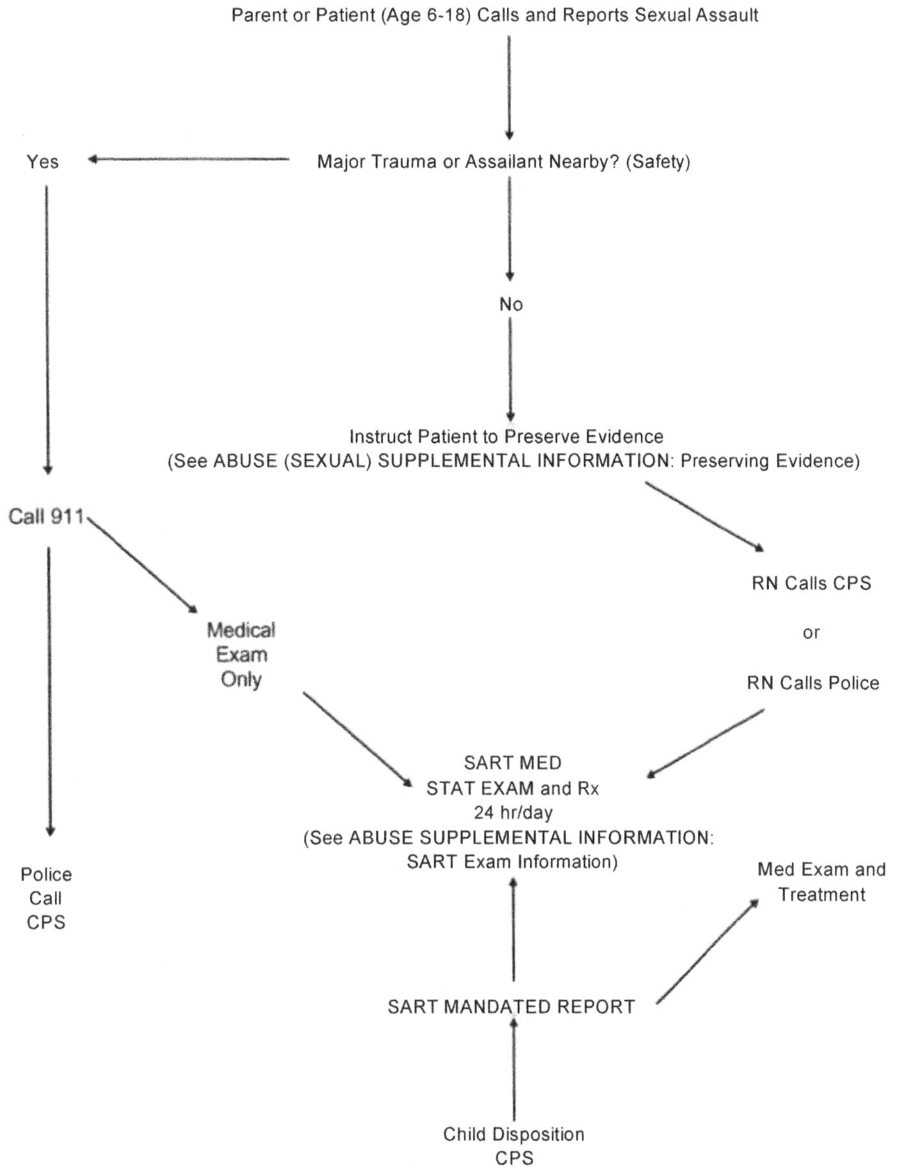

ABUSE 1 (SEXUAL) REPORTING TREE (AGE 0-6)

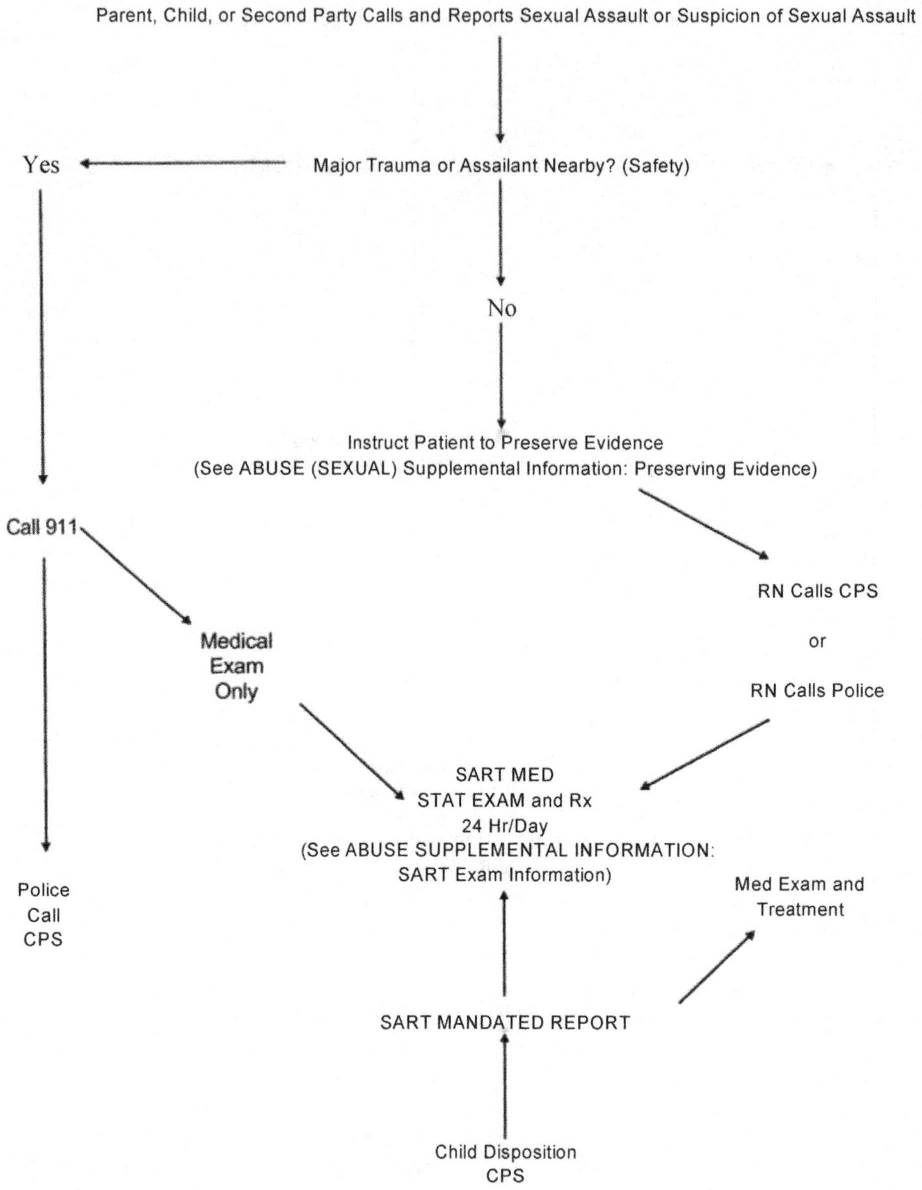

Abuse 1 (Sexual) Supplemental Information (All Ages)

AXIOMS

- Most sexual abuse is inflicted on survivor by people known to survivor.
- High-risk groups include: developmentally disabled, elderly, teen, and CHILD.
- High-risk groups are less likely to disclose abuse.
- As with ED visits, a high percentage of calls may have a hidden agenda of abuse.
- Abuse crosses all sexual, economic, cultural, and racial lines.

INSTRUCTIONS FOR PRESERVING EVIDENCE

- Comfort survivor.
- Do not shower, wash hands or face, or change clothes.
- Don't brush teeth.
- For women: Don't douche or remove tampon.
- Police may want to collect evidence in home or car (sheets, condom, etc.).
- Come with a friend.
- Bring change of clothes to ED. If you have changed, bring clothing worn at time of attack.

INFORMATION FOR THE SURVIVOR

Depending on the community, there may be a SART (Sexual Assault Response Team) or SANE (Sexual Assault Nurse Examiner).

- Examiner from SART, SANE or Forensic Examiner may be available 24 Hr for questions, intervention, advice, etc.
- Rape Crisis is called by SART, SANE or Forensic Examiner for every case. They take care of most of the psycho/social intervention and follow-up care.
- SART or SANE nurse handles the medical exam.
- < 72 Hr: Preserve evidence: Don't do <u>anything</u>. Come as you are!
- > 72 Hr: Survivor may have medical exam.
- Pt. will be referred: Physical injury; counseling; pubic lice.
- Follow-up appt w MD, SART coordinator, or CPS.
- STD RISK/IMMUNIZATION: If possible, go to be evaluated within 24 Hr.
  - Tests MAY be done for Gonorrhea, Chlamydia, and Syphilis. Follow-up tests for HIV and Hepatitis may be done.

- ANTIBIOTICS: You will be given antibiotics for STDs.
- A pregnancy test will be done.
- You will be given a pill to prevent pregnancy called "morning-after pill."

DOCUMENTATION AND REPORTING GUIDELINES

- **Consult with in-house counsel regarding developing written policies for reporting requirements to govern reporting of abuse suspected or verified through telephone triage.**
- Nurses are legally required to report any incidents that they reasonably suspect or are told about. If a report is made by another staff member, the nurse is not required to make a report.
- Failure to report abuse may result in disciplinary action against one's license, a misdemeanor, and being held liable for damages suffered by survivors.
- Nurses who negligently or recklessly report abuse cannot be held liable.
- Assess suspected abuse cases carefully. Take care not to be too direct, while still encouraging them to come in.
- ***Manage these calls carefully. Remember that patient safety is a priority.*** Survivors of abuse may be placed at greater risk if law enforcement personnel intervene.
- DOCUMENT in detail:
  - If survivor is in danger.
  - Name and relationship of person reporting suspected abuse.
  - Explicit details of in jury (where, when, how).
  - Name of assailant if possible.
  - Previous history of abuse.
  - ELDERS: Review medication history, level of mental acuity and physical mobility.
  - Use "survivor states" instead of "survivor alleges."
  - When referring to ED, you must inform ED of suspected abuse and have written documentation available.

REFERRAL SUPPORT GROUPS

- Self-defense classes.
- Community resources. (See Appendix D 2, 3, 6, 7, 8.)

SIGNS AND SYMPTOMS OF SEXUAL ABUSE: Sexual assault on and sexual exploitation of adult or CHILD. May be chronic or a single incident.

- STD symptoms in prepubescent child or any adult.
- GENITAL INJURIES: Bruises, lacerations of rectum or vagina.
- VAGINAL or URETHRAL discharge or lesions.
- RECTAL pain/bleeding.
- MOUTH/TONGUE: Bruising or tom tissue under tongue or between upper lip and teeth ("classic injury").

- BITE MARKS.
- Bloody underclothing.
- Excessive anxiety/fear: Nightmares, depression, withdrawal, aggressive behavior.
- Change in toilet habits: Bed-wetting, encopresis.
- Statements about sexual activities with parent or relatives, friend of family, or other adults.
- Survivor is known to be a survivor of other forms of abuse.
- CHILD: Early and/or exaggerated awareness of sex with either seductive interest or fearful avoidance of close contact with others.

References

See selected classic and current articles below for additional reading. For community-based in-services or consultation, contact your local Rape Crisis Hotline or Group Speaker's Bureau.

American Medical Association. (1992). Violence: A compendium from JAMA, American medical news and specialty journals of the AM A. *JAMA.* Chicago: AMA.

Briere, J. et al. (Eds.). (1997). *The APSAC handbook on child maltreatment.* London: SAGE.

Cowell, N.A. & Burgess, A.W. (Eds.). (1996). *Understanding violence against women.* Washington, D.C.: National Academy Press.

Lipscomb, G.H. et al. (1992). Male victims of sexual assault. *JAMA 267(22),* 3064-3066.

Markus, K. (1999). Reporting signs of abuse. *NurseWeek,* April 19, 13.

Reece. R.M. (1994). *Child abuse: Medical diagnosis and management.* Philadelphia: Lea & Febiger.

Winfrey, M.E. & Smith, A.R. (1999). The suspiciousness factor: Critical care nursing and forensics. *Critical Care Nursing 22* (1), 1-7. Gaithersburg, MD: Aspen.

Abuse 2 (Physical) Supplemental Information (All Ages)

COMMUNITY ALERT: Remain Aware of Precipitating Factors

- *Any* community celebration: Sport events (e.g.. Super Bowl), New Year's, etc., with or without alcohol or drug use.
- Natural disasters such as floods, earthquakes, hurricanes, etc.

CALL MANAGEMENT FOR PHYSICAL ABUSE (ALL AGES) *{Note: Refer to this section first, whether you are dealing with Spousal, Elder or Child Abuse.)*

ACTION PLAN

- When callers reveal that they have been abused: PATIENT'S SAFETY IS PRIMARY FOCUS.
  - Always tell the survivor that the police must and will be notified and will come to the site immediately.
  - Review escape plan. They should do the following:
    1. Collect money and credit cards.
    2. Get children.
    3. Collect important papers: Driver's License, Passports, Marriage Certificate, Birth Certificates, leases, deeds.
    4. Pack clothing.
    5. Call or go to a safe place or Shelter for Battered Survivors. (See Appendix D.)
- When referring to ED, you MUST inform them of suspected abuse situation and have written documentation available.

DOCUMENTATION AND REPORTING GUIDELINES

- Consult with in-house counsel regarding developing written policies for reporting requirements to govern reporting of abuse suspected or verified through telephone triage.
- Nurses are legally required to report any incidents that they reasonably suspect or are told about. If a report is made by another staff member, the nurse is not required to make a report.
- Failure to report abuse may result in disciplinary action against one's license, a misdemeanor, and being held liable for damages suffered by survivors.
- Nurses who negligently or recklessly report abuse cannot be held liable.
- Assess suspected abuse cases carefully. Take care not to be too direct, while still encouraging them to come in.
- ***Manage these calls carefully. Remember that patient safety is a priority.*** Survivors of abuse may be placed at greater risk if law enforcement personnel intervene.
- DOCUMENT (detailed documentation is essential):
  - If survivor is in danger.
  - Name and relationship of person reporting suspected abuse.
  - Explicit details of injury (where, when, how).
  - Name of assailant if possible.
  - Previous history of abuse.
  - Consult Policies and Procedures.
  - ELDERS: Review medication history, level of mental acuity and physical mobility.
  - Use "survivor states" instead of "survivor alleges."

PREVENTION/COUNSELING

- GOALS for prevention of Domestic Abuse:
  - Increase social support.
  - Decrease isolation.
  - Decrease burden of parenting and supporting family; encourage family to seek counseling.
- GOALS for prevention of Elder Abuse:
  - Respite care
  - Adult day care
  - Board and care
  - Conservatorships
- COUNSELING:
  - Express caring concern, e.g., "I do not want you (your child, your parent) to be hurt," "I am concerned for your (their) health and safety."

- Support survivor's decision to seek help.
- Be aware of the potential barriers to leaving an abusive situation (e.g., threats from the assailant, fear of poverty, failure of police and others to effectively intervene, hope that the abuse will stop, hope that child abuse will stop, fear of losing custody of the child, relationship can work, etc.).
- CHILD: Educate about impact of violence on children in home. Many abused people (usually women) believe themselves deserving of abuse but will respond to fears of harm to their children and will take action.
- CHILD: Remember that the child is often witness to the abuse—coordinate intervention with Pediatrics Services and/or Child Protective Services if child abuse is suspected or survivor describes such abuse in the course of giving own history.
- Explore ways to stay safe from future abuse. Provide a referral to self-help agencies.
- Have legal aid information and telephone number available.
- If possible, enhance parenting, caretaker, or spousal skills through classes or support groups. (See Appendix D.)

Abuse 2 (Physical) Child
Physical, Emotional, Neglect

AXIOMS

- Most common cause of death in infant age < 1 year is abuse inflicted by parent.
- All trauma involving any child is suspect for possible abuse.
- People who live with violence tend to normalize it. Abuse and denial go together. Be alert for minimization of injuries at all times (especially Head injuries).
- Possible indicators of abuse:
  - Frequent "accidents"
  - History of recurrent injuries
  - A delay in reporting
  - Inability to explain injury on the part of the parent
- Like ED visits, a high percentage of calls may have a hidden agenda of abuse.
- Abuse crosses all sexual, economic, cultural, and racial lines.
- Pregnancy (in teen) may either increase or decrease episodes of abuse (by boyfriend).

See CALL MANAGEMENT FOR PHYSICAL ABUSE (ALL AGES) at beginning of Abuse protocol.

SIGNS OF PHYSICAL CHILD ABUSE

- DEFINITION: "Any activity which results in a non accidental physical injury, unreasonable corporal punishment or unjustifiable punishment."*
  - ABDOMEN: Punch injuries, bruises.
  - ARMS: Circumferential bums, defensive injuries, or twisting breaks (mid ulna of arm). Bruising.
  - BACK: Whip/cord marks on back.
  - BITES, HUMAN: All sites, especially genitals/breast in sexual abuse.
  - BREAST: Bite injuries to breast, nipples.
  - EAR DRUM: Blood coming from ear due to blow to ear/head.
  - EYE: Injuries (all).
  - FACE: Bruises, lacerations, abrasions, fractured nose, broken or missing teeth, jaw or orbital fractures.
  - HAIR: Pulled out.
  - LEGS: Circumferential bums, twisting breaks.
  - MOUTH: Bruising, lacerations.
  - NECK: Bruising (from choking).
  - NEURO: Shaken baby syndrome: High pitched cry, bulging fontanelle, extreme irritability, child will not look at caretaker (retinal hemorrhage), bruises/handprint on trunk.

- GENITALIA: Vaginal/rectal bleeding/discharge/lesions, STD symptoms. (See ABUSE 1.)
- HIDDEN INJURIES: Internal injuries w or w/o hemorrhage: Ruptured spleen, liver. Bruising of muscles and bones. Cigarette bums: Genitals, soles of feet, abdomen.

■ OTHER:

- Belt buckle marks, handprints, pinches.
- Injuries on back of body from neck to knees on very young children.
- Excessively passive, compliant, or fearful child.
- Excessively aggressive or physically violent child.

RISK FACTORS

- Most abuse is committed by "normal people" during critical times in their lives. Causes include reactions to past problems, human frailty, vulnerability, unmet emotional needs, frequent crises, lack of parenting skills, social isolation, lack of experience leading to unrealistic expectations of normal childhood behaviors.

■ FACTORS IN PARENT:

- Parent abused as child.
- Past history of abuse of own child.
- Drug/alcohol abuse.
- History of family violence.
- Guns in home.
- Reaction to survivor defiance.
- Unemployment/homelessness/poverty.
- Gang activity: May have guns in home.
- Military service people may be subject to multiple stressors: Frequent geographical moves, lack of control over work hours, separations, dangerous work, masculine culture, downsizing.
- Abusive language.
- Anger: Poor impulse control, acts out anger, frustration through violence.
- Controlling behavior: Possessive, jealous; dictates dress, behavior, and with whom survivor may associate.
- Recent accident, car or other.

■ FACTORS IN CHILD:

- Prematurity.
- "Difficult child."
- Chronic illness.
- Physical disability.

- PRECIPITATING FACTORS IN CHILD:
  - Toilet training.
  - Colicky baby.
  - Temper tantrums.

SIGNS OF EMOTIONAL CHILD ABUSE

- DEFINITION: "Willful cruelty or unjustified punishment of a child including verbal abuse (constant taunting [humiliation]). Harder to prove or define."*
  - Withdrawn, depressed, apathetic child who "acts out."
  - Signs of emotional turmoil: Repetitive, rhythmic movement; no verbal or physical communication, regressive behavior like bed-wetting, rocking, thumb-sucking.
  - Parent continually refers to the child as "it."

SIGNS OF EMOTIONAL DEPRIVATION

- DEFINITION: "Parents do not provide the normal experiences which produce the feelings of being loved, secure and worthy."*
  - Refusing to eat enough food and becoming frail.
  - Overly exaggerated fears.
  - Continual seeking out and pestering of other adults for attention and affection.
  - Appearing normal but is unable to perform normal learned functions for a given age.

SIGNS OF NEGLECT

- DEFINITION: "Acts or omissions on the part of the responsible person include two categories: severe or general neglect. 'Severe neglect' is the failure of the parent or caregiver to protect the child from severe malnutrition or medically diagnosed non organic failure to thrive. 'General neglect' is the negligent failure to provide adequate food, clothing, shelter, medical care or supervision where no physical injury to the child has occurred."*
  - Unsanitary conditions in the home.
  - Spoiled food in the refrigerator or no food at all.
  - Untreated injuries that endanger the health of the child.
  - Unsafe home conditions and unsupervised young children left for long periods of time.

'Sources:

San Jose Police Department and Crime Prevention Unit.

Assault and Child Guidance Center, San Jose.

Dave Obrian, "Crimes Against Innocence," *San Jose Mercury News*, Sept. 7, 1991, p. l2C.

"Discipline or Abuse: The Fine Line," *Bay Area Parent,* August 1989, p. 24.

References:

(See selected classic and current articles below for additional reading. For community-based in-services or consultation, contact your local Domestic Abuse Speaker's Bureau.)

American Medical Association. (1992). Violence: A compendium from JAMA, American medical news and specialty journal of the AM A. *JAMA.* Chicago: AM A.

Briere, J. et al. (Eds.). (1997). *The APSAC handbook on child maltreatment.* London: SAGE.

Cowell, N.A. & Burgess, A.W. (Eds.). (1996). *Understanding violence against women.* Washington, D.C.: National Academy Press.

Jezierski, M. (1999). Family violence screening: Opportunities in prehospital settings. *Journal of Emergency Nursing* 25(3):201-205.

Lee, D. & Anderson, L.F. (1995). *Improving your community clinic s response to domestic violence.* Sacramento, CA: California Department of Health Services.

Markus, K. (1999). Reporting signs of abuse. *NurseWeek.* April 19, p. 13.

Reece, R.M. (1994). *Child abuse: medical diagnosis and management.* Philadelphia: Lea & Febiger.

Shea, C.A., Mahoney, M. & Lacey, J.K.M. (1997). Breaking through the barriers to domestic violence intervention. *AJN97(*6):26-33.

West, C.M. (1999). *Partner violence in military families.* University of New Hampshire, Family Research Laboratory.

Winfrey, M.E. & Smith, A.R. (1999). The suspiciousness factor: Critical care nursing and forensics. *Critical Care Nursing* 22(l):l-7. Gaithersburg, MD: Aspen.

Back Problem
(Upper & Lower)

BACK PROBLEM (UPPER & LOWER) (BIRTH-6 YR)

PAIN W OR W/O TRAUMA

ASSOC SX/SPECIFIC/CONSIDERATIONS	DISPOSITION/ADVICE
EMERGENT SYMPTOMS	**ED IN 0 MIN-1 HOUR**
• **TRAUMA (MAJOR): MVA, BLUNT TRAUMA/FALL/DIVING,** W OR W/O PAIN, Loss of Sensation/Ability to Move/Numbness & Tingling, **Incontinence? (Spinal Trauma)** → • **PAIN W/O TRAUMA** + FEVER, STIFF NECK, HEADACHE, N/V, Extreme Fatigue, ± Pinpoint Red Purplish Spots Progressing to Purple Patches, Extremely Irritable or Unresponsive, ± Seizure, 'Toxic Child" (See Toxicity Assessment), Infant-2 Yrs: High-pitched cry, bulging/tight fontanelle? (Meningitis) • Does RN feel Sx. are severe, extreme, emergent?	• **DON'T MOVE.**
URGENT SYMPTOMS	**ED/MD/APPT. IN 1-8 HOURS**
• **TRAUMA (MINOR-MOD.)** + SUSPICIOUS HX? (Abuse) **(See ABUSE)** → + BACK PAIN (Persistent)? (Vertebral Fx) • **BACK PAIN W/O TRAUMA** + FEVER, ± Limp? (Osteomyelitis, Diskitis) • **LOWER BACK PAIN W/O TRAUMA** + ± SEVERE, RADIATING FROM ABD./FLANK/BACK TO GROIN, Colicky Then Constant & Severe, FEVER/Chills, N/V, Dysuria, ± Hematuria, Frequency/Urgency? (Pyelonephritis) • **UPPER/MID BACK PAIN W/O TRAUMA** + FEVER, SHAKING, CHILLS, Cough, Substernal/Intercostal Retractions, Nasal Flaring, ± Wheezing, Rapid/Shallow Resp., N/V, ± Abd. Pain, Anorexia, Fatigue? (Pneumonia: Bacterial, Viral, Aspiration) • WORSENING SX After 24^18 Hr on Home Tx? • RECENT SURGERY or HOSPITALIZATION? (Poss. Complications) • Does RN feel Sx. are urgent?	• **BRING CHILD TO E.D. NOW.**
ACUTE SYMPTOMS	**ED/MD/APPT IN 8-24 HOURS**
• **BACK PAIN (CHRONIC)** + Gradual Onset, ± Trauma, Weakness, Fatigue, ± Headache, ± FEVER, ± Urinary Retention, Incontinence? (Neoplastic Disease) • AGE 3 MO-6 YR + MOD. SX + (AVED) = POSS. UPGRADE? • Does RN feel Sx. are acute?	
NON-ACUTE SYMPTOMS	**HOME TREATMENT W OR W/O APPT IN 24 + HOURS**
• **PAIN** + With Movement, w/o Assoc. Sx? (Muscle Strain/Overuse) • MINOR SELF-LIMITING SX EXISTING > 1 WK, NOT BECOMING MARKEDLY WORSE? • HOME TX ITEMS OR PHONE NOT AVAILABLE = POSS. UPGRADE? • Does RN feel Sx. are non-acute?	
CROSS-REFERENCES	**STANDARD FOLLOW-UP INSTRUCTIONS**
• ABUSE • RESPIRATORY PROBLEM 1; 2 • URINARY PROBLEM	PT TO CALL BACK: If symptoms become much worse or urgent or emergent symptoms arise (RN: review Protocol and advise caller). RN TO CALL BACK: If acute Sx in child AGE < 2 years. Routinely for Abdomen pain, Respiratory problems, Fever, Diarrhea, Marked change in ADL.

Behavioral Problems

Behavioral Problem (Eating; Sleeping; Elimination; Emotional; Developmental) Supplemental Information (Infant > 1 Mo, Toddler, School Age, and Teens)

Quick Reference:

(**NOTE:** Age < 1 mo: Regarding Newborn Problems, see Newborn Concerns.)

DEVELOPMENTAL MILESTONES (RANGE WHEN ACHIEVED)

- Laughs/coos/smiles: Age 1-2 mo
- Says Dada/Mama: Age 5-10 mo
- Rolls over: Age 2 to 4'A mo
- Sits w/o support: Age 4'A to 1A mo
- Drinks from a cup: Age 9-16 mo
- Tries to feed self: Age 4'A to 8 mo
- Cruises (walks holding on to furniture) Age 7 to 12'/2 mo
- Walks: Age 11-14 mo
- Says three words other than Mama/Dada: Age 11A to 20 mo

COLIC

See Newborn Concerns Behavior/Crying.

CRYING

Rule out toxicity or dehydration; see also Parent's Help in Appendix D.

Sleeping Requirements for Infants and Toddlers

- Causes: Physical discomfort, hunger, colic, need to be held, etc.
- Complication: Child abuse, shaken baby syndrome
- Prevention/Treatment: To help the child to become calm, try some of the following actions starting with the first item on the list.
  - -Make sure the baby is not wet, hungry, too hot/cold, or sick.
  - -Swaddle the newborn. It can calm and soothe the baby. It makes the infant feel like how he or she felt in the womb—firmly held and secure.

-Rock or walk with the baby in a "snugli" front-pack or your arms; try singing or talking to the baby.
-Play any soft music or classical music.
-Low, monotonous sounds can soothe the baby. Try putting the baby near the sound of a running shower/water or clothes dryer. Turn on the vacuum cleaner nearby the baby.
-Take the baby outdoors, if possible. Dress baby for the weather. Using a stroller, backpack, or front-pack, take baby for a walk for about 20 minutes. Babies like the fresh air and outdoors.
-Take the baby for a short ride in the car. Sometimes they will fall asleep. If the baby is sound asleep, and if you can, try to bring the baby into the house in the car seat, if the car seat is not too heavy.
-Call a friend, neighbor, or relative to talk or to take care of the baby for a few hours. If your baby cries a lot, try to get someone to watch the baby for a few hours between 4 PM and 9 PM, when both parent and baby are tired and irritable.
-Put the baby on his or her back in the crib, close the door, and check on him or her frequently.

DISCIPLINE

- Prevention—To prevent violent behavior:
  -Use firm, loving discipline.
  -The adults in the house should all agree on the rules and type of punishment if the child breaks them.
  -Be consistent.
  -Teach your child to use words when he or she is angry or upset.
  -Teach him or her not to kick, bite, or hit when angry.
  -Watch your own reactions. Learn to control your own temper. Express your anger quietly. Do not yell and scream.
  -Be very concrete in describing misbehavior: "Do not hit your sister." "Do not push Johnny."
  -Ignore your child when he or she acts out harmlessly such as tantrums, sulking, or whining.
  -Distract him or her with toys, foods, or games.
  -Praise and reward him or her for good behavior.
  -Set up your home so that it is safe; remove objects that cause problems w his or her behavior.
  -Use "time out" as a method of discipline. Rule of thumb: 1 min per 1 yr of age. Should not last more than 5 min. Put child in a boring place.

Breath-Holding Spells

- Definition: Child cries and holds his or her breath until his or her lips turn blue, then passes out. Usually starts breathing again and wakes up as soon as he or she passes out. Usually occurs in child age between 6 mo-5 yr. Usually does not happen more than 1-2 * a day. These episodes can end with a seizure-like movement. (See also Dizziness; Fainting Problem.)
- Cause: Spells usually follow periods of fear, anger, frustration, or temper tantrums.
- Complication: Breath holding, turning blue but not passing out; not abnormal (temper tantrum). Passing out can be followed by seizures.
- Prevention/Tx
  -Keep your child lying flat after the fainting spell to increase blood flow to the brain.
  -Apply a cold compress to his/her forehead (see Home Tx Ref).

-Try to remain calm during the episode.

-If a temper tantrum led to the spell, do not give in to your child's demands when s/he wakes up.

Temper Tantrums

- Definition: When a child throws a fit, kicking and screaming when he or she does not get his or her way.
- Cause: Normal part of growing up; usually happens because your child becomes frustrated and does not know how to express his or her frustration. Also a way of testing your limit setting.
- Prevention/Tx

  -Signs when a tantrum is coming. Child becomes moody and more irritable than usual; does not become distracted w a show of affection and w play; whines and becomes more demanding; does not respond to comforting; cries.

  -Make sure your child does not become too tired.

  -Provide for some "quiet time" when he or she is tired, sick, or has been very active.

  -Do not set rules/restrictions that are unrealistic.

  -Be loving, firm, and consistent.

  -Be calm when he or she is in the middle of a tantrum. Do not shout. Try to distract him or her.

  -If he or she is out of control, try holding him or her with a hug until he or she calms down.

  -Keep him or her safe.

EATING PROBLEMS

- Axioms

  -Children are interested in eating. They will eat when hungry.

  -Most children, esp. toddlers, won't eat new foods. With time and patience, they will learn to try different foods.

  -As a parent, you should try to choose and buy a variety of healthy foods. Feed your child at regular times. Your child is responsible for how much he or she eats.
- Causes: Many different causes

  -Normal part of development. Toddlers want to be independent, in control, and want to feed themselves. They are also learning to assert themselves and separate themselves from their parents by saying "no" to almost everything.

  -Children often lose their appetite when sick.
- Complications: Failure to thrive; poor eating habits; power struggle between parent and child
- Prevention/Tx

  -Do not give solid foods before age 4-6 mo. Infants don't know how to swallow very well until then.

  -Give solid foods when your baby can sit up by himself or herself and can hold his or her head steady.

  -Give finger foods at age 8 mo.

  -Allow him or her to feed himself w his or her fingers or spoon.

  -Do not force or trick your child into eating.

  -Do not threaten or punish your child for not eating or not finishing his or her plate.

  -Have regular and pleasant meals and snack.

  -Limit the amt. of juice (4-6 oz/day) and milk (16-24 oz/day for toddlers) that your child drinks. If he or she is thirsty, offer water instead.

-Give your child a multivitamin at least 1 x wk if your child is a picky eater.
-Give small servings in his or her plate. He or she is more likely to finish it and will feel good about himself/herself for finishing his or her meal. (Rule of thumb: 1 tablespoon for each year of the child's age = 1 serving.)
-Turn the TV off during mealtime.

- Daily servings needed
  -Milk or milk products: 2-3 cups
  -Fruits and vegetables: 4-6 servings
  -Breads and cereals: 4 servings
  -Meats, fish, poultry, or legumes: 2 servings
  -Vitamin A: Apricots, cantaloupe, carrots, spinach, greens, squash, sweet potatoes, broccoli, plums
  -Vitamin C: Broccoli, cabbage, cantaloupe, oranges, orange juice, squash

Food Allergies

- Definition: Allergic Sx after eating certain foods. May go w Hx of asthma, eczema, or hay fever, or family Hx of food allergies.
- Common Sx: Swelling around the mouth, lips, or tongue; diarrhea or vomiting; hives; itchy skin
- Prevention/Tx
  -Breastfeed for as long as possible (first year of life).
  -If possible, wait until age 5 mo before starting solid foods.
  -If strong family Hx, wait until age 6 mo before giving eggs and wheat.

ELIMINATION PROBLEMS

Bed-Wefting (Enuresis)

- Definition: Anytime there is bed-wetting after a few months of being dry, or after age 6-7 yr. It is more common in boys. Accidents while asleep are considered normal until age 6 yr. It is a very common problem in preschoolers.
  -It is normal for a child to wet his/her bed at night 2-3 times a wk right after he or she has been toilet trained (which is usually between age 2-4 yr). Most children outgrow it by the time they are teens.
- Causes: Small bladder, immature bladder, constipation, stressful events, such as physical or sexual abuse, new baby, divorce, or moving. If child continues to wet the bed after being dry for a few months, see MD. There might be an infection or a disease causing bed-wetting. Defects in bladder or diabetes can also cause bed-wetting.
- Complication: Emotional problems due to peer and/or family pressure. These causes are very rare through. Bed-wetting also often runs in families. Usually one parent has had it.
- Prevention/Tx
  -Always be kind and supportive to your child.
  -Don't use detergents or soap that are irritating to the skin.
  -Don't let child drink a lot of water or juice before bedtime.
  -Don't let child eat foods that cause irritation or increase urine output: citrus foods, caffeine.
  -Encourage fresh fruits and vegetables, which help to prevent constipation.
  -Encourage going to the bathroom before going to bed.

-Encourage your child to hold his or her urine for a little longer in the daytime to strengthen the bladder.
-Do not punish your child for wetting his or her bed. It is not his or her fault.
-Reward him or her for dry nights. Encourage him or her but don't pressure. It will get better in time.

- Make an appt w your pediatrician:

-If your child complains of burning or pain, cloudy or pink urine when going to the bathroom.
-If your child has blood or discharge on underpants.
-If your child still wets the bed, after following the above advice * 3 mo.
-If he or she wets his or her pants or bed even after going to the bathroom regularly.
-If he or she is straining or his or her urine dribbles out.
-Pink or red stains on his or her underpants or bedsheets.
-If bed-wetting is a new problem.

Soiling (Encopresis)

- Definition: Having small amounts of bowel movements in the child's underpants regularly; usually involves children age 4 yr or older. May have complaints of stomachache.
- Cause: Constipation, impaction, or child resisting toilet training by holding back bowel movements. Needs to see MD/RN if an ongoing problem x 2-5 days.
- Complication: Skin irritation; feeling ashamed of oneself; harsh toilet training techniques can lead to refusal/oppositional behavior; can lead to anxiety, withdrawal, depression, and poor self-esteem.
- Prevention/Tx

-Stool softeners to soften stools and make BMs easier.
-Give fruits and vegetables every day.
-Use bran as a natural laxative (e.g., bran flakes, bran muffins, whole wheat bread).
-Add good sources of fiber in the diet (e.g., beans, brown rice, popcorn, peas).
-Encourage regular toileting habits—sitting on the toilet for about 10 min each day. Do not force your child if he or she refuses or if he or she is busy with something.
-Encourage him or her to push while sitting on the toilet.
-Praise your child for success.
-Make an appt. w primary health care provider if no improvement in 1-2 wk.

Toilet Training: Most Children Are Ready To Be Potty Trained around 2 Yr.

- Signs of readiness

-You are ready to begin toilet training and keep it up every day for 3 months.
-He or she is able to walk to the toilet.
-He or she is able to pull his or her diapers/pants down.
-He or she can tell you he or she has to go "pee" or "potty" or use words both of you can understand.
-Your child understands what the potty chair or toilet is for.
-He or she prefers being dry or w clean diapers.
-Your child can tell when his/her bladder is full—jumps up and down, goes off to a corner to urinate or have a BM, or tells you "pee wants to come out."

- Ways to prepare your child for toilet training.

-Change his or her diaper often so that he or she becomes used to having a clean, dry diaper.
-Let your child watch you or his or her brothers or sisters use the bathroom.

-Buy your child a potty chair. Let him or her get used to it.
-Put your child on the potty chair every 2 hours. Stay with him or her. Read or talk to your child to help him or her relax.
-Usually, children will have a BM about 1 hour after eating.
-Let him or her practice using the potty chair when he or she acts like he or she is about to urinate or have a BM.
-Praise your child when he or she uses the potty chair successfully.
-It may take 3 months to get your child toilet trained. If they are not trained by then, talk with your doctor. He or she may not be ready to be trained yet.

SLEEPING PROBLEMS

- To avoid problems in the future, start early with good habits. While your child is still a baby:
  -Put your baby down when he or she is drowsy but still awake. You are teaching your baby how to fall asleep by him/herself.
  -The first 3 mo of life, hold your baby when he or she fusses; put him or her down when he or she calms down. This will teach your child to soothe him/herself to sleep.
  -Stop nighttime feeding by age 6 mo, esp. if he or she is eating solids.
  -Don't let your baby hold the bottle in bed or fall asleep w a bottle in his or her mouth.
  -If your child is still waking up at age 6 mo, make your visits brief and boring.
  -By age 1 yr, have a regular bedtime routine (bedtime stories).
  -Keep daytime naps short, no more than 2 hr.
  -Give him or her plenty of attention during the day, lots of hugs and kisses.
  -Keep regular, appropriate schedules for nap time and meal times. Avoid late or very early meals.
  -Don't let child play in crib. The crib is for sleeping *only.*
  -Create bedtime "rituals": Change diaper, change into nightie, have music.
  -Advice regarding child waking at night: Refer parents to books w standard behavioral techniques for helping child return to sleep on own.

Bedtime Resistance

- Definition: Child over age 2 yr who falls asleep while watching TV w parents; or who prolongs bedtime by stalling w crying, asking questions, or w temper tamtrums.
- Causes: Testing your limit setting; inability or difficulty controlling impulses
- Prevention/Tx
  -Start bedtime w a pleasant routine, which can include a bath, tooth brushing, and a bedtime story.
  -Make it a rule that your child cannot leave his or her room after bedtime.
  -Ignore requests for a drink. Do not carry on a conversation after you both have said your good nights.
  -Return your child to his or her bed if he or she comes out of the bedroom w/o lecturing/yelling. Tell him or her that you will have to keep the door closed if he or she comes out again.
  -Praise him or her in the morning if he or she stayed in his or her bedroom all night.

Early Morning Riser

- Definition: Usually child age 1-3 yr who wakes up at 5 AM fully rested and raring to go-

- Causes: The child usually had enough sleep and is not tired. Being put to bed too early or naps that are too frequent or too long. May not need as much sleep. (Average sleep required: 10-12 hr per night for age 1-10 yr.) Change of season—springtime when the sun shines bright and early.
- Prevention/Tx

-Shorten nap times or cut down on number of naps during the day.

-Don't put to bed until 8 or 9 PM.

-Give your child dinner a little later in the evening in case he or she is waking up because he or she is hungry.

-Set up strict rules: He or she has to stay in his or her room and play quietly until you get up.

-If still in a crib, put some quiet toys in the crib and leave him or her in the crib until 6 AM. Be careful not to put toys he or she can use to stand on.

-If your child cries, visit him or her for a very short time and give reassurance. Tell him or her that everyone else in the house is still sleeping.

-Praise your child when he or she does not wake people in the morning.

Nightmares

- Definition: Scary dreams that wake up the child. It can happen in toddlers but usually occurs in preschool children. Usually happens during the second half of the night. Child cries after waking up. He or she is afraid to go back to bed and may have trouble falling asleep. May talk about his or her dream.
- Causes: It may be the child's way of seeing his or her experiences that day. It may represent an aggressive feeling or fear that the child has. Stress due to separation from parent or start of daycare.
- Prevention/Tx

-Cuddle and reassure when it happens.

-Stay w your child until he or she calms down.

-Use a night light.

-Help him or her talk about any bad dreams during the day.

-Do not let him or her watch scary/violent movies or TV shows.

Night Terrors

- Definition: Occurs between ages 1-8 yr. Child screams and thrashes in his or her sleep and may have a look of panic w sweating and his or her heart beating fast. He or she does not wake up from sleep but may run around scared. Usually happens 1-2 hr after falling sleep. Your child may not be aware that you are there and push you away, screaming more when you try to restrain him or her. His or her eyes may be wide open and staring at you but he or she looks right through you. His or her fear and confusion disappear when he or she wakes up. He or she does not remember a dream or that he or she was yelling or thrashing around.
- Cause: Usually inherited. Being overtired can trigger it.
- Prevention/Tx

-Turn on the lights so that he or she does not become confused w shadows.

-Speak slowly and soothingly. "You're all right. You're home." Do not shake or shout at him or her.

-Protect your child from getting hurt. Keep him or her away from stairs, windows.

-Make sure that your child gets enough rest and sleep.

-An appt. should be made if the child has any drooling or jerky movements.

Bites

BITES 1 (HUMAN/ANIMAL) (SKIN PROBLEM 1) (ALL AGES)

HUMAN; CAT; DOG; BAT; HORSE; SQUIRREL; SKUNK; RACCOON; FOX

ASSOC SX/SPECIFIC/CONSIDERATIONS	DISPOSITION/ADVICE
EMERGENT SYMPTOMS	**ED IN 0 MIN-1 HOUR**
• **ALL BITES** ---------►	• IDENTIFY ANIMAL (Owner, History of Vaccination). • NOTIFY ANIMAL CONTROL.
+ PROGRESSIVELY: Anxious, Weak, Dizzy, Thirsty, N/V, SKIN: Pale. Blotchy/Discolored/Cool or Cold, Sweaty, LIPS/NAILBED: Blue, PULSE: Weak/Fast, BREATHING: Rapid/Shallow, Unresponsive, Loss of Consciousness? (Shock) (See SHOCK)	
• Does RN feel symptoms are severe, extreme, or emergent?	
URGENT SYMPTOMS	**ED/MD/APPT IN 1-8 HOURS**
• **BITE (HUMAN OR ANIMAL)** ---------►	• ALL BITES: Check Tetanus Status. + Lack of or outdated IMMUNIZATION => Risk tetanus.
+ HUMAN BITE + SUSPICIOUS HISTORY? (Abuse) (See ABUSE) ——— *-	• **COME TO E.D. NOW.**
+ Multiple or Large Wound, Face, Head, or Neck Laceration? (> Risk Infection, Hemorrhage) ---------►	• **COME TO E.D. NOW.**
+ PERSISTENT BLEEDING, History of Bleeding Disorder, Anticoagulants, Kidney/Liver Disease? (> Risk Hemorrhage) ---------►	• **COME TO E.D. NOW.**
+ HIGH RISK LOCATIONS: Hand, Wrist, Foot, Over Major Joint, Through Cheek, CHILD: Face or Scalp? (Infection, Fracture) ——►	• **COME TO E.D. NOW.**
+ HIGH RISK WOUNDS: All Punctures, Crushing (Horses, Cows), Over Vital Structure: Nerve, Joint, Artery? (Infection, Fracture) ——»	• **COME TO E.D. NOW.**
+ Sick, Rabid, Unprovoked Attack by Cat or Dog or Any Wild Animal: Raccoons, Squirrels, Bats, Foxes, Skunks, Rodents? (> Risk Rabies) «■	• **COME TO E.D. NOW.**
+ OVER KNUCKLES: "Fight Bite," Abraded, Lacerated, Punctured Skin from Teeth of Another Human? (> Risk Infection) ——»	• **See AXIOM Human Bite.**
+ Red ± Streaking, Swollen, Tender, Hot; ± Discharge, Often w FEVER, Swollen Nodes, History of Trauma/Bite/Local Infection? (Cellulitis)	
+ HIGH RISK PATIENTS: >50 YEARS, Asplenic, Diabetic. Alcoholic, AIDS/HIV, History of Chemotherapy, Steroid Therapy, Cardiac Valve Disease? (> Risk Infection)	
+ HIGH RISK SPECIES: Domestic or Large Cat, Human, Primates, Pigs? (> Risk Infection)	
+ Tetanus Immunization > 10 Yrs? (> Risk)	
• **BITE (CAT)**	
+ HAND: RAPIDLY PROGRESSING REDNESS/SWELLING (Pasteurella Multicedens Cellulitis) ——►	• **COME IN NOW**
• FAILURE TO IMPROVE on Antibiotics x 48 Hr? (Ineffective Rx)	
• MODERATE SYMPTOMS + RISK FACTORS (Age, Veracity, Emotional Distress, Debilitation/ Distance) = POSS. UPGRADE?	
• Does RN feel symptoms are urgent?	
ACUTE SYMPTOMS	**ED/MD/APPT IN 8-24 HOURS**
• **SCRATCH (CAT)**	See First Aid (Supplemental Information)
+ FEVER, Fatigue, Anorexia, Headache, Pustule at Site in 3-5 Days, Swollen/ Tender Lymph Nodes? (Cat Scratch Fever)	
• FAILURE TO IMPROVE on Home Treatment x 48 Hr?	
• Does RN feel symptoms are acute?	
NON-ACUTE SYMPTOMS	**HOME TREATMENT W OR W/O APPT IN 24 + HOURS**
• MINOR SELF-LIMITING SYMPTOMS EXISTING > 1 WK, NOT BECOMING MARKEDLY WORSE? • HOME TREATMENT ITEMS NOT AVAILABLE = POSS. UPGRADE? • Does RN feel symptoms are non-acute?	
CROSS-REFERENCES	**STANDARD FOLLOW-UP INSTRUCTIONS**
• ABUSE • SKIN PROBLEM 4 (LACERATION/WOUND)	PT TO CALL BACK: If symptoms become much worse or urgent or emergent symptoms arise (RN . Review Protocol and advise caller). RN TO CALL BACK: Routinely for Abdomen Pain, Respiratory Problems, Fever, Diarrhea, Marked change in ADL.

BITES 2 (SKIN PROBLEM 1) (ALL AGES)

SNAKE; JELLYFISH; SEA URCHIN; STINGRAY

ASSOC SX/SPECIFIC/CONSIDERATIONS	DISPOSITION/ADVICE
EMERGENT SYMPTOMS	**ED IN 0 MIN-1 HOUR**
• **SNAKE BITE** + PROGRESSIVELY: Anxious, Weak, Dizzy, Thirsty, N/V, SKIN: Pale, Blotchy/Discolored/Cool or Cold, Sweaty, LIPS/NAILBED: Blue, PULSE: Weak/Fast, BREATHING: Rapid/Shallow, Unresponsive, Loss of Consciousness? (Shock) (See SHOCK) • **MARINE ANIMAL STING** + SOB, WHEEZING, STRIDOR, Difficulty Swallowing, Agitation, Anxiety, Rash (Itchy, Raised, "Hive-Like"). Swelling of Face/Tongue, History of Allergies or Exp. to Allergen (Substance, Bite)? (Anaphylaxis) • Does RN feel symptoms are severe, extreme, emergent?	
URGENT SYMPTOMS	**ED/MD/APPT IN 1-8 HOURS**
• **SNAKE BITE** (w/o systemic manifestations) → + Rattlesnake? + Coral Snake? + Water Moccasin/Cottonmouth Snake? + Copperhead Snake?	• **CONTACT POISON CENTER** • **COME TO E.D. NOW.** • NEVER "CUT & SUCK," APPLY ICE, APPLY TOURNIQUET OR PRESSURE BANDAGE! + Move patient 20 feet from snake. + KEEP PATIENT CALM, WARM AND QUIET. + GENTLY Wash wound w soap & water. + Keep bite area ***below*** heart level. + Remove all jewelry, tight clothes, shoes as needed. + Splint area as for fracture.
• **JELLYFISH/PORTUGUESE MAN-OF-WAR STING?** (Neurotoxicity)-^	• **CONTACT POISON CENTER.** • **COME TO E.D. NOW** (See also FIRST AID below) • **FIRST AID (JELLYFISH STING):** Remove the tentacles/stingers. Relieve the pain. + PAIN: Soak w Vk sea water + % vinegar x 30 Min. Apply topical antihistamine (e.g.. Calamine lotion). + Pour flour or baking powder on affected area, remove stingers. + Do not rub the wound! It will make the stinging & pain worse! + JELLYFISH: No Antivenin.
• **SEA URCHIN SPINES?** (Toxicitvt →	• **CONTACT POISON CENTER. (See First Aid below)**
. **STINGRAY7** (Tnvirity) →	• **CONTACT POISON CENTER.** • **FIRST AID** (STINGRAY/SEA URCHIN) • STINGRAY/SEA URCHIN ADVICE + Remove spines. + Wash wound with any available water. + Place injured part in nonscalding hot water.
• **ALL BITES/STINGS** + PREVIOUS MEDICAL HISTORY: Bleeding Disorder, Kidney/Liver Disease, Anticoagulants? (> Risk Hemorrhage) →	• **COME TO E.D. NOW.**
+ PREVIOUS MEDICAL HISTORY: Asplenic, Diabetic, Alcoholic, AIDS/HIV, History of Chemotherapy, Steroid Therapy, Cardiac Valve Disease? (> Risk Infection) + AGE: > 50 Years, < 10 Years? (> Risk Toxicity) + Red ± Streaking, Swollen, Tender, Hot; ± Discharge, Often w FEVER, Swollen Nodes, History of Trauma/Bite/Local Infection? (Cellulitis/Infection) • Does RN feel symptoms are urgent?	
ACUTE SYMPTOMS	**ED/MD/APPT IN 8-24 HOURS**
NON-ACUTE SYMPTOMS	**HOME TREATMENT W OR W/O APPT IN 24 + HOURS**
CROSS-REFERENCES	**STANDARD FOLLOW-UP INSTRUCTIONS**
	PT TO CALL BACK: If symptoms become much worse or urgent or emergent symptoms arise (RN: Review Protocol and advise caller). RN TO CALL BACK: Routinely for Abdomen Pain, Respiratory Problems, Fever, Diarrhea, Marked change in ADL.

BITES 3 (SKIN PROBLEM 1) (ALL AGES)

BEE STINGS, YELLOW JACKET, HORNET, WASP; SPIDERS; SCORPIONS; FLEAS; TICKS

ASSOC SX/SPECIFIC/CON SIDE RATIONS	DISPOSITION/ADVICE
EMERGENT SYMPTOMS	**ED IN 0 MIN-1 HOUR**
• **ANY STING/BITE** + SOB, WHEEZING, STRIDOR, Retractions, Difficulty Swallowing, Agitation, Anxiety, Rash (Itchy, Raised, "Hive-Like"), Swelling of Face/Tongue, History of Allergies or Exp. to Allergen (Med., Drug, Food, Chemical, Substance, Bite)? (Anaphylaxis) (See SHOCK) ------► + PROGRESSIVELY: Anxious, Weak, Dizzy, Thirsty, NA/. SKIN: Pale, Blotchy/Discolored/Cool or Cold, Sweaty, LIPS/NAILBED: Blue, PULSE: Weak/Fast, BREATHING: Rapid/Shallow, Unresponsive, Loss of Consciousness? (Shock) (See SHOCK) • **SCORPION BITE** (Small. Silver White) + PAIN AT SITE, RESTLESSNESS, Roving Eye Movements, Difficult Speech, Loss of Bowel/Bladder Control, Difficult Breathing, Shaking, Resp. Distress? (Neurotoxicity) ——► • **BLACK WIDOW SPIDER BITE** + CRAMPS/PAIN, Abdomen/Chest/Back, Difficult Breathing, N/V, SOB. Weakness, Headache, Cardiac Arrhythmias, Boardlike Rigidity, Paralysis? (Neurotoxicity) ------*- • Does RN feel symptoms are severe, extreme, emergent?	• Epi kit as appropriate. + Benadryl (in any form) if immediately available. Dose: Age & wt. dependent. (See OTC REF) • **CONTACT POISON CENTER.** • **FIRST AID (SCORPION/BLACK WIDOW):** + Keep bite area below heart level. + Wash bite w soap & water. + Keep patient sitting quietly. + Remove all jewelry. + Splint affected area. + Place covered ice pack on bite. • **CONTACT POISON CENTER (SEE FIRST AID ABOVE).** * **AXIOM:** Black Widow bite symptoms may mimic MI or acute abdomen.
URGENT SYMPTOMS	**ED/MD/APPT IN 1-8 HOURS**
• **BROWN RECLUSE SPIDER BITE** ------»- + Painful, Burning Sensation within 10 Min, "Bull's Eye" Ulcer with Rash, FEVER, N/V, Jaundice (Neurotoxicity) • **BEE STINGS** + MULTIPLE STINGS, Near Eyes, on Face/Genitals, Generalized Itching, Raised Reddened Areas/Hives, CHILD or Elderly? (> Risk Toxicity) ——► • **ALL BITES (INSECT)** + Red ± Streaking, Swollen, Tender, Hot; ± Discharge, Often w FEVER, Swollen Nodes, History of Trauma/Bite/Local Infection? (Cellulitis/Infection) • WORSENING SYMPTOMS after 24-48 Hr on Home Treatment? • Does RN feel symptoms are urgent?	• **CONTACT POISON CENTER.** • **COME TO E.D. NOW.** • See First Aid above. • **COME TO E.D. NOW.**
ACUTE SYMPTOMS	**ED/MD/APPT IN 8-24 HOURS**
• **ALL OTHER SPIDER/SCORPION BITES?** • **ALL BITES (INSECT)** + Itchy, Honey-Colored Crusted Lesions? (Impetigo) • **HISTORY OF TICK BITE** + Present on Skin x 24-36 Hr? (> Risk Complications) + Parts of Tick Left in Skin After Removal? (Infection) + Red Rash That Looks Like Ring, 3-30 Days After Bite, ± Flu Symptoms, Aching Muscles, Fatigue, Headache? (Lyme Disease) • Does RN feel symptoms are acute?	
NON-ACUTE SYMPTOMS	**HOME TREATMENT W OR W/O APPT IN 24 + HOURS**
• BEE **STING** ------► + Moderate Local Swelling. Pain. Itching at the Site? (Localized Reaction) • **RASH** + Small Group Configuration, Itching, Animal Exposure? (Flea Bites) • **TICK BITE?** (See Supplemental Information) • MINOR SELF-LIMITING SYMPTOMS EXISTING > 1 WK, NOT BECOMING MARKEDLY WORSE? • HOME TREATMENT ITEMS/PHONE NOT AVAIL. = POSS. UPGRADE? • Does RN feel symptoms are non-acute?	• BEE STING TREATMENT: (See BITES SUPPLEMENTAL INFORMATION)
CROSS-REFERENCES	**STANDARD FOLLOW-UP INSTRUCTIONS**
• SKIN PROBLEM 6: RASH • SKIN PROBLEM 6: RASHES; CHILDHOOD RASHES • SUPPLEMENTAL INFORMATION	PT TO CALL BACK: If symptoms become much worse or urgent or emergent symptoms arise (RN: Review Protocol and advise caller). RN TO CALL BACK: Routinely for Abdomen Pain, Respiratory Problems, Fever, Diarrhea, Marked change in ADL.

Bites (Skin Problem 1) Supplemental Information (All Ages)

HUMAN BITES AXIOMS

- Human bites are often related to physical and sexual abuse. (See ABUSE 1 & 2.)
- Beware of "fight bites"—human bites over knuckles. Because of its location, this type of injury is high risk for serious joint infections.
- Whether accidental or intentional, all breaks in skin caused by human teeth = human bite.
- All human bites are potentially serious.

BITES (ALL) TREATMENT

- GOAL: Prevent infection.
  - Control bleeding by keeping bite area <u>above</u> heart (will decrease pain/swelling).
  - Flush with clean water from tap.
  - Wash with soap and water by filling large clean plastic bag with soap and water, poke hole in it with a knife or pin and squirt directly into wound x 3 minutes.
  - Cover with clean cloth or sterile dressing.
  - Tetanus must be given within 72 Hr.

ANIMAL BITES AXIOMS

- Treat all wild animals as rabid: wolves, foxes, skunks, bats, coyotes, woodchuck, bobcats, squirrels, feral or stray cats and dogs.
- CAT BITES: Up to 50% of all cat bites become infected.

RABIES

- SIGNS & SYMPTOMS: Depression, restlessness, fever. Progresses to muscle spasm, drooling, fear of water, coma, death.
- RABID WILD ANIMAL BEHAVIOR:
  - Daytime activity of nocturnal bats, raccoons, skunks, and foxes.
  - Wild animals who seem to lack normal fear of humans.
  - Any animal with furious behavior. (See below.)
- RABID DOMESTIC ANIMALS' & HUMAN'S BEHAVIOR:
  - Furious Rabies: Agitation and viciousness followed by paralysis and death within days.
- CAUSE: Virus. Incubation in humans 10 days-1 Yr (usually 6 Wk).

- PREVENTION:
  - DO NOT GO NEAR ANY WILD ANIMALS! Even in parks or campsites, deer, raccoons, chipmunks, and skunks are still WILD ANIMALS!
  - Never pick up sick or injured animals.
  - Never pet strange animals.
  - Never disturb eating animals.
  - Never stop animals from fighting.
  - Report all strays to police or animal control.

SNAKE BITE AXIOMS

- Treat all snakes as poisonous until proven otherwise.
- CHILD: 50% of all fatalities occur in children < 12 years old.
- CHILD: Bite victims are often young, intoxicated males who have been playing with snakes.

COMMUNITY ALERT

- Most snake bites occur in July and August. Snakes are active, and people are interacting with the outdoors.
- Snakes are more active at night.
- PREVENTION:
  - Stay alert at all times: Watch where you walk or put your hands.
  - Wear high boots, carry long pole to poke areas you cannot see.
  - If you see a snake, stay 20-30 feet away. Maximum strike distance is a few feet.
  - When it is hot, snakes seek cool places: under rocks, logs, caves, crevices, pools, water.
  - When it is cold, snakes seek warm places: warm rocks, sleeping bags, boots.
  - Never handle "dead" snakes; even after the snake is dead, accidental snake bites can happen.

INSECT BITES & STINGS

AXIOM: CHILD and Elderly are more sensitive to insect venom, thus are at greater risk for toxicity.

SPIDER BITES

- Black Widow: Shiny black body w red hourglass figure on belly.
  - Found in damp, cool places (woodpiles).
- Brown Recluse: Light brown color with violin-shaped marking on back.
  - Found in dark areas (basement, garage).

BEE STINGS

- BEE STING TREATMENT:
- GOAL: Remove stinger. Relieve the pain.

- Remove stinger: Scrape gently w fingernail or credit card. Touch w scotch tape.
- To reduce pain:
  - Baking Soda Paste. (See Home Treatment Ref.) **CAUTION:** Do not use Baking Soda or Meat Tenderizer near eyes or other sensitive skin.
  - *Cloth-covered* Ice Pack on affected area. (See Home Treatment Ref.)
  - Raise bite area above heart if possible.
  - Remove all jewelry, including rings, on affected hand, arm, ankle, or foot as needed.
  - Tylenol as appropriate. (See OTC Ref.)
  - Itching: Benadryl. (Dose: Age & wt. dependent)

■ BEE STING PREVENTION:

- Don't wear bright colors.
- Wear shirt and shoes.
- Use care when drinking from cans (bees may go inside).
- Avoid using perfume when outdoors.

■ INSECT BITES CARE

- Wash with soap and water.
- Cover with clean bandage or band-aid.
- Don't scratch the bite—it can become infected.
- Cut nails; keep clean and short.
- Itching: Antihistamines. Calamine lotion. Hydrocortisone.
- Watch for signs of infection (review).

TICK BITES

COMMUNITY ALERT

■ General information about ticks:

- Tick season: December-June.
- In endemic areas, only 1-2% of ticks are infected w Lyme Disease. However, there are "pockets" where the rate is much higher.

■ TICK BITES CARE

■ GOAL: Remove tick. Prevent complications.

- TICK REMOVAL:
  - Use tweezers (pointed are best).
  - Grab tick's mouth as close to skin as possible.
  - Gently but firmly pull tick straight out. Do not twist or jerk.
  - Don't touch or squeeze the tick.
  - See instructions below for saving tick for Lyme Disease test.

- Mark date of bite on calendar. Mark a circle w ink around bite and check it daily x 3-4 days.
- Observe for complications.

LYME DISEASE

Infection caused by bacteria carried by ticks and transmitted by tick bites.

- SIGNS & SYMPTOMS: (See BITES 3)
- COMPLICATIONS:
  - (Week-Months) Heart rhythm problems, facial drooping, impaired walking, moving.
  - (1 Month to 1-2 Yrs) Arthritis, joint swelling (knees).
- PREVENTION:
  - Where found: Grasses and brush in country and city.
  - How they get to humans: Ticks climb to tips of weeds and plants. They wait for humans or animals to brush against the plants and will jump on them. They do not fly.
  - When walking in woods, tuck pants into boots or socks. Tuck shirt in.
  - Wear light-colored clothes. You can see the tick better that way.
  - Stay out of grassy areas.
  - Stay on wide clear trails.
  - Check yourself and CHILD often. Look behind ears, in armpits, back, and in belly button.
  - Shower or bathe with soap and washcloth after being in woods.
  - Carry "needle-nosed" pointed tick tweezers on hikes.
  - Mow grass along trails, buildings.
  - Check pets for ticks. Use tick collar or Rx.
  - Put special tick repellent on pants, socks, shoes.
- TREATMENT:
  - Antibiotics work well if they are taken when the rash is first seen.
  - If the tick has Lyme Disease, then antibiotics are given.
- LYME DISEASE TEST
  - (FOR HUMAN): Most accurate if done 4-6 Wks after tick bite.
  - (FOR TICK): SAVE TICK: To save tick for future (when symptoms appear): Put tick in wet paper towel in baggie, in glass jar in refrigerator. To get test results, mail tick in wet towel and baggie to local Public Health Dept.

ROCKY MOUNTAIN SPOTTED FEVER

- SIGNS & SYMPTOMS: Resistant FEVER, headaches, fatigue, joint pain; red flat rash progressing to red/purple pinpoint, starts on wrist/ankles; periorbital edema w conjunctivis, meningismus, coma.
- INCUBATION PERIOD: 2-14 days.

References

Auerbach, P.S. (Ed.)- (1995). *Wilderness medicine: Management of wilderness and environmental emergencies.* (3rd ed.). Si. Louis, MO: Mosby.

Clawson, J.J., M. D., & Dernocoeur, K.B. (1998). *Principles of emergency medical dispatch.* (2nd ed.). Salt Lake City, UT: Priority Press.

Manhoff, D. (1996). *Mosby's outdoor emergency medical guide.* (1st ed.). St. Louis, MO: Mosby.

Olson, K.R. (Ed.). (1990). *Poisoning and drug overdose.* San Mateo, CA: Appleton & Lange.

Bowel Problem

BOWEL PROBLEM 1 (BIRTH-6 YR)

DIARRHEA (SEVERE/MODERATE/MILD); BLOODY STOOL

ASSOC SX/SPECIFIC/CONSIDERATIONS	DISPOSITION/ADVICE
EMERGENT SYMPTOMS	**ED IN 0 MIN-1 HOUR**
• **BLOODY STOOL** + BLACK/BLOODY OR TARRY BMs? (Lower GI Bleeding)	
URGENT SYMPTOMS	**ED/MD/APPT. IN 1-8 HOURS**
• **BLOODY STOOL** + ± ABD. PAIN, DISTENTION, ± Hx Antibiotics? + (Pseudomembranous Colitis, Hemolytic Uremic Syndrome) + WITHOUT SX OF SHOCK? (Internal Bleeding/Meckel's Diverticulum) ---*	• **BRING CHILD TO E.D. NOW.**
+ AGE < 2 YR: SUDDEN ONSET, RECURRENT, COLICKY, SHARP ABD. PAIN, ± Vomiting Thick, Bright Green Bitter Tasting Fluid, ± Bloody Mucus Stool (Currant Jelly Stool), 'Toxic Child" ± Sev. Dehydration? (See Toxicity/Dehydration Assessment) (Intussusception) -- ▶	• **BRING CHILD TO E.D. NOW.**
• **DIARRHEA (± SEV.-MOD.)** + "TOXIC" or "VERY ILL" CHILD, Sev.-Mod. Dehydration (See Toxicity/ Dehydration Assessment)? (Toxicity/Dehydration) ------------------------------------*	• **BRING CHILD TO E.D. NOW.** • SA: Pinch skin briefly and release. Describe; if skin stays pinched-looking = tenting or + for dehydration.
+ ABD. PAIN, SUDDEN, Colicky, Vomiting, Abd. Distention, Hx of Major Change in Bowel Habits? (Bowel Obstruction) ——————-------------->	• **BRING CHILD TO E.D. NOW.**
+ CRAMPY ABD. PAIN; Watery Stools ± Blood/Mucous/Pus, Alternating w Normal Stools, ± N/V, FEVER, Recent Immigration, Hx of Foreign Travel, Exp. to Contaminated Water, Undercooked Meat/ Seafood/Poultry/Improperly Stored Food? (Infectious Diarrhea, "Food Poisoning") + Hx Antibiotics? (Clostridia difficile) • **AGE < 3 MO + FEVER > 38°C or 100.4°F@?** -- ▶	• **BRING CHILD TO E.D. NOW.**
• FEVER >40°C or 104°F? • AGE < 3 MO + MOD. SX + RISK FX (AVED)? • FAILURE TO IMPROVE on Antibiotics X 24-48 Hr? (Ineffective Rx) • WORSENING SX After 24-48 Hr on Home Tx? • RECENT SURGERY or HOSPITALIZATION? (Poss. Complications) • Does RN feel Sx. are urgent?	
ACUTE SYMPTOMS	**ED/MD/APPT IN 8-24 HOURS**
• **DIARRHEA (MILD)** + "Sick Child," Mild Dehydration (See Toxicity/Dehydration Assessment)? (Mild Dehydration) • AGE 3 MO-6 YR + MOD. SX + (AVED) = POSS. UPGRADE? • Does RN feel Sx. are acute?	

continues

BOWEL PROBLEM 1 (BIRTH-6 YR)

continued

ASSOC SX/SPECIFIC/CONSIDERATIONS	DISPOSITION/ADVICE
NON-ACUTE SYMPTOMS	**HOME TREATMENT W OR W/O APPT IN 24+HOURS**
• **DIARRHEA (MILD)** + On Antibiotics or Antacids? (Drug Side Effects) (See Supplemental Information) + Chronic Diarrhea + Hx of HIV/AIDS? (See Supplemental Information) + Related to Milk Products? (Lactose Intolerance) + Related to Diet Change, > Fruit, Juices? (Dietary Disturbance) + Crampy Abd. Pain, w/o Dehydration Sx: NA/, ± FEVER ± Headache? (Gastroenteritis) + (MILD), > AGE 4 Yr, Frequent Soiling, Hx Constipation, Vague Abd. Pain, Hx Toilet Training Prob? (Encopresis) • **LARGE/OILY/FOUL BMs** + Hx of Bowel Surgery? (Malabsorption Syndrome) + Hx Recurrent Resp. Infections, Poor Growth? (Cystic Fibrosis) • MINOR SELF-LIMITING SX EXISTING > 1 WK, NOT BECOMING MARKEDLY WORSE? • HOME TX ITEMS OR PHONE NOT AVAILABLE = POSS. UPGRADE? • Does RN feel Sx. are non-acute?	• DIARRHEA TX GOAL: Rest the bowels. Stop diarrhea. Prevent dehydration. (See Dehydration Assessment) + Rest as much as possible. + Watch for signs & Sx of dehydration. (Review)
CROSS-REFERENCES	**STANDARD FOLLOW-UP INSTRUCTIONS**
• ABDOMEN PROBLEM • BOWEL PROBLEM 2 • Dehydration Assessment/Rehydration Guidelines • FEVER • RECTAL PROBLEM • VOMITING/NAUSEA	PT TO CALL BACK: If symptoms become much worse or urgent or emergent symptoms arise (RN: review Protocol and advise caller). RN TO CALL BACK: If acute Sx in child AGE < 2 years. Routinely for Abdomen pain, Respiratory problems, Fever, Diarrhea, Marked change in ADL.

BOWEL PROBLEM 2 (BIRTH-6 YR)

CONSTIPATION; STOOL COLOR CHANGE

ASSOC SX/SPECIFIC/CONSIDERATIONS	DISPOSITION/ADVICE
EMERGENT SYMPTOMS	**ED IN 0 MIN-1 HOUR**
URGENT SYMPTOMS	**ED/MD/APPT. IN 1-8 HOURS**
• **CONSTIPATION** + PAIN ± SEVERE, Colicky, Vomiting, Abd. Distention, Hx of Major Change in Bowel Habits? (Bowel Obstruction) ---------- *- + NEWBORN: Failure To Pass Meconium in 1st 72 Hr? (Hirschsprung's Disease) + INFANT/CHILD W HX CONSTIPATION, Abd. Distention, ± Vomiting, Failure to Thrive/Grow? (Hirschsprung's Disease) • HX VIRAL INFECTION, ± < Food Intake, Sev.-Mod. Dehydration (See Dehydration Assessment)? (Viral Illness w Ileus) • **AGE < 3 MO + FEVER > 38°C or 100.4°F®?**........ → • FEVER >40°C or 104°F? • AGE < 3 MO + MOD. SX + RISK FX (AVED)? • WORSENING SX After 24-48 Hr on Home Tx? • RECENT SURGERY or HOSPITALIZATION? (Poss. Complications) • Does RN feel Sx. are urgent?	• **BRING CHILD TO E.D. NOW.** • **BRING CHILD TO E.D. NOW.**
ACUTE SYMPTOMS	**ED/MD/APPT IN 8-24 HOURS**
• **CONSTIPATION (CHRONIC)** + AGE < 1 MO: Poor Feeding, Sluggish, Hypoactive, Weak Cry? (Congenital Hypothyroidism) + ± Failure to Respond to Home Tx? (Hirschsprung's Disease) • **COLOR CHANGE** + FEVER, NA/, Anorexia, Yellow Skin, Yellow Sclera, Fatigue, Swollen Glands, Clay-Colored Stools, Dark Urine, ± Exp. to Hepatitis? (Hepatitis) (See APPENDIX A) • AGE 3 MO-6 YR + MOD. SX + (AVED) = POSS. UPGRADE? • Does RN feel Sx. are acute?	
NON-ACUTE SYMPTOMS	**HOME TREATMENT W OR W/O APPT IN 24 + HOURS**
• **CONSTIPATION** + Hx of Chronic Constipation (Hard/Dry Stools, Frequent Soiling), Mentally Challenged or Immobilized? (Impaction) + Hx Spinal Cord Injury? (Autonomic Hyperflexia) + (MILD), AGE > 4 Yr, Frequent Soiling, Hx Constipation, Vague Abd. Pain, Hx Toilet Training Prob? (Encopresis) + INFANT AGE > 1 MO: w Hx of Infrequent BM, Hard Stools, w/o Blood, Crying/Straining w BM? (Normal Newborn Stooling) + Hx New Rx or OTC Med? (Drug Side Effect) • **BLEEDING/PAIN** + Sm. Amt., Bright Red, on Outside of BM or Toilet Paper or Toilet Bowl; Hx of Constipation? (Anal Fissure, Hemorrhoid/Polyp) • **COLOR CHANGE** + BM Color Change/Food Related? (See SUPPLEMENTAL INFORMATION) + BM Color Change/Med Related? (See SUPPLEMENTAL INFORMATION) • MINOR SELF-LIMITING SX EXISTING > 1 WK, NOT BECOMING MARKEDLY WORSE? • HOME TX ITEMS OR PHONE UNAVAILABLE = POSS. UPGRADE? • Does RN feel Sx. are non-acute?	

continues

BOWEL PROBLEM 2 (BIRTH-6 YR)

continued

ASSOC SX/SPECIFIC/CONSIDERATIONS	DISPOSITION/ADVICE
CROSS-REFERENCES	**STANDARD FOLLOW-UP INSTRUCTIONS**
• ABDOMEN PROBLEM • BEHAVIORAL PROBLEM • BOWEL PROBLEM 1 • HEPATITIS (APPENDIX A) • RECTAL PROBLEM	PT TO CALL BACK: If symptoms become much worse or urgent or emergent symptoms arise (RN: review Protocol and advise caller). RN TO CALL BACK: If acute Sx in child AGE < 2 years. Routinely for Abdomen pain, Respiratory problems, Fever, Diarrhea, Marked change in ADL.

Bowel Problem Supplementary Information (Birth-6 Yr)

QUICK REFERENCE: BM Color Change
Breastfed Baby's Stools
Constipation
Dehydration
Diarrhea
Drug Side Effect (Constipation)
Drug Side Effect (Diarrhea)
HIV or AIDS Patients w Diarrhea
Infectious Diarrhea ("Food Poisoning")
Lactose Intolerance

AXIOM

Diarrhea that lasts more than 2 wk may be a sign of a more serious problem.

BM COLOR CHANGE

- Food Effect: Foods and juices that may cause BM color change: Red—Grape juice, beets, tomatoes; Black—Licorice, spinach; Red and Green—Jello, red and green.
- Disease Effect
  - Hepatitis (clay-colored stools) (See Hepatitis.)
- Drug Effect
  - Antacids (yellow/white stools)
  - Iron supplements (black stools)

BREASTFED BABY'S STOOLS

See Newborn Concerns.

CONSTIPATION

See also Behavioral Problem, Toilet Training

- Axioms
  - There is a wide variety of normal frequency for bowel movements (from once every 3 days to 3 x /day).
  - Constipation is unusual in the newborn. If suspected, needs immediate evaluation.
- Definition: Hard, dry, infrequent BMs that are hard to pass
- Causes: Age > 4 mo: Introduction of solids or new foods. Lack of fiber in diet (raw fruit and vegetables). Not drinking enough water. Not doing enough exercise. Sometimes, travel and stress cause constipation. Iron therapy. May be due to behavioral or emotional problem.
- Complication: Bowels get clogged and stretched.
- Prevention/Tx
  - Age 1-5 mo: 2-4 oz. water w 2-3 tsp. apple or prune juice
  - Age>4yr: Drink 2-3 additional glasses of water or juice daily.

- More fiber in diet. Eat raw fruits, vegetables, cereals 3 x /day. (Fruit: prunes, dates, raisins, kiwi, all fruit w skin. Vegetables: lettuce, all veg. raw. Cereals: bran flakes, muffins, whole wheat bread, shredded wheat, popcorn.)
- Don't feed child too much dairy (milk, cheese, yogurt, ice cream). It is constipating.
- Exercise daily. Walk, vigorous outdoor play, or sports 3 x/wk.
- Try to get child to have BM at a regular time each day; e.g., have child sit x 5 min on toilet w book after each meal.

DEHYDRATION

See also Dehydration Assessment/Rehydration Guidelines.

- Definition: Not enough water in body. May be very serious in the very young.
- Complications: Loss or imbalance of salt, potassium in the circulatory system.
- Prevention/Tx: Offer sips of clear liquids, ice chips, or water every 15 min. Increase as tolerated (see also Home Tx Ref, Clear Liquids).

DIARRHEA

See also Dehydration above.

- Causes: Infection, inflammation, irritation of bowel. Usually caused by bacteria, virus, food poisoning, or parasite.
- Complication: Dehydration. (See Dehydration Assessment/Rehydration Guidelines.)
- Prevention/Teaching
  - Diarrhea can be made worse or will last longer if the child eats the wrong foods. Avoid fatty/fried foods. Limit juice to Vfe glass per day.
  - Cook and refrigerate foods well. Wash your hands to prevent spread of infection.
  - Don't drink any water from creeks or streams (see Home Tx Ref, Clear Liquids and Soft Diet).
  - Antibiotics can cause mild diarrhea. Don't stop taking them. If diarrhea is more than every 2-3 x /hr, then call your M.D. Eat yogurt to help soothe bowels.

DRUG SIDE EFFECT: CONSTIPATION

(Possible explanation: accidental ingestion)
Drugs that may cause constipation:

- antacids w aluminum (also yellow/white stools)
- antihistamines
- diphenhydramine (Benadryl, Nytol, Sominex, Sleep-Eze)
- calcium
- carafate (Sulcrafate)
- codeine
- cough mixtures
- morphine and other opiates
- verapamil (Isoptin)
- vitamins or supplements w iron (also black stools)

DRUG SIDE EFFECT: DIARRHEA

(Possible explanation: accidental ingestion)

May still occur 1-10 days after antibiotic Rx. Most common drugs and classes of drugs that may cause Diarrhea

- antibiotics (all)
- ampicillin
- antacids, magnesium-based
- erythromycin
- tetracyclines

HTV OR AIDS PATIENTS W DIARRHEA

- Axiom: Patients w HIV or AIDS often have chronic diarrhea (any amount). Always watch for dehydration.
- Causes: HIV virus, secondary infection (1 or more germs).
- Complications: Dehydration, weight loss (see Dehydration above)

INFECTIOUS DIARRHEA ("FOOD POISONING")

- Signs and Sx: see Protocol
- Causes: Parasites in food, water, stool
- Complications: Dehydration; weight loss. (See Dehydration above.)
- Prevention
  - Handwashing before eating.
  - Avoid contaminated water, raw or uncooked seafood.
  - Eat only well-cooked foods.
- Tx: Medications prescribed by M.D.

LACTOSE INTOLERANCE

- Axiom: All milk products can cause diarrhea.
- Definition: Inability to digest milk, cheese, etc.
- Cause: Lacks enzyme for digestion of milk products.
- Complications: Diarrhea, weight loss, poor nutrition (See Diarrhea above.)
- Prevention: Don't drink milk or eat ice cream, cheese, yogurt. Use products w added lactase. Drink "lactate" milk or soy formula for infants.

Breastfeeding Problem

Breastfeeding Initial Assessment Questions (All Ages)

QUICK REFERENCE: General Appearance
Intake
Urine Output
Stools
Cross-Reference

RED FLAG

Always rule out toxicity and dehydration in newborn (See Toxicity/Dehydration Assessment).

GENERAL APPEARANCE

Elicit as Detailed Information as Is Possible. If infant exhibits any of the following Sx, BRING BABY IN NOW.

- Age < 3 mo: Fever (> 38°C or 100.4°F®)?
- Is baby jaundiced/yellow?
- Weak cry?
- "Floppy" baby?
- Lethargic?
- "Shrivelled" appearance "like old man"?

INTAKE

- Breast only? How often? Number of min/feeding? Both breasts offered?
- Who initiates feeding? Who ends feeding?
- Mom's perception of baby's suck: Strong? Weak?
- How long does baby sleep at one time?

URINE OUTPUT

- Age > 3 days: When mother's milk is in, baby should have 6-8 wet diapers/24 hr. Urine should be pale with minimal odor.
- Number of soaked, heavy wet diapers/past 24 hr? Color: Dark? Pale?
- Type of diaper: Cloth? Disposable? Caution: Difficult to assess with disposable diapers.
- Red Flag: Orange-looking urine/crystals in diaper = Possible Dehydration

STOOLS

- Number and characteristics of stools/past 24 hr:
- Normals:
  - First few days after birth: Dark, tarry stool (meconium)?
  - 24-48 hr after milk "comes in": Loose, wet, yellow, yellow-green, or tan? (2-5 stools/24 hr is normal.)

- Green stool? (Occasional green stool also normal.)
- Red Flag: Continually green or brown stool = Possible Dehydration

CAUTION

Assess all mothers calling with breastfeeding problems for adjustment to motherhood

- How are you feeling? (Does affect match self-description?)
- Are you able to take care of yourself (i.e., sleeping, eating, drinking when thirsty, showering)?
- Is someone available to help you? (Assess support system.)
- How are you feeling about the baby?

CROSS-REFERENCE

Post-Partum Emotional Problem *(See Adult or Age 6-18 Protocols.)*

BREASTFEEDING PROBLEM (ALL AGES)

PAIN W OR W/O FEVER; SORE NIPPLES; PAINFUL BREASTS

ASSOC SX/SPECIFIC/CONSIDERATIONS	DISPOSITION/ADVICE
EMERGENT SYMPTOMS	**ED IN 0 MIN-1 HOUR**
(See BREASTFEEDING INITIAL ASSESSMENT QUESTIONS)	
URGENT SYMPTOMS	**ED/MD/APPT IN 1-8 HOURS**
• **PAIN W FEVER** + SUDDEN ONSET: FEVER > 38.5°C or 101.3°F, Localized Red, Hot, Swollen Area on Breast, Usually Unilateral, Intense Pain, Flu-Like Sx? (Mastitis) + RED, SWOLLEN, Tender Area, ± FEVER, Nausea, Dizziness, Aching Muscles, Fatigue? (Abscess) • FEVER >40°C or 104°F? • FAILURE TO IMPROVE on Antibiotics x 24-48 Hr? (Ineffective Rx or Abscess) • RECENT SURGERY or HOSPITALIZATION? (Poss. Complications) • Does RN feel Sx. are urgent?	
ACUTE SYMPTOMS	**ED/MD/APPT IN 8-24 HOURS**
• **PAIN W/O FEVER** + Burning During Breastfeeding, Red or Pink Nipples/Areola, Hx of Mom/Baby on Antibiotics or C-section, ± Baby w Thrush? (Thrush) • MOD SX + RISK FX (AVED) = POSS. UPGRADE? • FAILURE TO IMPROVE on Home Tx x 48 Hr? • Does RN feel Sx. are acute?	
NON-ACUTE SYMPTOMS	**HOME TREATMENT** W **OR W/O APPT IN 24 +HOURS**
• **LUMP IN BREAST** + Plug or White Bump on Nipple, ± Tenderness, + Pressure Around Plug, No Fever/Flu-like Sx? (Plugged Duct) • **SORE NIPPLES** + Pain on Nipples While Breastfeeding, ± Cracks on Nipples? (Fissures)	
+ Blisters on the Nipple? (Nipple Trauma) -- ►	• Apply very warm compresses before feeding to soften blister. <X>- **REVIEW LATCH-ON TECHNIQUE** <X>-
+ Nipples Tender, Achy, Red, Abrasions, Pain Throughout Feeding? (Poss. Improper Latch-On) -- ►	• <X> **REVIEW LATCH-ON TECHNIQUE** <X>_
+ Nipples Sting, More Painful Between Feedings, in Shower, When Exposed to Air Immediately Following Feeding? (Dermatitis)------------------ ►	• 1 % Cortisone ointment to nipples sparingly after each feeding
+ Blanched Nipple Tips 5-10 Min After Feeding/Between Feeding, Worse w Contact to Cold Air, Better in Warm Shower or While Baby Nursing? (Vasospasm) -- *-	• Home Tx: + Apply Warm Compress to nipple. (See HOME TX REF) + Take Ibuprofen. (See OTC REF) + Close bra flaps immediately after feeding.
• **PAINFUL BREASTS W/O FEVER** + Feeling of Fullness, ± Swelling, ± Hard, ± Tender, Warm? (Engorgement) • QUESTIONS RE: COMMONLY USED MEDS FOR BREASTFEEDING MOMS • HOME TX ITEMS OR PHONE NOT AVAILABLE = POSS. UPGRADE? • Does RN feel Sx. are non-acute?	

continues

BREASTFEEDING PROBLEM (ALL AGES)

continued

ASSOC SX/SPECIFIC/CONSIDERATIONS	DISPOSITION/ADVICE
CROSS-REFERENCES	**STANDARD FOLLOW-UP INSTRUCTIONS**
• BREASTFEEDING PROBLEM SUPPLEMENTAL INFORMATION • POST-PARTUM CONCERNS, *Age 6-18* and *Adult* • POST-PARTUM EMOTIONAL PROBLEM, *Age 6-18* and *Adult* • TOXICITY & DEHYDRATION ASSESSMENT	PT TO CALL BACK: If symptoms become much worse or urgent or emergent symptoms arise (RN: review Protocol and advise caller). RN TO CALL BACK: If acute Sx in child < 2 years. Routinely for Abdomen pain, Respiratory problems, Fever, Diarrhea, Marked change in ADL.

Breastfeeding Problem Supplemental Information (All Ages)

QUICK REFERENCE:
- Latch-on Technique
- Abscess
- Engorgement
- Feeding Problems
- Inadequate Milk Supply
- Lactation Suppression
- Mastitis
- Mother Care
- Plugged Duct
- Sore Nipples
- Taking Medication While Breastfeeding
- Thrush
- Weaning from Breast
- Referrals

LATCH-ON TECHNIQUE

- Baby's tummy turned toward mother's tummy
- Baby's legs even with rest of body and baby held snugly against mother
- Mother supporting breast with free hand. Her hand or fingers should not cover any part of the areola
- Stroke baby's lower lip with nipple to encourage baby to open his mouth, like a yawn
- Mother quickly brings the baby onto her breast pulling him in close
- Baby taking breast 1 to lVfe inches back from nipple
- Baby's lips rolled out and relaxed against breast
- Baby's jaw movement visible with little or no cheek movement
- Mother can hear swallowing (clicking sound—not smacking of lips)
- Baby's chin and the top of his nose touch the breast during the entire nursing
- Nipples should not be sore. If they are, you need to check for proper poSi'.i-jiu,.b

ABSCESS

- Definition: Infection. A collection of pus w nowhere to drain
- Signs and Sx: Fever, flu-like Sx (nausea, dizziness, aching muscles, fatigue); : „ len and tender area
- Causes: Mastitis that has gone untreated or has not responded to antibiotics
- Prevention/Tx
  - May require surgical drainage
  - Antibiotics
  - Rest
  - Warm soaks
  - Complete emptying of breast every 2-4 hr
  - Breastfeeding can continue if the incision/drain is far enough from the areola
  - If breastfeeding is not temporarily stopped, watch the baby closely for signs of infection

ENGORGEMENT

- Definition: Swelling and fullness of the breasts due to blood vessels dilating and the milk ducts filling w milk
- Signs and Sx: Moderately severe: Breasts feel full, hard, and tender. Severe: Hard, tense and warm, generalized aching and/or throbbing pain. Both breasts are usually affected
- Causes: Infrequent or missed breastfeedings. Inadequate letdown. Hard, overfull, heavy breasts due to short feedings or "sleepy baby." Breast makes more milk than baby is taking, causing swelling of breast tissue
  - Usually happens when you first begin breastfeeding new baby. Usually lessens in 24-48 hr.
  - Swelling and discomfort may get worse if you don't nurse often or long enough.
- Complications
  - Slow infant weight gain if unable to latch on to breast
  - Sore nipples if breast too firm to grasp
  - Mastitis due to poor milk flow
  - Decreased milk supply
- Tx Goal: Reduce engorgement and pain. Prevent complications.
  - Breastfeed often around the clock. Feed baby as often as possible.
  - Apply cold, fresh *green* cabbage leaf to breast.
  - Tylenol as appropriate for pain relief
- Before Feeding
  - Before feeding, put a warm cloth on breasts or take hot shower.
  - Baby must be positioned and latched on well. (See Latch-on Technique above.)
  - Hold breast between palms and gently squeeze breast while moving hands toward nipple to express small amount of milk. This softens breast and makes it easier for baby to latch on.
  - Massage breasts prior to and during breastfeeding.
- After Feeding
  - Cold compresses between feedings to reduce pain and swelling
  - Wear a well-fitting and supportive bra.
  - Do not pump breasts.

FEEDING PROBLEMS

- Foods causing fussiness: Keep a 2-7 day diary of food and drinks and dates/times of infant fussiness. Call back to discuss.
- "Fussy about breast": Some newborns are "disorganized" nursers—slow to latch on, frantic, or agitated. Start baby off sucking on your little finger. Then, when sucking is strong and consistent, transfer to breast.

INADEQUATE MILK SUPPLY ("NOT ENOUGH MILK")

- How do I know I'm producing enough milk?
  - The amount of milk you produce depends on how often you breastfeed and how effectively your baby sucks.
  - When the baby is bom, you produce colostrum. This is a very thick, concentrated liquid that the baby gets the first 3-5 days of life.
  - 3-5 days after giving birth, your milk will begin to "come in."
  - During the first few weeks, breastfeed at least 8-12 x a day. Nurse for at least 10-15 min on each breast.
  - Your baby should have 6-8 wet diapers/day after your milk has come in (day 3-4); the urine should be pale yellow in color.
  - Your baby's stool after day 2-3 should be loose and seedy; and may be yellow to yellowish green to tan in color.
  - In first month of life, your baby should have at least 2 stools each day.

LACTATION SUPPRESSION

- Tx Goal: To reduce swelling/pain of breasts when a mother does not wish to breastfeed or must stop quickly for some reason
- Do the following for 1-2 days:
  - Fold large bath towel or sheet in half lengthwise.
  - Wrap snugly around breasts, pinning in front.
  - Tuck Ice Pack or Cold Pack (see Home Tx Ref, Ice Pack or Cold Pack) between layers of towel or sheet against breasts for 24-48 hr.
  - Change Ice Packs q 1 hr.
  - Don't nurse, touch, or wash breasts in warm water.

MASTITIS

- Definition: A serious infection of the whole breast
  - Mastitis: Can turn into an abscess if you don't take antibiotics.
  - Abscess: Pus collects in a pocket with nowhere to drain.
- Signs and Sx: Fatigue, localized breast tenderness, flu-like Sx, fever, appearance of a hot, reddened, and tender area on breast (usually unilateral and in upper outer breast quadrant).
- Causes: Can occur as a result of an untreated plugged duct, cracked or fissured nipple, constriction due to tight bra, engorgement, stress, or abrupt change in feeding pattern.
- Complication: Abscess
- Prevention/Tx
  - Bedrest
  - Antibiotics
  - Increased fluid intake

- Moist heat applications
- Breastfeed frequently on the affected side
- Loosen constrictive clothing/bra
- Nurse the baby in different positions (cradle hold, football hold, lying down)
- Check for proper latch-on technique (make sure the baby has part of or your whole areola in his/her mouth)
- Tylenol as appropriate for fever

MOTHER CARE

- Continue to take prenatal vitamins until you have stopped breastfeeding.
- Eat more foods w calcium: Milk, yogurt, cheese, ice cream, carrots.
- Water is very important when you are breastfeeding. Drink 6-8 glasses of water, juice, milk, or decaf herbal tea every day.
- Eat lots of fruits, vegetables, meat, eggs, fish, poultry.
- Rest when baby rests. Ask friends/family to help w housework, cooking, care of older children. Mother should care for baby and self.

PLUGGED DUCT

- Definition: Milk forms a plug. New milk backs up behind it.
- Signs and Sx: A plug or "white head" on nipple; feeling of tenderness and pressure around the plug; no fever or flu-like Sx
- Causes: Missed or shortened feedings leaving the breast overfull; poor positioning during feeding; lack of rest; breasts are too full; pressure on breast; infection from cracked nipple
- Complications: Mastitis, serious infection, and abscess
- Tx Goal: Comfort. Unplug duct. Prevent Mastitis.
    - Put warm, damp cloths to area 5 min before feeding and while nursing to > milk flow and drainage.
    - Nurse on side w plug. Begin each feeding w side that is affected.
    - Massage area in gentle but firm circular motion before and during feeding.
    - Increase fluid intake.
    - Do not use underwire or tight-fitting bra.
    - Bedrest
- Prevention: Adequate rest; nurse often; let baby finish feeding; wear supportive bra; avoid tight bra or clothes.
- Pain/Fever: Tylenol as appropriate

WEANING FROM BREAST

- Start by substituting bottle/cup feeding for one breast feeding.
- Wait until breasts adjust (not engorged), then substitute bottle/cup feeding for an additional breastfeeding.
- Continue until baby is entirely on bottle/cup feeding.
- If engorgement occurs, express only enough milk to relieve pressure. *(See also* Lactation Suppression above.)

REFERRALS

- See Appendix D7, Parents' Help, and D8, Pregnancy.
- La Leche League
- Approved Texts (See Bibliography)
- In-House Parenting Support Group

Burn

BURN 1 (SKIN PROBLEM 2) (BIRTH-6 YR)

THERMAL; CHEMICAL; ELECTRICAL

ASSOC SX/SPECIFIC/CONSIDERATIONS	DISPOSITION/ADVICE
EMERGENT SYMPTOMS	**ED IN 0 MIN-1 HOUR**
• **ALL ELECTRICAL BURNS** ----------▶ + +/- CHEST PAIN, Palpitations, > Heart Rate, Fainting, Hx of Lightning Strike? (Cardiac Dysrhythmia)	• **AXIOM:** ALL ELECTRICAL BURNS HAVE POTENTIAL FOR PROGRESSIVE INJURY. May be worse than it looks!
• **ALL THERMAL BURNS** ----------▶ • **BURN W DECREASED CONSCIOUSNESS** + Weak, Dizzy, Cold/Mottled/or Pale Skin, Blue Lips/ Nailbeds, Rapid/Shallow Breathing, Unresponsive, Loss of Consciousness? (Shock) (See SHOCK) • **BURN W RESPIRATORY SYMPTOMS** + Hoarseness, Cough, Wheezing, SOB, Singed/Black Nares, Facial Bum, Smoke Inhalation, Black Sputum? (Inhalation Injury) • **BURN (DEEP)** + White, Dark, Charred Appearance, Loss of Skin, Regardless of Size? (3RD DEGREE) • **BURN (OVER 9%)** + Red, Mottled, Blisters, Extreme Pain? (2ND DEGREE, MAJOR) • **BURN OF FINGER(S) (CIRCUMFERENTIAL)** + Unable to Remove Rings? (> Risk Circ.) • **FACIAL/NECK BURN?** (Retinal, Inhalation Burn)	• **ALL THERMAL BURN FIRST AID:** • SA: Estimate using one palm of *victim's* hand (not including fingers) = 1%. (See BURN SUPPLEMENTAL INFORMATION) • IF CLOTHING STICKS TO SKIN, do not remove clothing! Immerse burned area for no more than 3 min in cool tap water. • IF CLOTHING DOES NOT STICK TO SKIN, remove it. + IF > 5%, do not immerse. Cover with clean wet sheet + plastic wrap. + IF < 5%, immerse immediately in cool tap water x 10 min. • **DO NOT PUT butter, oil or creams on burn!** • **DO NOT PUT ice on burn: could lead to** > **skin damage,** > **shock.**
• **ALL CHEMICAL BURNS** ----------▶	• **AXIOM:** ALL CHEMICAL BURNS HAVE POTENTIAL FOR PROGRESSIVE INJURY. May be worse than it looks! SECONDS COUNT!
+ On Skin and/or Eyes? ----------▶	• **CONTACT POISON CENTER IMMEDIATELY AND QUICKLY DO THE FOLLOWING:** + WET CHEMICALS: RINSE skin/eyes w cool tap water. + DRY CHEMICALS: BRUSH OFF from skin/eyes. + BRING SUBSTANCE TO E.D. W YOU.
• Does RN feel Sx. are severe, extreme or emergent?	
URGENT SYMPTOMS	**ED/MD/APPT. IN 1-8 HOURS**
• **BURN:UNUSUAL PATTERN** + BURN PATTERN: Cigarettes, Groin, Genitals, Feet, Hands, Circumferential Inj. or SUSPICIOUS EXPLANATION? (Abuse) (See ABUSE)----------▶	• See FIRST AID above. **BRING CHILD IN TO E.D. NOW.** + For transport: Wrap bum in clean plastic wrap to keep warm, clean and reduce pain.
• **BURN (CIRCUMFERENTIAL)** + Face/Neck/Hands/Feet/Arms/Legs/Perineum/Any Joint? (Circ. Obstruction) ----------«-	• See FIRST AID above. **BRING CHILD IN TO E.D. NOW.**
• **BURN W BLISTERS** + Red, Mottled, Extreme Pain, 5-9%? (2ND DEGREE)-*-	• See FIRST AID above. **BRING CHILD IN TO E.D. NOW.** + Remove all jewelry only *IF* it can be done *easily.*
• **BURN HX** + FAILURE TO IMPROVE on Antibiotics x 48 Hr? (Ineffective Rx) • FEVER >40°C or 104°F? • Does RN feel Sx. are urgent?	

continues

BURN 1 (SKIN PROBLEM 2) (BIRTH-6 YR)

continued

ASSOC SX/SPECIFIC/CONSIDERATIONS	DISPOSITION/ADVICE
ACUTE SYMPTOMS	**ED/MD/APPT IN 8-24 HOURS**
• **BURN HX** + Foul Smelling, Purulent Discharge, > Swelling, > Streaks and Pain, FEVER? (Infection) • **BURN (MODERATE)** + Tetanus Immunization > 10 Yr? (> Risk Infection) + Red, Blisters, Pain 1-5%? (2ND DEGREE) + > Pain/Swelling: Worsening or Failure to Improve on Home Tx x 48 Hr = POSS. UPGRADE? • MOD SX + RISK FX (AVED) = POSS. UPGRADE? • Does RN feel Sx. are acute?	• Check Tetanus Status. • See FIRST AID above.
NON-ACUTE SYMPTOMS	**HOME TREATMENT W OR W/O APPT IN 24 + HOURS**
• **BURN (MINOR)** + Reddened, Mild, Swelling, Moderate Pain, No Blisters? (1ST DEGREE) + Red, Mottled, Blisters, Pain, < the Size of One Hand (1 %)? (2ND DEGREE) • MINOR SELF-LIMITING SX EXISTING > 1 WK, NOT BECOMING MARKEDLY WORSE? • HOME TX ITEMS NOT AVAILABLE = POSS. UPGRADE? • Does RN feel Sx. are non-acute?	
CROSS REFERENCES	**STANDARD FOLLOW-UP INSTRUCTIONS**
• ABUSE • BURN 2 (SKIN PROBLEM 2)	PT TO CALL BACK: If symptoms become much worse or urgent or emergent symptoms arise (RN: review protocol and advise caller). RN TO CALL BACK: If acute Sx in child AGE < 2 years. Routinely for Abdomen pain, Respiratory Problems, Fever, Diarrhea, Marked change in ADL.

BURN 2 (SKIN PROBLEM 2) (BIRTH-6 YR)

RADIATION (SUNBURN)

ASSOC SX/SPECIFIC/CONSIDERATIONS	DISPOSITION/ADVICE
EMERGENT SYMPTOMS	**ED IN 0 MIN-1 HOUR**
• **SUNBURN W < CONSCIOUSNESS** + FEVER (HIGH), Sev. Fatigue, Confusion, Fainting, Hot, Dry Red Skin, Rapid Shallow Breathing? (See HEAT EXPOSURE) • Does RN feel Sx. are severe, extreme or emergent?	
URGENT SYMPTOMS	**ED/MD/APPT. IN 1-8 HOURS**
• **SUNBURN (SEVERE-MOD)** QIIQPir.IOUR FYPLANATION? f Ahn<w>/NIAnlprt\ (See ABUSE) →	• **BRING CHILD IN TO E.D. NOW.**
+ EYE PAIN, Photophobia, < Vision? **(Retinal Involvement)** →	• **BRING CHILD IN TO E.D. NOW.**
+ EXTENSIVE, DEEP SUNBURN, FEVER, Pain (Sev.-Mod.), Dehydration Sx., Generalized Swelling of Burned Area? (Sun Poisoning) →	• **BRING CHILD IN TO E.D. NOW.**
• **RED, MOTTLED, BLISTERS** > 5%, Extreme Pain? (2ND DEGREE) • **SUNBURN HX** + FOUL SMELLING, PURULENT DISCHARGE, Worsening Swelling or Pain, Streaks, FEVER? (Infection) • FEVER >40°C or 104°F? • FAILURE TO IMPROVE on Antibiotics X 48 Hr? (Ineffective Rx) • Does RN feel Sx. are urgent?	
ACUTE SYMPTOMS	**ED/MD/APPT IN 8-24 HOURS**
• **SUNBURN W BLISTERS** + Red, Mottled, Tender, Covering 5% of Body? (> Risk Infection) • **OPEN BUSTERS,** + Discharge, ± FEVER? (> Risk Infection) • MOD SX + RISK FX (AVED) = POSS. UPGRADE? • FAILURE TO IMPROVE on Home Tx X 48 Hr? • Does RN feel Sx. are acute?	
NON-ACUTE SYMPTOMS	**HOME TREATMENT W OR W/O APPT IN 24 + HOURS**
• **SUNBURN** + PAIN/Tendemess, Deeply Pigmented Skin Types? (1ST DEGREE) + Red, Mild Swelling, Moderate Pain, No Blisters? (1ST DEGREE) • HOME TX ITEMS NOT AVAILABLE = POSS. UPGRADE? • Does RN feel Sx. are non-acute?	
CROSS REFERENCES	**STANDARD FOLLOW-UP INSTRUCTIONS**
• ABUSE • DEHYDRATION ASSESSMENT • HEAT EXPOSURE	PT TO CALL BACK: If symptoms become much worse or urgent or emergent symptoms arise (RN: review protocol & advise caller). RN TO CALL BACK: Routinely for Abdomen pain, Respiratory Problems, Fever, Diarrhea, Marked change in ADL.

Burn (Skin Problem 2) Supplemental Information (Age 6-18)

QUICK REFERENCE:	Blister Care Burn Assessment (Rule of Nines) Burn Care Sunburn Treatment

BLISTER CARE

- Don't break blisters. They are like "nature's band aids" and will protect your skin from infection
- If they break, leave them alone. Do not peel off skin from broken blisters.
- Cover w clean, dry dressing. Change as needed.
- Watch for signs and symptoms of infection. (See Bum Care below and review with caller.)

BURN ASSESSMENT

RULE OF NINES: A useful, quick method to estimate percentage of body surface areas that were burned. (See also Bums Estimation, Rules of Nines, or the Lund-Browder chart in *The Merck Manual*, (16th Ed.), page 2503.)

- Palm of victim's hand, not including fingers = 1 %
- Arm = 9%
- Leg = 14%
- Head = 18%
- Ant. Trunk =18%
- Post. Trunk =18%

BURN CARE

Immediate Care

- Pain: Tylenol
- Pain/Swelling: Cold compress QID. (See HOME TX REF.)
- Remove rings, bracelets, etc., only if you can do so easily. If not, you need to come in to have the items removed.
- Pain/Swelling: Raise the bum area above heart level.
- Don't use "Caines" or Benadryl sprays for bum—may cause a reaction.
- Check Tetanus Status. If you have a clean bum and your last tetanus shot was > 10 years ago, you need a tetanus shot within 72 hrs.

Prevention Of Infection

- Keep bum clean and dry. Cover w sterile dressing (nonsticky if possible).
- Polysporin or Bacitracin ointment.

- Use Warm Soapy Soak for small bums (<1 %). (See HOME TX REF)
- Change dressing daily. Remove dressing by first soaking in warm water x 5 min.
- Healed Bum: Apply skin cream to healing skin. Do not expose bum to sunlight for more than 1 hr. Use sunblock.
- Despite the greatest care, bums can become infected. Call if any of the following signs of infection develop:
  - Increasing pain, swelling or tenderness after the first 24 hr.
  - Pus
  - Red streaks
  - Fever/chhills
  - Numbness
  - Bad smell

SUNBURN TREATMENT

Treatment Goal: Relieve Pain. Provide comfort; prevent more damage

Pain

- Tylenol (Pain is worse 6-48 hours after initial bum)
- Cool bath: Aveeno, oatmeal, baking soda. (See HOME TX REF)
- Cool compresses QID. (See HOME TX REF)
- Steroid cream .5%; do not use on face
- May use Benadryl or "Caine" sprays

Prevention of Infection

- Blister care (see above)
- Check Tetanus Status

Preventing Sunburn and Skin Cancer

- The best way to prevent sunburns and skin cancer is to not sunbathe, swim or spend long periods of time in sun between 10 A.M.-4 P.M. That is when the sun's rays are the strongest and most harmful. If possible, stay in the shade. If you must sunbathe, wear sunscreen and do it before 10 A.M. or after 4 P.M.
- Always wear #30 sunscreen. Cover arms & legs completely. Use waterproof sunscreen when you swim. Always follow instructions on package about how often to reapply.
- REMEMBER: Always use sunscreen every time and avoid the sun between 10 A.M. and 4 P.M. If you are red-headed, blond or very fair skinned, DO NOT rely only on sunscreen for protection. Sunburns and spending long periods of time in the sun, *even with sunscreen,* may lead to serious skin cancers.

REFERENCES

Berkow, R., et al. (Eds.). (1992). *The Merck Manual of Diagnosis and Therapy,* Whitehouse Station, NJ: Merck & Co., Inc.

Manhoff, D. (1996). *Mosby's Outdoor Medical Guide,* St. Louis: Mosby.

Settle, J. A. (Ed). (1996). *Principles and Practice of Burn Management,* (pp. 199-201; 203-207; 355-365). New York: Churchill Livingstone.

Tangley, L. (1998, March 2). Deadly rays may pierce the screen. *U.S. News & World Report,* 124 (8), 37.

Chest Pain

CHEST PROBLEM (BIRTH-6 YR)

PAIN W OR W/O TRAUMA

ASSOC SX/SPECIFIC/CONSIDERATIONS	DISPOSITION/ADVICE
EMERGENT SYMPTOMS	**ED IN 0 MIN-1 HOUR**
• **PAIN W OR W/O TRAUMA (MAJOR): MVA, FALL, BLUNT** + SUDDEN ONSET, SHARP CHEST PAIN, Dyspnea, Dry Hacking Cough, Cyanosis, Hx Cystic Fibrosis/Asthma? (Pneumothorax) + PENETRATING OBJECT? ---------- ►	• **DO NOT REMOVE IMPALED OBJECT.**
• **PAIN W/O TRAUMA** + ASSOC. W VIGOROUS ACTIVITY, Color Change, Fainting, Dizziness, c/o Irregular Heartbeat, ± Cardiac Disease? (Cardiac Disease) • Does RN Feel Sx. are severe, extreme, emergent?	
URGENT SYMPTOMS	**ED/MD/APPT IN 1-8 HOURS**
• **TRAUMA (MINOR-MOD.)** + SUSPICIOUS HX? (Abuse) **(See ABUSE)** ──────►	• **BRING CHILD TO E.D. NOW.**
• **PAIN W/O TRAUMA** + SUSPICIOUS HX? (Rib Fracture) (See ABUSE)---------- ►	• **BRING CHILD TO E.D. NOW.**
+ ± SEVERE CRUSHING, SHARP, SOB, > Resp., Hx Sickle Cell Disease? (Sickle Cell Crisis)----------*-	• **BRING CHILD TO E.D. NOW.**
+ FEVER, SHAKING, CHILLS, COUGH, Substernal/Intercostal Retractions, Nasal Flaring, ± Wheezing, Rapid/Shallow Resp., ± Abd. Pain, Anorexia, Fatigue? (Pneumonia: Bacterial, Viral, Fungal)---------- ►	• **BRING CHILD TO E.D. NOW.**
+ SOB, ANXIETY, ± Hx Cardiac Disease? (> Risk Cardiac Complications)----------*-	• **BRING CHILD TO E.D. NOW**
+ HX CHRONIC COUGH, FB Aspiration? (Foreign Body) + SHARP/DULL, ± Radiates to Neck/Shoulder, > w Inspiration Movement/Cough, Repeat Viral Infection? (Pericarditis)	
• **AGE < 3 MO + FEVER > 38°C or 100.4°F®?**---------- ►	• **BRIN. NOW.**
• FEVER >40°C or 104°F? • AGE < 3 MO + MOD. SX + RISK FX (AVED)? • FAILURE TO IMPROVE on Antibiotics x 24-48 Hr? (Ineffective Rx) • WORSENING SX After 24-48 Hr on Home Tx? • RECENT SURGERY or HOSPITALIZATION? (Poss. Complications) • Does RN feel Sx. are urgent?	
ACUTE SYMPTOMS	£i>/Mu^PPT **IN 8-24 HOURS**
• **PAIN W TRAUMA** + Worse w Inspiration or After Coughing Spasm? (Rib Fx) ---------- ►	• SA: Press on pair-f«! •,-•a. Pain =+)
• **PAIN W/O TRAUMA** + Substemal, Worse w Eating or Lying Down, ± Vomiting, Fullness After Eating, Regurgitation, Relieved by Antacids? (Esophagitis, Hiatal Hernia, GE Reflux) • AGE 3 MO-6 YR + MOD. SX + (AVED) = POSS. UPGRADE? • Does RN feel Sx. are acute?	
NON-ACUTE SYMPTOMS	**HOME TREATMENT W OR W/O APPT IN 24+HOURS**
• **PAIN W/O TRAUMA** + Dull, Steady, > w Breathing/Movement? (Costochondritis) ----------*-	• SA: Press on painful area. (> Pain = +)
• MINOR SELF-LIMITING SX EXISTING > 1 WK, NOT BECOMING MARKEDLY WORSE? • HOME TX ITEMS OR PHONE NOT AVAILABLE = POSS. UPGRADE? • Does RN feel Sx. are non-acute?	

continues

CHEST PROBLEM (BIRTH-6 YR)

ASSOC SX/SPECIFIC/CONSIDERATIONS	DISPOSITION/ADVICE
CROSS-REFERENCES	STANDARD FOLLOW-UP INSTRUCTIONS
• ABUSE • RESPIRATORY PROBLEM 1; 2	PT TO CALL BACK: If symptoms become much worse or urgent or emergent symptoms arise (RN: review Protocol and advise caller). RN TO CALL BACK: If acute Sx in child AGE < 2 years. Routinely for Abdomen pain, Respiratory problems, Fever, Diarrhea, Marked change in ADL.

Chest Problem Supplemental Information (Birth-6 Yr)

QUICK REFERENCE: Costochondritis
Pleuritis
Retractions (Intercostal)

COSTOCHONDRITIS

(Inflammation of rib cartilage; rib pain)

- Signs and Sx: see Protocol
- Causes: Inflammation due to trauma or virus
- Complications: None
- Prevention/Tx
  - Goal: Prevent pain/complications. Patient will seek medical Tx.
  - Pain: Tylenol as appropriate
  - Heat, rest. Don't do anything that hurts.
  - If Sx persist or >, call for appt.

PLEURITIS

(Inflammation of pleura, membrane surrounding lungs)

- Signs and Sx: see Protocol
- Causes: Infection—Viral, bacterial, fungal
- Complications: Chronic pleurisy, pneumonia
- Prevention/Tx
  - Antibiotic Tx
  - Bedrest
  - > Fluids

RETRACTIONS (INTERCOSTAL)

(Skin between ribs being pulled back, w each expiration. "Marked" vs. "mild") Marked: Extends throughout upper and lower rib cage. Mild: Extends to upper rib cage only.

- Signs and Sx: Labored breathing, "can see ribs" when breathing. May be accompanied by nasal flaring, SOB.
- Causes: Poor air exchange, secondary to infection/trauma
- Tx
  - Goal: Change breathing pattern.
  - Fever: Give Tylenol as appropriate.
  - Asthma: Suggest bronchodilatation.

Cold Exposure

COLD EXPOSURE (ALL AGES)

HYPOTHERMIA; FROSTBITE

ASSOC SX/SPECIFIC/CONSIDERATIONS	DISPOSITION/ADVICE
EMERGENT SYMPTOMS	**ED IN 0 MIN-1 HOUR**
• **COLD EXPOSURE** ---------------------► + *Progressive Picture*—Shivering, Feeling Numb, Fatigue, Apathy, Drowsiness; SKIN: Cold, Gray/Blue/Pale, SPEECH: Slurred or Difficult, ACTIVITY: Slow Uncoordinated Movements, Clumsiness; Sitting/Lying; GAIT: Staggering/Uncoordinated; COLOR: Generalized Blue/Gray Coloring, Slow Breathing/Pulse, Rigid Muscles/Posture, No Shivering, Temp. <35° C or 95°F, LOC: Stuporous, Coma? (Profound Hypothermia) + CHILD: Lethargic, Rigid Child, SKIN: Reddened, Swelling of Extremities, Temp. <35°C or 95°F? (Hypothermia) • Does RN feel symptoms are severe, extreme, emergent?	• **FIRST AID:** + HANDLE COMATOSE PATIENT VERY LITTLE OR NOT AT ALL! Hypothermia = > Risk dysrhythmias. + Keep warm, dry and protected from wind, cold, rain. + *Carefully* remove wet or constrictive clothing/shoes. + Wrap in warm blankets, sleeping bag. + Cover with plastic sheet/garbage bag to keep heat in. + Give warm fluids only if person is conscious. + Do not massage skin. + Do not give alcohol or caffeine.
URGENT SYMPTOMS	**ED/MD/APPT IN 1-8 HOURS**
• **COLD EXPOSURE** + SUSPICIOUS HISTORY? (Poss. Abuse/Neglect) (See ABUSEf- • **COLD EXPOSURE** + **RISK FACTORS?** (Urban Hypothermia) ➔ + CHILD: Newborn, Infant; ADULT: All Elderly? + MEDICATION: Drug Use/Overdose: Beta Blockers, Sedatives Recreational Use/Overdose: Cocaine-Induced Hypothermia? + PREVIOUS MEDICAL HISTORY: Any Chronic Disease Esp. Hypothyroidism, Heart Disease, Diabetes, Homelessness, Malnutrition, Anorexia Nervosa? + PREVOUS INJURY, ILLNESS: Extreme Physical Exertion, Exhaustion; Burn History?	• **COME TO E.D. NOW.** • **COME TO E.D. NOW.** • **FIRST AID:** + HANDLE INJURY AS LITTLE AS POSSIBLE! + Keep area warm, dry and protected from wind, cold, rain. + *Carefully* remove wet or constrictive clothing/shoes. + Wrap in warm blankets or sleeping bag. + Cover area with plastic sheet/garbage bag to keep heat in. + Give warm fluids. + Do not massage or rub the affected area. + Do not give alcohol, tobacco or caffeine. + Do not break any blisters.
• UULU inJUfxT ^finger, iucb, rduc, INUDC, cdibj r ———————^ + Blisters, Numbness/Tingling, Cold, White, Waxy Appearance, Firm/Hard to "Frozen Feeling." Swelling of Entire Extremity? (Deep or Late Cold Injury) • Does RN feel symptoms are urgent?	• **COME TO E.D. NOW.** • **FIRST AID:** (see above)
ACUTE SYMPTOMS	**ED/MD/APPT IN 8-24 HOURS**
• **COLD INJURY** (Finger, Toes, Face, Nose, Ears)? ———————► + Blanching, < Feeling/Sensation, Skin Soft? (Superficial or Early Cold Injury) • MODERATE SYMPTOMS IN HIGH-RISK PATIENT (Age, Veracity, Emotional Status, Debilitation/Distance) = POSS. UPGRADE? • FAILURE TO IMPROVE on Home Treatment after 48 Hr? • Does RN feel symptoms are acute?	• **FIRST AID:** + Warm soak (temp, tolerable to rescuer's elbow). + Do not rub or massage area. + Raise area on pillows to cut down on swelling. + Pain: Tylenol prn. • Check Tetanus Status.
NON-ACUTE SYMPTOMS	**HOME TREATMENT W OR W/O APPT IN 24 + HOURS**
• HOME TREATMENT ITEMS NOT AVAILABLE = POSS. UPGRADE? • Does RN feel symptoms are non-acute?	
CROSS-REFERENCES	**STANDARD FOLLOW-UP INSTRUCTIONS**
• ABUSE	PT TO CALL BACK: If symptoms become much worse or urgent or emergent symptoms arise (RN: review Protocol & advise caller). RN TO CALL BACK: Routinely for Abdomen Pain, Respiratory Problems, Fever, Diarrhea, Marked change in ADL.

Cold Exposure Supplemental Information (All Ages)

QUICK REFERENCE Hypothermia
High-Risk Groups for Urban Hypothermia
Frostbite

COMMUNITY ALERT: "Urban hypothermia" increases during extreme cold weather conditions. See list below for at-risk populations.

HYPOTHERMIA AXIOMS

- Extremes of age add to the risk of hypothermia. Err on the side of caution with Children < 10 and Adults > 60.
- Extreme cold temperatures may aggravate other medical problems. Don't overlook other possible medical conditions that may be present.
- The longer the cold exposure, the higher the risk for hypothermia; although any patient can develop hypothermia in a very short time.
- Hypothermia can be fatal within several hours.
- Hypothermia may be misinterpreted as drug/alcohol intoxication.
- Profound Hypothermia (see below): The heart is extremely sensitive to ventricular fibrillation and standstill. Handle stuporous and comatose patients with extreme caution and care.
- "No one is dead until warm and dead." EMD Axiom. Until patient is wanned to 35°C or 95°F, they may be successfully resuscitated.
- Unlike frostbite, hypothermia can occur at temperatures well above freezing, due to wind and rain.

HYPOTHERMIA

- Definitions:
  - Mild hypothermia: Core temperature is 90-96.8°F (32°C).
  - Profound hypothermia: Core temperature is below 90°F.
- Signs and Symptoms: (See Protocol)
- Causes: There are two ways hypothermia can happen:
  - In healthy people: Overexposure to cold temperatures due to lack of preparation.
  - When any condition or disease lowers the body temperature, like a near drowning, head or spinal cord injury, sepsis, drug ingestion, shock, or diseases such as hypothyroidism, heart disease, diabetes.
- Complications: Coma, death.

HIGH-RISK GROUPS FOR URBAN HYPOTHERMIA

- AGE
  - Newboms/infants
  - Elderly (all)

- MEDICATIONS
  - Alcohol related illness/injury
  - Drug use/overdose
  - Cocaine-induced hypothermia
- MEDICAL CONDITIONS
  - Diabetes
  - Hypothyroidism
  - Heart disease
  - Malnutrition
  - Anorexia Nervosa
  - Any chronic disease
  - Homelessness
  - Any injury
  - Burn History

Adapted from McSwain, N.E., Jr., Paturas, J.L., & Wertz, E. (Eds.). (1990). *Pre-hospital trauma life support* (3rd ed.). St. Louis, MO: Mosby.

FROSTBITE AXIOMS

- Initial appearance and sensation may not correlate well with extent of injury. Always consider contributing factors such as temperature, duration of exposure, dampness of environment and/or clothing.
- Do not attempt to rewarm deep frostbite, unless a lengthy transport is anticipated. It may be hazardous, and should be performed under controlled conditions.

FROSTBITE

- Signs and Symptoms: (See Protocol)
- Causes: Prolonged exposure to damp, cold temperatures. Other conditions or diseases may also lower the body temperature: drowning, head or spinal cord injury, sepsis, drug ingestion, shock or diseases such as hypothyroidism, heart disease, diabetes.
- Complications: Blister formation, nerve damage, infection, gangrene, amputation of extremities.
- Prevention/Treatment:
  - Remove wet clothing.
  - Wear loose-fitting, layered wool or synthetic clothing. Wool retains heat when wet.
  - Wear waterproof outer clothing to protect from wind and rain.
  - Keep your head warm at all times. A lot of heat may be lost from your head. Wear a wool stocking cap.
  - FOR CHILDREN, ESPECIALLY INFANTS < 3 Mo.: In cool weather, they need knit caps because their body's ability to stay warm is not well developed.

References

Auerbach, P.S. (Ed.). (1995). *Wilderness medicine: management of wilderness and environmental emergencies.* (3rd ed.). St. Louis, MO: Mosby.

Clawson, J.J., M. D., & Democoeur, K.B. (1998). *Principles of emergency medical dispatch.* (2nd ed.). Salt Lake City, UT: Priority Press.

Goold, G.B. & Vahradian, S. (1997). *Basic first response.* Upper Saddle River, N.J.: Prentice-Hall.

Manhoff, D. (1996). *Mosby's outdoor emergency medical guide.* (1 st ed.). St. Louis, MO: Mosby.

McSwain, N.E., Jr., Paturas, J.L., & Wertz, E. (Eds.). (1990). *Pre-hospital trauma life support* (3rd ed.). St. Louis, MO: Mosby.

Confusion

CONFUSION (ALL AGES)

SUDDEN; CHRONIC

ASSOC SX/SPECIFIC/CONSIDERATIONS	DISPOSITION/ADVICE
EMERGENT SYMPTOMS	**ED IN 0 MIN-1 HOUR**
• CONFUSION (SUDDEN ONSET) W OR W/O TRAUMA	
+ PROGRESSIVELY: Anxious, Weak, Dizzy, Thirsty, NA/, SKIN: Pale, Blotchy/Discolored/Cool or Cold, Sweaty, LIPS/NAILBED: Blue, PULSE: Weak/Fast, BREATHING: Rapid/Shallow, Unresponsive, Loss of Consciousness? (Shock) (See SHOCK)	
+ DRUG INGESTION: ACCIDENTAL/PURPOSEFUL, Street Drugs/Rx/ Barbiturates, Poisonous Plant, Toxic Chemical or Pesticide? (Toxic Exposure/Ingestion) →	• [illegible] PLANT/POISON/PILLS/CHEMICAL TO E.D. [illegible]
+ HEADACHE, SUDDEN/SEVERE, Pupil Changes, N/V, Respiratory Changes, Stupor, Disorientation, Slurred Speech, Blurred/Double Vision, Unsteady Gait, Confusion, Numbness/Weakness/Tingling in Extremities, Loss of Urine or Bowel Control, Tongue Biting, History of BCP/Atrial Fib/> BP? (CVA, Aneurysm, Lesion, Abscess)	
+ HEADACHE ± TRAUMA (Sudden/Sharp or Gradual/Dull/Throbbing), Neck Pain/Stiffness, Resp. Changes, Progressing: Irritable/Lethargic/ ± Loss of Consciousness; Visual Changes, Weakness, NA/, Staggering, Slurred Speech? (Intracranial Hemorrhage, Lesion, Abscess)	
+ CHILD/INFANT-2 yrs: FEVER, Stiff Neck, Headache, NA/, Extreme Fatigue, ± Pinpoint Red Purplish Spots Progressing to Purple Patches, Extremely Irritable or Unresponsive, High-Pitched Cry, Bulging/Tight Fontanelle, "Toxic Child," ± Seizure? (Sepsis, Meningitis, Encephalitis)	
+ HEADACHE, Neck Pain, Photophobia, FEVER/Chills, N/V, ± Confusion, Restlessness, Somnolence, ± History of HIV? (Meningitis, Encephalitis)	
+ FEVER >40°C or 104°F? (Delirium)	
+ HISTORY OF HEAD INJURY? (See HEAD PROBLEM 1)	
[illegible] →	• If conscious, give glass of fruit juice, or water with 3 Tbsp. table sugar.
• Does RN feel symptoms are severe, extreme, emergent?	
URGENT SYMPTOMS	**ED/MD/APPT IN 1-8 HOURS**
• CONFUSION (SUDDEN)	
+ TRAUMA + SUSPICIOUS HISTORY? (Abuse/Neglect) (See ABUSE) →	• [illegible]
+ POOR ATTENTION SPAN, Changing (Fluctuating) Level of Consciousness, Overactive, Visual Hallucinations, Impaired Judgment? (Delirium) →	• **COME TO E.D. NOW.**
+ DETERIORATION OF THOUGHT PROCESS, Affective Response and Ability To Be in Touch w Reality? History of Psychiatric Disorder, Failure to Take Psych. Meds.? (Relapse, Noncompliance, Psychosis) →	• SA: Hearing voices = + Combative behavior = + Delusions = +
+ Headache, Dizziness, N/V? (Carbon Monoxide Poisoning)	
+ FRAIL ELDERLY? (Pneumonia, Sepsis, Overmedication, Drug [illegible]) →	• **AXIOM:** In elderly persons, confusion may be the only sign of underlying pneumonia, sepsis, overmedication.
+ HISTORY: Recent Seizure? (Postictal State)	
+ HISTORY: Renal Failure, or Hepatic Failure? (Encephalopathy)	
• Does RN feel symptoms are urgent?	

continues

ASSOC SX/SPECIFIC/CONSIDERATIONS	DISPOSITION/ADVICE
ACUTE SYMPTOMS	**ED/MD/APPT IN 8-24 HOURS**
• **CONFUSION (CHRONIC)** + Any Major Change from Everyday Behavior = POSS. UPGRADE? • **PAIN W TRAUMA (MOD.-MINOR)** + History of Trauma (Days-Months), Dizziness, Confusion, ± N/V, Sensitivity to Noise/Light? (Post-Concussive Syndrome) • Moderate Symptoms + Risk Factors (Age, Veracity, Emotional Distress, Debilitation/Distance) = POSS. UPGRADE? (> Risk) • Does RN feel symptoms are acute?	
NON-ACUTE SYMPTOMS	**HOME TREATMENT W OR W/O APPT IN 24 + HOURS**
• **CONFUSION (CHRONIC)** → + Slow Onset, Increases Over Time, Impaired Judgment, No Underlying Disease, Sleep/Wake Cycle Disruption, Progressive Memory Loss, HIV History? (Chronic Dementia) • Does RN feel symptoms are non-acute?	• SA: Does patient know: Own name? Caretaker's name? Can patient perform personal care activities?
CROSS-REFERENCES	**STANDARD FOLLOW-UP INSTRUCTIONS**
• ABUSE • DIZZINESS • EMOTIONAL PROBLEMS • FAINTING • HEAD PROBLEM 2 • SEIZURES • SUBSTANCE ABUSE	PT TO CALL BACK: If symptoms become much worse or urgent or emergent symptoms arise (RN: Review Protocol & advise caller). RN TO CALL BACK: Routinely for Abdomen Pain, Respiratory Problems, Fever, Diarrhea, Marked change in ADL.

Confusion Supplemental Information (All Ages)

QUICK REFERENCE Infection
Chronic Conditions
Drug Side Effects

AXIOMS

- CHILD: With confusion, severe agitation, or hallucinations should be seen immediately.
- CHILD: Accidental ingestion of alcohol, IV/street drugs, poisonous plants, pesticides, toxic chemicals is common under age 6 yr.
- CHILD/ADOLESCENT: Always rule out possible accidental or purposeful ingestion or inhalation.
- ALL AGES: Severe confusion with agitation is most often caused by accidental or purposeful inhalation or ingestion.
- ELDERLY: All sudden confusion in frail elderly is urgent.

INFECTION

- ELDERLY: Confusion may be only sign of underlying pneumonia, sepsis, other infection
- Meningitis
- Herpes encephalitis
- Cat scratch fever
- Lyme disease/Rocky Mountain Spotted Fever
- CHILD: Reyes syndrome
- CHILD: Measles, encephalitis
- INFANT: Sepsis in newborn

CHRONIC CONDITIONS PRESENTING WITH CONFUSION

- Congestive heart failure (congenital heart disease)
- Endocrine disorders (adrenal/thyroid disease)
- Hypernatremia (severe dehydration secondary to diarrhea/vomiting)
- Diabetes (hypoglycemia, insulin overdose)
- Liver/kidney disease (hepatic/hypertensive/uremic encephalopathy)

DRUG SIDE EFFECT: CONFUSION

This is not an exhaustive list of substances causing confusion. Most commonly known are:

PRESCRIPTION/OTC DRUGS:	*TOXINS:*	*ILLICIT STREET DRUGS:*
Adrenal Steroids	Chemical poisons	Alcohol
Anticonvulsants	C02	Amphetamines
Antidepressants	Glue	Cocaine

PRESCRIPTION/OTC DRUGS:	*TOXINS:*	*ILLICIT STREET DRUGS:*
Antipsychotics	Lead	LSD
Barbiturates	Paint thinner	Marijuana
Insulin overdose	Pesticides	Mescaline
Isoniazid (INH)	Poisonous plants	
Salicylate:	Mushrooms	
Aspirin		
Bismuth subsalicylate (Pepto Bismol)		
Tranquilizers		
Tricyclic antidepressants		

References

Goold, G.B. & Vahradian, S. (1997). *Basic first response.* Upper Saddle River, N.J.: Prentice-Hall.

Dizziness and Fainting

DIZZINESS (BIRTH-6 YR)

W OR W/O TRAUMA

ASSOC SX/SPECIFIC/CONSIDERATIONS	DISPOSITION/ADVICE
EMERGENT SYMPTOMS	**ED IN 0 MIN-1 HOUR**
• **DIZZINESS W OR W/O TRAUMA (MAJOR): MVA, FALL, BLUNT** + HEADACHE (Sudden/Sharp or Gradual/Dull/Throbbing), Neck Pain/ Stiffness, Resp. Changes, Progressing: Irritable/Lethargic/± Loss of Consciousness; Visual Changes, Weakness, N/V, Staggering, Slurred Speech? (Intracranial Hemorrhage) + HX EXP. TO STREET DRUGS/RX, Poisonous Plant or Inhalation/ Ingestion of RX, OTC Med, Toxic Chemical or Pesticide? (Toxic Exposure) ------------------------------ *■ + SEIZURES? (See SEIZURES) + HEAD TRAUMA? (See HEAD PROBLEM 1) • Does RN feel Sx. are severe, extreme, emergent?	• **AXIOM:** Accidental ingestion of Rx/street drugs, poisonous plants, pesticides, toxic chemicals is very common in this age group (mouthing/tasting = developmental stage). • **CONTACT POISON CENTER.** BRING SUBSTANCE TO E.D. W YOU.
URGENT SYMPTOMS	**ED/MD/APPT IN 1-8 HOURS**
• **DIZZINESS W TRAUMA (MINOR-MOD.)** + SUSPICIOUS HX? (Poss. Abuse) (See ABUSE)------------------ ► + ANY RECENT TRAUMA?------------------ ► • **DIZZINESS W/O TRAUMA** + (GRADUAL ONSET), N/V, Fatigue, Anorexia? (Lead Toxicity)------------------ ► + HEADACHE, CONFUSION? (Carbon Monoxide Poisoning) ------------------*- + HEADACHE, ABD. PAIN, Falling? (Partial-Complex Seizure) (See SEIZURES) + SUDDEN ONSET, N/V, Jerky Eye Movement, ± Hx URI, ± Hearing Loss? (Labyrinthitis, Vestibular Neuronitis) ------------------ ► • **AGE < 3 MO + FEVER > 38°C or 100.4°F®?**------------------ ► • FEVER > 40°C or 104T? • AGE < 3 MO + MOD. SX + RISK FX (AVED)? • RECENT SURGERY or HOSPITALIZATION? (Poss. Complications) • Does RN feel Sx. are urgent?	• **BRING CHILD TO E.D. NOW.** • **BRING CHILD TO E.D. NOW.** • **BRING CHILD TO E.D. NOW.** • **BRING CHILD TO E.D. NOW.** • **BRING CHILD TO E.D. NOW.** • **BRING CHILD TO E.D. NOW.**
ACUTE SYMPTOMS	**ED/MD/APPT IN 8-24 HOURS**
• **DIZZINESS W/O TRAUMA** + (GRADUAL ONSET), Persistent, ± Headache, ± Seizures? (Mass/Lesion) + Hx Ototoxic Drugs? ------------------ ► + (SUDDEN ONSET), Pallor, Vomiting, Sweating, Jerky Eye Movement, Child Appears Frightened, w/o Hx infection? (Benign Paroxysmal Vertigo) + Hx or Suspected FB/Impacted Ear Wax? (FB) • AGE 3 MO-6 YR + MOD. SX + (AVED) = POSS. UPGRADE? • Does RN feel Sx. are acute?	• Stop med.
NON-ACUTE SYMPTOMS	**HOME TREATMENT W OR W/O APPT IN 24 + HOURS**
• **DIZZINESS W/O TRAUMA** + Assoc, w Car, Plane, Boat Travel, ± N/V? (Motion Sickness) • MINOR SELF-LIMITING SX EXISTING > 1 WK, NOT BECOMING MARKEDLY WORSE? • HOME TX ITEMS OR PHONE NOT AVAILABLE = POSS. UPGRADE? • Does RN feel Sx. are non-acute?	

continues

DIZZINESS (BIRTH-6 YR)

continued

ASSOC SX/SPECIFIC/CONSIDERATIONS	DISPOSITION/ADVICE
CROSS-REFERENCES	**STANDARD FOLLOW-UP INSTRUCTIONS**
• ABUSE • BEHAVIORAL PROBLEM • CONFUSION • EAR 1; 2 • FAINTING • HEAD PROBLEM 2 • SEIZURES	PT TO CALL BACK: If symptoms become much worse or urgent or emergent symptoms arise (RN: review Protocol and advise caller). RN TO CALL BACK: If acute Sx in child AGE < 2 years. Routinely for Abdomen pain, Respiratory problems, Fever, Diarrhea, Marked change in ADL.

FAINTING (BIRTH-6 YR)

ASSOC SX/SPECIFIC/CONSIDERATIONS	DISPOSITION/ADVICE
EMERGENT SYMPTOMS	**ED IN 0 MIN-1 HOUR**
• FAINTING/SUDDEN BRIEF LOSS OF CONSCIOUSNESS?------------------------ ►	• **FIRST AID** + Lie child flat. Elevate legs higher than heart. + Loosen tight clothing. + Remove noxious stimuli. + Apply cool cloth. + Do not slap or shake. + Don't let child stand up.
[Listed Below Are POSSIBLE CAUSES of FAINTING]	
DYSRHYTHMIA: + HX HEART DISEASE, Chest Pain, Irregular Heartbeat?	
HYPOVOLEMIA: + TRAUMA? (Hemorrhage) + "TOXIC CHILD"? (See Toxicity Assessment) (Toxicity) + Severe N/V, Diarrhea? (See Dehydration Assessment/Rehydration Guidelines) (Dehydration)	
NEUROGENIC: + HX OF EXP. TO STREET DRUGS/Rx, Poisonous Plant, or Inhalation/Ingestion of Toxic Chemical or Pesticide? (Toxic **Exposure**) ———►	• CONTACT POISON [illegible] BRING [illegible] SUBSTANCE TO E.D. W YOU.
+ HEADACHE ± TRAUMA (Sudden/Sharp or Gradual/Dull/ Throbbing), Neck Pain/Stiffness, Resp. Changes, Progressing: Irritable/Lethargic/± Loss of Consciousness; Visual Changes, Weakness, N/V, Staggering, Slurred Speech? (Intracranial Hemorrhage)	
+ **POSS. SWALLOWED FB? (FB Aspiration)** ———►	• [illegible]
METABOLIC: + HUNGER, PALLOR, Sweating, Confusion? (Hypoglycemia) —►	• If conscious, give small amt. of sugar.
+ THIRST, VOMITING, Flushed Skin, > Resp., Fruity Breath, Confusion, > Urination? (Hyperglycemia, Diabetes w Acidosis, Dehydration)	
+ TREMORS, Sweating, Headache, Hx DM? (Insulin Reaction) —►	• If conscious, give small amt. of sugar.
• Does RN feel Sx. are severe, extreme, emergent?	
URGENT SYMPTOMS	**ED/MD/APPT IN 1-8 HOURS**
• **TRAUMA (ALL)** + SUSPICIOUS HX? (Abuse) (See ABUSE) -------------------►	• **BRING CHILD TO E.D. NOW.**
• **FAINTING** **[Listed Below Are POSSIBLE CAUSES of FAINTING]** + HX SUDDEN PAIN/FRIGHT, Preceded by Nausea, Yawning, Weakness, Blurred Vision? (Vasovagal Syncope) + ASSOC. W COUGH/URINATION or Bearing Down During BM? (Valsalva, < Venous Return) + STANDING FOR LONG PERIOD W/O MOVING, ± Heat Exp.? ("Parade Square Faint," Venous Pooling) + ± HX PROLONGED BEDREST? (Venous Pooling) + HEAT EXPOSURE? (Heat Syncope) + > RESP, DIZZINESS, Anxiety, Tingling Fingers/Lips? (Hyperventilation Syndrome)	

continues

FAINTING (BIRTH-6 YR)

continued

ASSOC SX/SPECIFIC/CONSIDERATIONS	DISPOSITION/ADVICE
ACUTE SYMPTOMS	**ED/MD/APPT IN 8-24 HOURS**
NON-ACUTE SYMPTOMS	**HOME TREATMENT W OR W/O APPT IN 24 +HOURS**
• **FAINTING** + Hx Recurrent Temper Tantrum/Breath Holding? (Temper Tantrum, Breath Holding) (See BEHAVIORAL PROBLEM INFOSHEET)	
CROSS-REFERENCES	**STANDARD FOLLOW-UP INSTRUCTIONS**
• ABUSE • BEHAVIORAL PROBLEM • CONFUSION • DIZZINESS • SEIZURES	PT TO CALL BACK: If symptoms become much worse or urgent or emergent symptoms arise (RN: review Protocol and advise caller). RN TO CALL BACK: If acute Sx in child AGE < 2 years. Routinely for Abdomen pain, Respiratory problems, Fever, Diarrhea, Marked change in ADL.

Ear

EAR PROBLEM 1 (BIRTH-6 YR)

PAIN W TRAUMA; FB; HEARING LOSS; RINGING; EARLOBE TRAUMA

ASSESSMENT	ACUITY LEVEL		DISPOSITION/ADVICE
Key Questions		**Emergent Symptom Patterns**	**ED 0 Min -1 Hr.**
Major Trauma	+	Clear or Bloody Drainage? (See Head Problem 1)	
Chemical in Ear?		-->	Contact Poison Center. Bring substance to ED w you.
Does RN feel that symptoms are severe, extreme, or emergent?			

Key Questions		**Urgent Symptom Patterns**	**ED/UCC/Office 1-8 Hr.**
Trauma	+	Suspicious History? (Abuse) (Possible Abuse)-------------------->	Come to ED Now!
Pain w Trauma	+	Penetrating (Q-Tip, Pencil), +/- Bloody Drainage? (Laceration/Perforation/Ruptured TM)	
	+	Sudden Onset Hearing Loss, Failure to Respond to Voice/Noise, Behavior Change, N/V, Dizziness? (Hemorrhage, Blood behind Ear Drum)	
Trauma/Laceration Pain		Of Earlobe/Pinna? ------------------------------------>	Apply cool compress, firm pressure. (See Home Tx Ref)
Pain	+	< Hearing, +/- Discharge, "Digging at Ear"? (Foreign Body)-->	Do not try to remove object!
Age < 3 mo	+	Fever > 38°C or 100.4°F? ---------------------------->	Bring child to ED Now!
Toxicity/Dehydration	+	School Age? (See Toxicity/Dehydration Assessment)	
Pain/Symptoms	+	Fever > 40°C or 104°F?--- >	Come to ED Now!
Unusual Pain/Symptoms	+	Post-Op or Postprocedure? (Poss. Complications/Infection)	
Symptoms of Infection	+	Failure to Improve on Antibiotics x 48 Hr? (Ineffective Rx)	
Does RN feel that symptoms are urgent?			

Key Questions		**Acute/Nonacute Symptom Patterns**	**FA 8+ Hr. +/- Home Tx**
Pain	+	Following Blast of Noise? (Ruptured TM)	
Hearing Loss (Acute Onset)	+	Hx Ototoxic Meds, Failure to Respond to Voice/Noise, Behavior Change, Discipline Problem? (Drug Side Effect, OM, Hearing Loss, Earwax)	
Ringing	+	Hx Prolonged Use of ASA, Other RX? (Drug Side Effect) (See SI)	

continues

continued

Key Questions		Acute/Nonacute Symptom Patterns	FA 8+ Hr. +/- Home Tx
Hearing Loss (Gradual Onset)	+	Hx of Long Exposure to Loud Noise?	
	+	Hx of Excessive Earwax? (Impacted Earwax)	
Moderate Symptoms	+	High-Risk Patient: Extremes of Age, Communication Barrier, Emotional Distress, Hx Chronic Illness, Far from Hospital? (+/- Upgrade to Urgent)	
Minor Symptoms	+	Self-Limiting, Existing > 1 Week, Not Becoming Markedly Worse?	
	+	Failure to Improve on Home Treatment?	

Cross-References

Abuse

Dizziness

Ear Problem 2

Head Problem 1

EAR PROBLEM 2 (BIRTH-6 YR)

PAIN W/O TRAUMA; DISCHARGE; CONGESTION; EARLOBE SWELLING

ASSESSMENT		ACUITY LEVEL	DISPOSITION/ADVICE
Key Questions		**Emergent Symptom Patterns**	**ED 0 Min -1 Hr.**
Pain	+	Resp. Distress, Nasal/Pharyngeal Infection, Throat/Neck Swelling/Pain, Fever, Difficulty Swallowing, Drooling, Neck Pain W Movement? (Retropharyngeal Abscess)-- >	Axiom: Meningitis is most common in children age < 2 years and is often preceded by respiratory infection or otitis.

Does RN feel that symptoms are severe, extreme, or emergent?

Key Questions		Urgent Symptom Patterns	ED/UCC/Office 1-6 Hr.
Pain (+/- Severe)	+	Persistent, Throbbing, In or behind Ear, Fever, Creamy/Profuse Discharge, Hx of OM, Tenderness, Redness and Swelling behind Ear, < Hearing? (Mastoiditis)-->	SA: Apply pressure behind ear. Describe results. (Exquisite pain = +)
	+	Fever, Fussiness, Ear Pulling, Difficulty Sleeping, Irritability, +/- N/V, +/- Diarrhea, **+/-** Hx URI? (Otitis Media)	
Swollen Earlobe	+	Red **+/-** Streaking, Tender, Hot; **+/-** Discharge, Often w Fever, Swollen Nodes, Hx of Trauma/Bite/Local Infection, Recent Ear Piercing? (Auricular Cellulitis)	
Age < 3 mo	+	Fever > 38°C or 100.4°F®?--- >	Bring child to ED Now!
Toxicity/Dehydration	+	School Age? (See Toxicity/Dehydration Assessment)	
Pain/Symptoms	+	Fever > 40°C or 104°F?--->	Come to ED Now!
Unusual Pain/Symptoms	+	Post-Op or Postprocedure? (Poss. Complications/Infection)	
Symptoms of Infection	+	Failure to Improve on Antibiotics x 48 Hr? (Ineffective Rx)	

Does RN feel that symptoms are urgent?

continues

continued

Key Questions	Acute/Nonacute Symptom Patterns	FA 8+ Hr. +/- Home Tx
Pain	+ Without Fever, "Very Ill Child" (See Toxicity Assessment)? (Otitis Media)	
	+ With Discharge, Foul Odor, Hx of Seborrhea, Swimmer? (Otitis Externa)--	> SA: Pull on child's earlobe. (> Pain = +)
	+ With Hot, Cold Foods, Chewing? (Dental Inflammation)	
Pain/Congestion	+ Hx URI, Congestion? (Viral Syndrome)--------------------------------------	> Ear Pain Tx Goal: Relieve pain. Relieve congestion.
	+ Post Flight, Worse on Descent? (Otitic Barotrauma)	
	+ Temporary, Due to Cold Wind, Lack of Cover? (See Ear SI)	
Moderate Symptoms	+ High-Risk Patient: Extremes of Age, Communication Barrier, Emotional Distress, Hx Chronic Illness, Far from Hospital? (+/- Upgrade to Urgent)	
Minor Symptoms	+ Self-Limiting, Existing > 1 Week, Not Becoming Markedly Worse?	
	+ Failure to Improve on Home Treatment?	

Cross-References

Dizziness | Ear Problem SI | Face/Jaw

Ear Problem Supplemental Information (Birth-6 Yr)

AXIOMS

- Children may get mild earaches in cold, windy weather. Always put warm hats that cover ears on all children in cold weather (also see below).
- Pain from other areas such as the jaw or teeth often gets referred to the ear.

GENERAL ADVICE

- Never insert anything in ear (may perforate eardrum).
- Avoid blowing nose too hard.
- After swimming dry ears; turn head to side, and pull ear lobe for drainage.
- Don't expose child to loud noise; it may be harmful.

AIR TRAVEL WITH CHILDREN AND INFANTS

- Young child: Chew gum (age appropriate), swallow, or yawn w nose pinched closed while plane lands.
- Infant: Encourage nonnutritive sucking while plane lands.

DRUG SIDE EFFECT—HEARING LOSS AND TINNITUS

(Possible explanation: accidental ingestion.) Drugs and classes of drugs that may cause tinnitus and hearing loss:

- antibiotics
  -gentamicin
  -neomycin
  -streptomycin
  -tobramycin
  -vancomycin
  -ethacrynic acid
- diuretics (all)
- quinine
- salicylates
  -aspirin
  -Pepto Bismol (bismuth subsalicylate)

EARACHE

- Damp, warm compress to ear pm (see Home Tx Ref)
- Tylenol as appropriate
- Increase fluids. Take 2-3 extra glasses of fluids daily.

EAR INFECTION

- Signs and symptoms:
  -Age birth-3 yr: Fever, fussiness, ear pulling, irritability, N/V, diarrhea
  -Age > 3 yr: All above + ear pain, bloody or purulent discharge, stomachache
- Cause: Bacterial or viral
- Complication: Hearing loss, sepsis, meningitis
- Prevention/Tx:
  -Follow-up appointment after infection is important.
  -Take all antibiotic medicine until gone.
  -Discourage "bottle propping." Hold baby upright when feeding.

EARWAX INSTRUCTIONS

- Earwax instructions are not to be given prior to being seen and diagnosed (i.e., advice for follow-up visits only).
- For earwax: apply Debrox, or 1:1 mineral oil and H_20_2—2 gtts. in ear 2 * day.
- Do not use ear drops in the following conditions:
  -After ear surgery
  -Drainage
  -Pain
  -Irritation
  -Rash
  -Dizziness
- General instructions for earwax removal
  -Tilt head to the side. Apply 2 to 3 drops Debrox (or other brand name) into the ear that has wax in it.
  -Keep head tilted to side for a few minutes, or place cotton in ear to keep drops in ear.
  -Put drops in 2 x a day. Use them before you come to see MD as directed.
  -Ear drops are sold over the counter.

HEARING LOSS

- Signs and symptoms: Child complains of < hearing or sensation of fullness; parent/caretaker notices child has < hearing.
- Causes: Foreign body or impacted wax; trauma
- Tx: Needs appt.

RINGING IN EAR (TINNITUS)

- Signs and symptoms:
  -Sensation of "ringing" or buzzing in ear.
  -Behavior changes
  -Language delay/changes
- Causes
  -Chronic exposure to loud noise
  -Head trauma
  -Damage to eardrum
  -Abnormalities of the auditory nerve and its connection within the brain
  -Drug side effect; one of the first symptoms produced by an ototoxic drug
- Complication: Possible hearing loss. Persistent and severe tinnitus can interfere w the ability to perform daily activities. Can prevent pt. from getting sufficient sleep/rest. Can be incapacitating, cause speech delay, behavioral problems.

- Tx: Try to determine underlying cause and treat the cause.
- Referral: American Tinnitus Association, RO. Box 5, Portland, OR 97207

SWIMMER'S EAR (EXTERNAL EAR INFECTION)

- Signs and symptoms: Itching, pain, swelling, foul smell, drainage
- Cause: Bacteria or fungus, from getting water or other irritant into the canal. Irritation from cleaning or scratching canal can start the infection.
- Complication: Severe pain, < hearing. Can lead to frirther infection (spreading cellulitis).
- Prevention

  -Dry ears completely with hair dryer after swimming.

  -Q-Tip w 14 + 14 vinegar and water into outer ear canal to dry.

  -Keep ears dry/clean.

  -Wear ear plugs when swimming.

  -Do not try to clean inside the ear. Ears are "self-cleaning."

Extremities

EXTREMITIES (UPPER) (BIRTH-6 YR)

PAIN W OR W/O TRAUMA; SWELLING; LACERATIONS; FRACTURES

ASSOC SX/SPECIFIC CONSIDERATIONS	DISPOSITION/ADVICE
EMERGENT SYMPTOMS	**ED IN 0 MIN-1 HOUR**
• **TRAUMA (MAJOR): MVA, FALLS, BLUNT, ASSAULT** + ALL AMPUTATIONS? (See SHOCK)------------ ▶	• CONTROL BLEEDING: Apply firm pressure (see Supplemental Information). Save body part, wrap in clean cloth. (Place in plastic bag & place on ice.)
+ WEAK, DIZZY, Cold/Mottled/or Pale Skin, Blue Lips/Nailbeds, Rapid/Shallow Breathing, Unresponsive, Loss of Consciousness? (Shock) (See SHOCK) + OPEN WOUND w Bone Visible? (Compound Fracture, > Risk Infection) ------------ ▶	• COVER W CLEAN CLOTH. KEEP VERY STILL, DO NOT MOVE.
+ 2 OR MORE FX? (> Risk Hemorrhage) • Does RN feel Sx. are severe, extreme, emergent?	
URGENT SYMPTOMS	**ED/MD/APPT IN 1-8 HOURS**
• **TRAUMA (MINOR-MOD.)** + SUSPICIOUS HX? (Abuse) (See ABUSE) ------------ ▶	• **BRING CHILD TO E.D. NOW.**
• **SWELLING/PAIN W TRAUMA (MOD.-SEVERE)** + LACERATIONS (ALL) w Persistent Bleeding, Hx of Bleeding Disorder, Kidney/Liver Disease, Anticoagulants? (> Risk Hemorrhage) ------------ ▶	• **BRING CHILD TO E.D. NOW.** • CONTROL BLEEDING. + Cover w clean cloth. + Apply firm pressure to wound (see Supplemental Information). + Elevate injured area.
+ SWELLING, Deformity, Discoloration, < ROM or Refusal to Use? (Fracture) ------------ ▶	• **BRING CHILD TO E.D. NOW.** • SA: With fingers, gently press along bone to find injury. + Take off all jewelry on injured part (possible swelling). + Ice Pack to injured part. (See HOME TX REF) + Do not move injured part. + Do not eat or drink. (Pre Op)
+ (SEV.) PAIN, Numb, Pale Skin, Hx of Recent Trauma/Surgery, Cast Application, Pain Unrelieved by Ice, Elevation, Pain Meds? (Cast Problem/Compartment Syndrome) ------------ ▶	• **BRING CHILD TO E.D. NOW.**
+ (ELBOW) Hx of Lifted by or Sudden Pulling of Arm, Refusal to Move/Use Arm, Point Tenderness? (Nursemaid Elbow) • **SWELLING/PAIN W/O TRAUMA** + RED ± STREAKING, Tender, Hot; ± Discharge, Often w FEVER, Swollen Nodes, Hx of Trauma/Bite/Local Infection? (Cellulitis/ Lymphangitis) + ± FEVER, POINT TENDERNESS, Unilateral, Non-Use, Hx of Recent Infection? (Osteomyelitis) • **AGE** < 2 **WK: LUMP** (CLAVICULAR), < MOVEMENT on Affected Side? (Erb's Palsy)	
• **AGE** < **3 MO** + **FEVER** > **38°C** or **100.4°F®?**------------ ▶ • FEVER >40°C or 104°F? • AGE < 3 MO + MOD. SX + RISK FX (AVED)? • FAILURE TO IMPROVE on Antibiotics x 24-48 Hr? (Ineffective Rx) • WORSENING SX After 24-48 Hr on Home Tx? • RECENT SURGERY or HOSPITALIZATION? (Poss. Complications) • Does RN feel Sx. are urgent?	• **BRING CHILD TO E.D. NOW.**

continues

ASSOC SX/SPECIFIC/CONSIDERATIONS	DISPOSITION/ADVICE
ACUTE SYMPTOMS	**ED/MD/APPT IN 8-24 HOURS**
• **PAIN** + (FINGER) Hx Trauma, Blood Under Nail, Discoloration? (Subungual Hematoma) + (FINGER) Dull, Red, Swelling of Cuticle, Nail-Fold? (Paronychia) • AGE 3 MO-6 YR + MOD. SX + (AVED) = POSS. UPGRADE? • Does RN feel Sx. are acute?	
NON-ACUTE SYMPTOMS	**HOME TREATMENT W OR W/O APPT IN 24 + HOURS**
• **SWELLING** (Mild) + Trauma, ± Discoloration? (Hematoma) • **AGE** < **2 WK: LUMP** (CLAVICULAR), < Movement on Affected Side? (Clavicular Fx) (See EXTREMITIES SUPPLEMENTAL INFORMATION) • **CAST CARE** Instructions? • MINOR SELF-LIMITING SX EXISTING > 1 WK, NOT BECOMING MARKEDLY WORSE? • HOME TX ITEMS OR PHONE NOT AVAILABLE = POSS. UPGRADE? • Does RN feel Sx. are non-acute?	
CROSS-REFERENCES	**STANDARD FOLLOW-UP INSTRUCTIONS**
• ABUSE • EXTREMITIES (LOWER) (As Appropriate) • JOINT PROBLEM • SKIN PROBLEM 4: LACERATIONA/VOUND • SKIN PROBLEM 5: LESION/LUMP/SWELLING	PT TO CALL BACK: If symptoms become much worse or urgent or emergent symptoms arise (RN: review Protocol and advise caller). RN TO CALL BACK: If acute Sx in child AGE < 2 years. Routinely for Abdomen pain, Respiratory problems, Fever, Diarrhea, Marked change in ADL.

EXTREMITIES (LOWER) 1 (BIRTH-6 YR)

PAIN W TRAUMA; SWELLING; LACERATIONS; FRACTURES

ASSOC SX/SPECIFIC CONSIDERATIONS	DISPOSITION/ADVICE
EMERGENT SYMPTOMS	**ED IN 0 MIN-1 HOUR**
• **PAIN W TRAUMA (MAJOR): MVA, FALLS, BLUNT, PENETRATING** + ALL AMPUTATIONS? (Shock) (See SHOCK) ▶	• CONTROL BLEEDING, APPLY FIRM PRESSURE (See Supplemental Information). Save body part, wrap in clean cloth. (Place in plastic bag on top of ice.)
+ WEAK, DIZZY, Cold/Mottled/or Pale Skin, Blue Lips/Nailbeds, Rapid/Shallow Breathing, Unresponsive, Loss of Consciousness? (Shock) (See SHOCK)	
+ OPEN WOUND w Bone Visible? (Compound Fracture, > Risk Infection)	• COVER W CLEAN CLOTH. KEEP VERY STILL, DO NOT MOVE.
+ ALL FEMUR FX? (> Risk Hemorrhage) ▶ + 2 OR MORE FX? (> Risk Hemorrhage)	• SA: W fingers, gently press along bone to find injury. (> Pain = +) SA: Unable to bear weight? (Yes = +) + Take off all jewelry on injured part (possible swelling). + Ice Pack to injured part. (See HOME TX REF) + Do not move injured part. + Do not eat or drink. (Pre Op)
• Does RN Feel Sx. are severe, extreme, emergent?	
URGENT SYMPTOMS	**ED/MD/APPT IN 1-8 HOURS**
• **PAIN/SWELLING W TRAUMA (MINOR-MOD.)** + SUSPICIOUS HX? (Abuse) (See ABUSE) ▶	• **BRING CHILD TO E.D. NOW.**
+ (SEV.) PAIN, Numb, Pale Skin, Hx of Recent Trauma/Surgery, Cast Application, Pain Unrelieved by Ice, Elevation, Pain Meds? (Cast Problem/Compartment Syndrome)	• **BRING CHILD TO E.D. NOW.**
+ LACERATIONS (ALL) w Persistent Bleeding, Hx Bleeding Disorder, Kidney/Liver Disease, Hx Anticoagulants? (> Risk Hemorrhage)	• **BRING CHILD TO E.D. NOW.** • CONTROL BLEEDING. + Direct pressure to wound (See Supplemental Information). + Elevate injured area. + Cover w clean cloth, apply firm pressure. Keep very still, do not move.
+ LIMP, Refusal to Walk or Crawl, Deformity? (Fracture) ▶	• SA: W fingers, gently press along bone to find injury. (> Pain = +) SA: Unable to bear weight? (Yes = +) + Take off all jewelry on injured part (possible swelling). + Ice Pack to injured part. (See HOME TX REF) + Do not move injured part. + Do not eat or drink. (Pre Op)
• **AGE** < **3 MO** + **FEVER** > **38°C** or **100.4°F®?** ▶ • FEVER > 40 °C or 104°F? • AGE < 3 MO + MOD. SX + RISK FX (AVED)? • WORSENING SX After 24-48 Hr on Home Tx? • RECENT SURGERY or HOSPITALIZATION? (Poss. Complications) • Does RN feel Sx. are urgent?	• **BRING CHILD TO E.D. NOW.**

continues

EXTREMITIES (LOWER) 1 (BIRTH-6 YR)

continued

ASSOC SX/SPECIFIC/CONSIDERATIONS	DISPOSITION/ADVICE
ACUTE SYMPTOMS	**ED/MD/APPT IN 8-24 HOURS**
• **LIMP** + Gradual Onset, ± Trauma, Painful Gait? (Legg-Calv6-Perthes Disease) • AGE 3 MO-6 YR + MOD. SX + (AVED) = POSS. UPGRADE? • Does RN feel Sx. are acute?	
NON-ACUTE SYMPTOMS	**HOME TREATMENT W OR W/O APPT IN 24 + HOURS**
• **SWELLING** (MILD) + Trauma, ± Discoloration? (Hematoma) • **LACERATION/CUT/BRUISE (MINOR)?** (See SKIN PROBLEM 4) • **CAST CARE** Instructions? • MINOR SELF-LIMITING SX EXISTING > 1 WK, NOT BECOMING MARKEDLY WORSE? • HOME TX ITEMS OR PHONE NOT AVAILABLE = POSS. UPGRADE? • Does RN feel Sx. are non-acute?	
CROSS-REFERENCES	**STANDARD FOLLOW-UP INSTRUCTIONS**
• ABUSE • EXTREMITIES (LOWER) 2 • JOINT PROBLEM • SKIN PROBLEM 4: LACERATION/WOUND	PT TO CALL BACK: If symptoms become much worse or urgent or emergent symptoms arise (RN: review Protocol and advise caller). RN TO CALL BACK: If acute Sx in child AGE < 2 years. Routinely for Abdomen pain, Respiratory problems, Fever, Diarrhea, Marked changed in ADL.

EXTREMITIES (LOWER) 2 (BIRTH-6 YR)

PAIN W/O TRAUMA; SWELLING; WEAKNESS/NON-USE; LIMP

ASSOC SX/SPECIFIC/CONSIDERATIONS	DISPOSITION/ADVICE
EMERGENT SYMPTOMS	**ED IN 0 MIN-1 HOUR**
URGENT SYMPTOMS	**ED/MD/APPT IN 1-8 HOURS**
• **PAIN (SEVERE)** + NUMB, PALE SKIN, Hx of Recent Surgery/Cast Application, Pain Unrelieved by Ice, Elevation, Pain Meds? (Compartment Syndrome) ————————————	• **BRING CHILD TO E.D. NOW.**
• **LIMP/NON-USE** + ± FEVER, POINT TENDERNESS, Unilateral, Non-Use, Hx of Recent Infection? (Osteomyelitis) • **WEAKNESS/STAGGERING/DIFFICULTY WALKING** + ± PAIN, ± Bowel/Bladder Changes, Numbness, Tingling? (Acute Cerebellar Ataxia, Spinal Cord Tumor) + TOE WALKING, Fatigues Easily, ± Muscle Thinning? (Neuromuscular Disease) • **SWELLING (LEG)** + RED ± STREAKING, Tender, Hot; ± Discharge, Often w FEVER, Swollen Nodes, Hx of Trauma/Bite/Local Infection? (Cellulitis/ Lymphangitis) • **AGE < 3 MO + FEVER > 38°C or 100.4°F®?**--------------------------------	• **BRING CHILD TO E.D. NOW.**
• FEVER > 40°C or 104°F? • AGE < 3 MO + MOD. SX + RISK FX (AVED)? • FAILURE TO IMPROVE on Antibiotics x 24-48 Hr? (Ineffective Rx) • WORSENING SX After 24-48 Hr on Home Tx? • RECENT SURGERY or HOSPITALIZATION? (Poss. Complications) • Does RN feel Sx. are urgent?	
ACUTE SYMPTOMS	**ED/MD/APPT IN 8-24 HOURS**
• **LIMP** + > 24 Hr, ± FEVER? (Poss. Unwitnessed Accident, Infection) + Painful to Walk, Hip Tenderness? (Avascular Necrosis) + Unable to Bear Full Wt. ± Knee Pain? (Septic Arthritis, Toxic Synovitis of Hip) + Gradual Onset, ± Trauma, Painful Gait? (Legg-Calv6-Perthes Disease) • AGE 3 MO-6 YR + MOD. SX + (AVED) = POSS. UPGRADE? • Does RN feel Sx. are acute?	
NON-ACUTE SYMPTOMS	**HOME TREATMENT W OR W/O APPT IN 24 + HOURS**
• **LIMP** + Hx of Cut, Splinter, Foreign Body on Plantar Surface of Foot? (Laceration) (See SKIN PROBLEM 4) • **INTERMITTENT C/O PAIN IN CALVES, THIGHS,** at Night, > w Activity? (Growing Pains) + MINOR SELF-LIMITING SX EXISTING > 1 WK, NOT BECOMING MARKEDLY WORSE? + HOME TX ITEMS OR PHONE NOT AVAILABLE = POSS. UPGRADE? + Does RN feel Sx. are non-acute?	

continues

EXTREMITIES (LOWER) 2 (BIRTH-6 YR)

continued

ASSOC SX/SPECIFIC/CONSIDERATIONS	DISPOSITION/ADVICE
CROSS-REFERENCES	**STANDARD FOLLOW-UP INSTRUCTIONS**
• DIZZINESS • EXTREMITIES (LOWER) 1 • EXTREMITIES (UPPER) • JOINT PROBLEM • SKIN PROBLEM 4: LACERATION/WOUND	PT TO CALL BACK: If symptoms become much worse or urgent or emergent symptoms arise (RN: review Protocol and advise caller). RN TO CALL BACK: If acute Sx in child AGE < 2 years. Routinely for Abdomen pain, Respiratory problems, Fever, Diarrhea, Marked change in ADL.

Extremities (Upper and Lower) Supplementary Information (Birth-6 Yr)

AXIOMS

- Due to the accelerated rate of growth, injuries to extremities will more often result in fractures than in sprains or strains.
- Certain lower extremity deformities are common in this age group: Bow legs, pigeon toes, knock knees. They frequently correct themselves w time.

CAST CARE

- Never let a cast get wet. Use a hair blow dryer if it does get wet.
- Wait 48 hr for the cast to get strong. Don't walk or use the casted arm or leg until it is strong.
- Raise cast up on pillows, above heart level if possible, to stop swelling.
- Wiggle toes or fingers, if it does not cause pain. It will help prevent swelling.
- If the hand or foot swells or gets cold, blue, or numb, or very painful, bring child in to be seen right away.

FRACTURE

- Signs and Sx: Severe pain/swelling, obvious deformity, point tenderness, audible snap at time of injury, lack of ROM, refusal to bear weight, inability to move limb, "favoring" arm or leg
- Causes: Trauma, pathological fractures, birth trauma
- Complications: Tetanus, neurovascular compromise, and compartment syndrome, hemorrhage, infection
- Prevention/Tx: (See Cast Care above; See Tx Goal for Fracture/Bruise below)

HEMATOMA (BRUISE)

- Definition: Blood clotted in the tissue
- Signs and Sx: Discoloration of skin, swelling, mild to moderate pain
- Causes: Trauma, bleeding problem
- Complications: Infection/abscess (only if massive)

- Tx Goal: Relieve pain, prevent complication. (See also Tx Goal for Fracture/Bruise below.)
  - Warm Compress or Ice Pack—not directly on skin (See Home Tx Ref)
  - NSAIDS w Rx only
  - Raise injured part above level of heart.

LEG CRAMPS/PAIN

- Causes
  - Lack of calcium to muscle
  - Excessive exercise
  - Frequently occurs in this age group due to activity and rapid growth rate. "Normal growing pains."
- Prevention/Tx
  - Child needs calcium: Drink milk; eat carrots, broccoli; take Turns.
  - Take warm baths at bedtime.
  - Avoid pointing your toes.
  - Try to pull toes toward you.
  - Put a pillow under the covers at the foot of bed to keep weight of covers off feet.

NEWBORN—CLAVICULAR FRACTURE

- Definition: Hard bump is the bone healing. It will go away in a few weeks.
- Cause: Large baby, difficult delivery
- Tx: Do not pull baby up by arms. No Tx required.

PRESSURE POINTS

- Raise injured part above heart to < bleeding.
- Arm wound: Apply pressure (firm and continuous) to pulse point inside the upper arm. Use four fingers. Apply pressure firmly against bone until you can no longer feel pulse.
- Leg wound: Place victim on back and feel for pulse in groin area—at top of leg where leg bends. Use the heel/palm of hand, keep arm straight, press artery against bone. If you need to, use both hands.

SPRAIN

- Signs and Sx: Pain, swelling, difficult to use joint
- Causes: Trauma, wrenching or twisting of a joint, w or w/o partial tear of ligaments
- Complications: Damage to nearby blood vessels, muscles, tendons, and nerves
- Prevention/Tx: (See Tx Goal for Fracture/Bruise below)

STRAIN

- Signs and Sx: Pain w/o swelling following overexertion of a muscle
- Causes: Overstretching of a muscle
- Complications: Rare
- Prevention/Tx: (See Tx Goal for Fracture/Bruise below)

TX GOAL FOR FRACTURE, BRUISE

- Prevent swelling, pain. Prevent complications.
  - Raise the injured part above heart to reduce swelling. Use pillows or blankets for comfort.
  - Ice packs help cut down on swelling in the first 48 hr. (See Home Tx Ref, Ice Pack)
  - Warm compress after 48 hr may relieve persistent Sx. (See Home Tx Ref, Warm Pack)
  - If swollen, use Ace bandage.
  - If you use an Ace (elastic) bandage, don't wrap it too tight. Always take it off when you sleep.
  - Keep off injured area. Keep part still.
  - Pain medication: Tylenol as appropriate

Eye

EYE 1 (BIRTH-6 YR)

PAIN W TRAUMA; BURN; FB; VISION CHANGES; BLOOD IN

ASSOC SX/SPECIFIC/CONSIDERATIONS	DISPOSITION/ADVICE
EMERGENT SYMPTOMS	**ED IN 0 MIN-1 HOUR**
• **TRAUMA (MAJOR): MVA, BLUNT, FALL?** (See HEAD PROBLEM) • **TRAUMA** (MOD) + PENETRATION INJURY/Flying Object/FB, ± Leaking Fluid/Pain? (Globe Trauma, Hyphema) ----------▶	• DO NOT REMOVE IMPALED OBJECT. DO NOT PATCH. Shield w paper cup & tape.
+ (FACE/HEAD/EYE) + VISION CHANGE (ALL) ----------▶ + SUDDEN Painless Partial or Complete Loss of Vision (Veil, Shadow, Tiny Dots)? (Detached Retina, Hemorrhage, Subluxated Lens)	• Do not lie down or bend over. Have child sit up.
• **BURN** + CHEMICAL, Toxic Gas? (Corneal Bum) ----------▶ • Does RN feel Sx. are severe, extreme, emergent?	• **CONTACT POISON CENTER.** BRING SUBSTANCE TO E.D. W YOU. • Eyewash. (See HOME TX REF)
URGENT SYMPTOMS	**ED/MD/APPT. IN 1-8 HOURS**
• **TRAUMA (MINOR-MOD.)** + SUSPICIOUS HX? (Abuse) (See ABUSE) ----------*>	• **BRING CHILD TO E.D. NOW.**
• **EYELID LACERATION?** ----------▶	• **BRING CHILD TO E.D. NOW.** + APPLY DRY COMPRESS gently (w clean folded cloth—not cotton ball).
• **PAIN W TRAUMA** + RED EYE, Blurred Vision, Hx of Scratch, Contact Lens, FB? (Corneal Ulceration/Abrasion) ----------*-	• **BRING CHILD TO E.D. NOW.**
• **FB/CONTACT LENS,** Unable to Remove at Home? (> Risk of Abrasion) ——————▶	• DO NOT RUB OR TOUCH EYE.
• **AGE** < 3 **MO + FEVER** > **38°C or 100.4°F®?** ----------▶ • FEVER >40°C or 104°F? • FAILURE TO IMPROVE on Antibiotics x 24-48 Hr? (Ineffective Rx) • WORSENING SX After 24-48 Hr on Home Tx? • RECENT SURGERY or HOSPITALIZATION? (Poss. Complications) • Does RN feel Sx. are urgent?	• **BRING CHILD TO E.D. NOW.**
ACUTE SYMPTOMS	**ED/MD/APPT IN 8-24 HOURS**
• **TRAUMA** + Bruising Eye Area w/o Vision Change? (Lid Contusion, "Black Eye") • AGE 3 MO-6 YR + MOD. SX + (AVED) = POSS. UPGRADE? • Does RN feel Sx. are acute?	
NON-ACUTE SYMPTOMS	**HOME TREATMENT W OR W/O APPT IN 24 + HOURS**
• **FOREIGN BODY** (Sand, Dust, Dirt, Hair)? ----------▶ • **PHOTOPHOBIA?** (See EYE 2) • **BLEEDING IN CONJUNCTIVA** + Without Pain, ± Hx of Straining, Coughing, Sneezing, Birth Trauma? (Subconjunctival Hemorrhage) • MINOR SELF-LIMITING SX EXISTING > 1 WK, NOT BECOMING MARKEDLY WORSE? • HOME TX ITEMS OR PHONE NOT AVAILABLE = POSS. UPGRADE? • Does RN feel Sx. are non-acute?	• FB TX GOAL: Remove FB. Comfort. Prevent further injury. • TX: Clean gently around eye. Eyewash. (See HOME TX REF) • PAIN: + Tylenol as appropriate. + Cool Compress. (See HOME TX REF)
CROSS-REFERENCES	**STANDARD FOLLOW-UP INSTRUCTIONS**
• ABUSE • EYE 2	PT TO CALL BACK: If symptoms become much worse or urgent or emergent symptoms arise (RN: review Protocol and advise caller). RN TO CALL BACK: If acute Sx in child AGE < 2 Years. Routinely for Abdomen pain, Respiratory problems, Fever, Diarrhea, Marked change in ADL.

EYE 2 (BIRTH-6 YR)

PAIN W/O TRAUMA; PHOTOPHOBIA; BLOOD IN; DISCHARGE; SWELLING; VISION CHANGES

ASSOC SX/SPECIFIC/CONSIDERATIONS	DISPOSITION/ADVICE
EMERGENT SYMPTOMS	ED IN 0 MIN-1 HOUR
URGENT SYMPTOMS	ED/MD/APPT. IN 1-8 HOURS
• EYELID SWELLING (± EXTREME) + FACIAL SWELLING, FEVER, Redness/Tendemess, Fatigue, or Pain w Pressure on Globe or Eye Movement? (Periorbital Cellulitis)-- ——————»	• BRING CHILD TO E.D. NOW.
+ RED ITCHY EYES, Hx Exp. to Poison Oak or Exp. to Irritant/ Allergen? (Allergic Reaction) -- ▶	• Benadryl (in any form) if immediately available. Dose: Age & wt. dependent.
• **PAIN/PHOTOPHOBIA** ——————————————————►	• BRING CHILD TO E.D. NOW. + Topical corticosteroids contraindicated.
+ FB SENSATION, Constant Tearing, Blinking, Redness? (Corneal Ulcer/Herpes Keratitis) + HEADACHE (SEV.-MOD.), THROBBING, ± Unilateral, N/V, Abd. Pain, > Sensitivity to Light & Noise, ± Dizziness/Staggering, ± Preceded by Aura (See HEAD PROBLEM)? (Migraine) (See HEAD PROBLEM 2) • EYELID DROOP + ± DOUBLE VISION, Progressive Muscle Weakness, Trouble Chewing/Swallowing, Slurred Speech? (Myasthenia Gravis)	
• **AGES < 3 MO + FEVER > 38°C or 100.4°F®?** ——————————►	• BRING CHILD TO E.D. NOW.
• FEVER >40°C or 104T? • AGE < 3 MO + MOD. SX + RISK FX (AVED)? • FAILURE TO IMPROVE on Antibiotics x 24-48 Hr? (Ineffective Rx) • WORSENING SX After 24-48 Hr on Home Tx? • RECENT SURGERY or HOSPITALIZATION? (Poss. Complications) • Does RN feel Sx. are urgent?	
ACUTE SYMPTOMS	ED/MD/APPT IN 8-24 HOURS
• DISCHARGE + Red or Pink Eye, Yellow Discharge, Eyelids Stick Together/Esp. After Sleeping; Dried Eye Discharge on Face, ± URI? (Conjunctivitis: Bacterial, Viral, Allergic, Chemical) • AGE 3 MO-6 YR + MOD. SX + (AVED) = POSS. UPGRADE? • Does RN feel Sx. are acute?	

continues

EYE 2 (BIRTH-6 YR)

continued

ASSOC SX/SPECIFIC/CONSIDERATIONS	DISPOSITION/ADVICE
NON-ACUTE SYMPTOMS	**HOME TREATMENT W OR W/O APPT IN 24 + HOURS**
• **DISCHARGE** + Irritation, Hx of Recent Swimming? ("Swimming Pool" Conjunctivitis) + AGE < 6 MO: Chronic or Intermittent, Purulent or Clear/Watery w/o Irritation, Unilateral? (Blocked Tear Duct) (See EYE SUPPLEMENTAL INFORMATION) + (WATERY), Itching, Swollen Lid, ± Hx of Allergy? (Allergic Conjunctivitis) • **BLEEDING IN CONJUNCTIVA** + Concurrent Viral Infection? (Subconjunctival Hemorrhage) • **PUSTULE ON EYELID,** Swelling, Redness, Tenderness, + ± Discharge on Eyelid? (Stye/Chalazion) (See EYE SUPPLEMENTAL INFORMATION) • **EYE TWITCHING?** (Fatigue, Tic) • **NEWBORN: EYE IRRITATION** in First 2 Days of Life? (Chemical Conjunctivitis) • **WANDERING EYE** + Newborn? (Newborn Normal Strabismus) + AGE > 6 MO? (Strabismus) • MINOR SELF-LIMITING SX EXISTING > 1 WK, NOT BECOMING MARKEDLY WORSE? • HOME TX ITEMS OR PHONE NOT AVAILABLE = POSS. UPGRADE? • Does RN feel Sx. are non-acute?	
CROSS-REFERENCES	**STANDARD FOLLOW-UP INSTRUCTIONS**
• EYE 1 • FACE/JAW • HEAD PROBLEM 2 • NEWBORN CONCERNS	PT TO CALL BACK: If symptoms become much worse or urgent or emergent symptoms arise (RN: review Protocol and advise caller). RN TO CALL BACK: If acute Sx in child AGE < 2 Years. Routinely for Abdomen pain, Respiratory problems, Fever, Diarrhea, Marked change in ADL.

Eye Supplemental Information (Birth-6 Yr)

QUICK REFERENCE: Allergic Response
Black Eye
Blocked Tear Ducts
Conjunctivitis
Corneal Abrasion
Spontaneous Subconjunctival Hemorrhage
Stye

GENERAL AXIOM

- Eye Medication: Don't let tip of dropper touch the eye. It may spread infection to other eye.
- Eyepatch: Affects ability to see well. Leave eyepatch on as directed by M.D. May need mittens; may be off while sleeping.

ALLERGIC RESPONSE

- Signs and Sx: Discharge, tearing, itching, reddened, crusted, swollen eyelids, URI Sx
- Causes: Pollens, irritants (chronic), mechanical or chemical
- Complications: Worsening of Sx; chronic irritation; possible vision loss
- HomeTx
  - antihistamines
  - compresses, warm or cool (see Home Tx Ref)
  - natural tears
- Prevention: Elimination of irritating factors

BLACK EYE

- Signs and Sx: Bruising, swelling, pain, tenderness
- Cause: Injury
- Complications: Orbital Fx, infection
- Home Tx: Cold Compresses (See Home Tx Ref); Tylenol as appropriate

BLOCKED TEAR DUCTS

- HomeTx
  - Massage inner eyelid gently q 2 hr while awake. Wash hands w soap and water before massaging eye.
  - Moist, warm compresses to area for 10 Min, 3-4 x /day.

CONJUNCTIVITIS

- Tx Goal: Comfort; treat infection; prevent further infection or passing on to others
- Signs and Sx: see Protocol
- Causes: Bacterial, viral, allergic, chemical, or physical cause

- Complication: None
- Home Tx: Natural tears. Cool Compresses (See Home Tx Ref)
- Prevention
  - Don't let child share towel/washcloth with others who have conjunctivitis.
  - Caretaker + child: Wash hands frequently with soap.
  - Don't let child rub eyes.
  - Wash child's eye with warm washcloth. Don't use on the other eye.

CORNEAL ABRASION

- Signs and Sx: Tearing, severe pain, unilateral redness, and often refusal to open eye
- Causes: Scratch or trauma
- Complication: Possible vision loss
- Home Tx: Needs to be seen by M.D.

SPONTANEOUS SUBCONJUNCTIVAL HEMORRHAGE

- Definition: Leaking of blood into the white of the eye w pie-shaped area of blood
- Causes: Cough, sneeze, vomiting, standing on head or straining (constipation,, ,11th trauma
- Home Tx: No Tx. Will disappear in 2 wks. Reassurance.

STYE

- Signs and Sx: Pain, pimple-like lesion on the eyelid that may be at base of lid or deep within lid
- Cause: Inflammation of one or more of the sebaceous glands of the eyelid
- Complication: Infection spreads
- Home Tx: Warm Compresses for 15 min q 2 hr to promote drainage and help localize infection (See Home Tx Ref)

Face/Jaw

FACE/JAW PROBLEM (ALL AGES)

PAIN W OR W/O TRAUMA; DROOPING; SWELLING; WEAKNESS

ASSESSMENT	ACUITY LEVEL	DISPOSITION/ADVICE
Key Questions	**Emergent Symptom Patterns**	**ED 0 Min - 1 Hr.**
All Penetrating Trauma	--->	Do not remove penetrating object.
Major Trauma	--->	Axiom: Always consider head/neck injury w face/ jaw trauma.
	+ Assoc. Cervical Spine Trauma? (See Neck Problem)--->	Do not move patient.
Pain (Jaw) w/o Trauma	+ Chest Pain: +/- Exertion (Dull Ache, Pressure, Squeezing, Crushing, Radiates to Neck/Jaw/Arms), SOB, Sweating, Dizziness, Lightheaded, N/V, Pale, Anxiety, Sense of Impending Doom? (MI/Angina)	
Facial Drooping w/o Trauma (Unilateral)	+ Slurred Speech, +/- Headache, Sudden/Severe, Unsteady Gait, Confusion, +/- Incontinence, Hx of BCP/Atrial Fib/> BP? (CVA, Cerebral Hemorrhage, Embolus)	
Facial Swelling w/o Trauma	--->	Benadryl.
	+ SOB, Wheezing, Stridor, Difficulty Swallowing, Agitation, Anxiety, Rash (Itchy, Raised, "Hive-Like"), Swelling of Face/Tongue, Hx of Allergies or Exp. to Allergen (Med., Drug, Food, Chemical, Substance, Bite)? (Anaphylaxis)	

Does RN feel that symptoms are severe, extreme, or emergent?

Key Questions	Urgent Symptom Patterns	ED/UCC/Office 1-8 Hr.
Trauma	+ Suspicious History? (Abuse) (Possible Abuse)----------->	Come to ED Now!
Facial Trauma	--->	Axiom: Always consider head/neck injury w face/jaw trauma.
	+ Asymmetry, Severe/Sharp Pain, Swelling, Improper Bite? (Fx Mandible/Maxilla/Zygoma)------------------------>	Come to ED Now!
Facial Movements (Unusual)	+ Involuntary (Sudden Onset) Grimacing, Chewing, Wormlike Tongue, Drooling, Hx Phenothiazines? (Tardive Dyskinesia)-->	Come to ED Now!
Face/Jaw Pain w/o Trauma	+ Prolonged URI Sx, Nasal Discharge (Any Color), Cough, +/- Periorbital Swelling, Bad Breath, Headache, +/- Fever, Sinus Tenderness, Swollen Glands, Esp. in Teen? (Sinusitis)	

continues

continued

Key Questions	Urgent Symptom Patterns	ED/UCC/Office 1-8 Hr.
Face/Jaw Pain w/o Trauma continued	+ Swelling, Tenderness, Hx Toothache, Redness, Fever (> 38.5°C/101.3°F), Warm to Touch, Drainage? (Dental Abscess)	
	+ (Skin) Red +/- Streaking, Swollen, Tender, Hot; +/- Discharge, Often w Fever, Swollen Nodes, Hx of Trauma/Bite/Local Infection? (Cellulitis) (See also Eye)	
	+ Jabs of Pain around Eye, "Triggers" Cause Pain, Severe Spasms, Brief, Shooting Pain, Unilateral, Female, Age > 50 Yr? (Trigeminal Neuralgia, Tic Douloureux)--->	SA: Does touching certain areas of face cause painful spasm? (Yes = +)
Facial Weakness/Numbness w/o Trauma	+ Sudden Onset, Unilateral Drooping (Face & Mouth), Drooling, Feeling of Fullness, Swelling, Pain, "Crooked Smile," Irritated/Dry/Tearing Eye, Hx of Viral Infection, Unable to Close Eye? (Bell's Palsy)	
"Sick Infant/Child"	+ Toxicity/Dehydration Symptoms (See Toxicity/Dehydration Assessment)	
Pain/Symptoms	+ Fever > 40°C or 104°F?-->	Come to ED Now!
Unusual Pain/Symptoms	+ Post-Op or Postprocedure? (Poss. Complications/Infection)	
Symptoms of Infection	+ Failure to Improve on Antibiotics x 48 Hr? (Ineffective Rx)	
Fever	+ Age < 3 Mo + Fever > 38°C or 100.4°F? -------------->	Bring child to ED Now!

Does RN feel that symptoms are urgent?

Key Questions	Acute/Nonacute Symptom Patterns	FA 8+ Hr. +/- Home Tx
Facial Pain	+ (Skin) Lesion, Linear/Painful, Follows the Path of Nerve, Unilateral, Begins as Cluster of Bumps, Becomes Blisters, Then Dry Crust, +/- Sev. Itching? (Herpes Zoster/Shingles)	
Jaw Pain	+ Dizziness, Tinnitus, Popping Crackling Sound While Chewing, < Hearing, Itching/FB Sensation in Ear, Jaw Click? (TMJ Syndrome)-------------------------------->	SA: Clicking sound when opening mouth = + Chewing > pain = +
Facial Swelling	+ (Area below Ear on Cheek), Chills, Mod. Fever, Anorexia, Malaise, Pain on Chewing/Swallowing Acidic Fluids, Exp. to Mumps? (Mumps, Anterior Cervical Adenitis)	

continues

continued

Key Questions	Acute/Nonacute Symptom Patterns	FA 8+ Hr. +/- Home Tx
	+ Hx of Steroids, "Moon Face"? (Addison's Disease, Cushing's Syndrome)	
	+ Any Trimester of Pregnancy? (See Pregnancy Problems)	
Moderate Symptoms	+ High-Risk Patient: Extremes of Age, Communication Barrier, Emotional Distress, Hx Chronic Illness, Far from Hospital? (+/- Upgrade to Urgent)	
Minor Symptoms	+ Self-Limiting, Existing > 1 Week, Not Becoming Markedly Worse?	
	+ Failure to Improve on Home Treatment?	

Cross-References

Abuse
Ear Problem 2
Eye Problem 2
Neck Problem
Pregnancy Problems
Skin Problem 4
Skin Problem 5

Face/Jaw Problem Supplemental Information

Quick Reference:	Bell's Palsy	Trigeminal Neuralgia (Tic Douloureux)
	Cellulitis	Tutorial
	TMD (Temporomandibular Jaw)	References

BELL'S PALSY

- Definition: Facial paralysis due to damage to the facial nerve. There also may be pain, tearing, drooling, or hypersensitivity to sound in the affected ear and impaired taste ability.
- Bell's Palsy is more common in pregnant women and people with diabetes, influenza, a cold, or upper respiratory infection.
- Signs and symptoms: Facial weakness/numbness, feeling of fullness, swelling, pain, "crooked smile," irritated/dry/tearing eye, sudden onset, unilateral drooping (face and mouth), drooling, Hx of viral infection, unable to close eye
- Cause: Temporary nerve damage caused by virus
- Cause: The common cold sore virus, herpes simplex, and other herpes viruses are common causes of Bell's palsy.
- Tx Goals
  - -Steroid and pain medications
  - -Treatment is given to protect the eye from drying when sleeping.
  - -Even without treatment, patients begin to get better within a few weeks.
  - -Eighty percent recover completely within 3 months.
- Complications: In a rare case, the symptoms may never completely disappear.

CELLULITIS

See Skin Problem 3 (Lesion/Lump/Swelling).

TMD (TEMPOROMANDIBULAR [JAW] DISORDERS, ALSO CALLED TMJ SYNDROME)

- Definition: A disorder of the jaw muscles and joint. Symptoms include painful clicking, popping, or grating sounds when opening or closing the mouth, the jaw "locks," or there is limited jaw movement or a change in the "bite."
- Cause
  - -Severe injury to the jaw
  - -A fracture of the jaw
  - -Arthritis in the jaw joint
  - -Bad bite
  - -Stress may cause or worsen TMD.
  - -People with TMD often clench or grind their teeth at night, which can tire the jaw muscles and lead to pain.
  - -Women develop TMD twice as often as men.
- Signs and symptoms: Pain, popping or crackling sounds in ear when chewing; pain on side of face, tinnitus, < hearing, itching, or sensation of FB in ear

- Cause:
  -"Bad bite"
  -Dental work
  -Grinding teeth at night
- Definition: Damage to the facial nerve causing a sudden, severe, electric shock-like or stabbing pain on one side of the jaw or cheek.
  -Talking, brushing teeth, touching the face, chewing, or swallowing may trigger pain.
  -Trigeminal neuralgia is more common in women and people over age 50.
- Complications: > Pain and symptoms
- Prevention/Tx:
  -Limit yawning and movement of jaw.
  -Heat or ice to area
  -Pain: Tylenol or NSAIDs
  -"Nightguard" to prevent grinding
  -Biofeedback
  -Correction of "bite"
  -Surgery and injections are usually a last resort.

TRIGEMINAL NEURALGIA (TIC DOULOUREUX)

- Signs and symptoms: Severe pain in jaw lasting seconds to minutes, one-sided painful spasms
- Cause: Uncertain, possible compression of nerve by veins
- Prevention/Tx: Needs appt. w MD
  -Chew on unaffected side.
  -Gently brush teeth on affected side or not at all.
  -Use drinking straw.
  -Avoid cold drafts, chewing, drinking cold liquids, brushing hair, washing face.
- Tx: Anticonvulsant medication
  -If medication fails to relieve pain, surgical treatment may be recommended.
- Complications
  -Trigeminal neuralgia may come and go throughout the day.
  -The pain may last for days, weeks, or months.
  -Symptoms may disappear for months or years.
  -It may become worse.

TUTORIAL

Red Flags

Populations and symptoms that increase risk (SAVED: Severe symptoms, high-risk populations: Age, Veracity, Emotional distress, Debilitation)

- Symptoms
  -Severe, sudden, or suspicious pain.
  -Beware of pain that is more severe than expected or unrelenting.
  -Beware of any pain that awakens patient or keeps him or her awake at night.
- Age
  -Very young and very old patients have increased risk of infection and fracture.
- Veracity: All calls regarding infant/children are second party calls.
- Recent Injury

-Local joint trauma predisposes for infection.
-Remain alert for possible abuse.

Rules of Thumb

- All severe pain must be seen within 8 hours or less.
- Infant/Child: Atypical or novel presentation may be more common. Unlike adults, children may not display classic presentations of many conditions.
- Infant/Child: Subtle (or marked) changes in behavior or activities of daily living parameters in infants and young children may be the only indicators of serious illness/injury.
- Minority callers may fail to recognize acute symptoms, report fewer symptoms, or attribute them to other causes.

Red Herrings

"Red Herrings[11] are common distractions (symptoms or situations) that lead the nurse astray, away from the main problem.

- Remain vigilant to possible patient, parent, or caretaker denial, and minimization or misinterpretation of symptoms.
- Regard with suspicion: All unusual sounding presentations, including symptoms described as "the flu" or symptoms described as "new," "sudden," or "unexpected."
- Patients who have been "seen recently" may still need to be seen today.
- Do not be misled by concurrent complaints or patient self-explanation.
- Patients "on medication" may be on the wrong medication (antibiotics).
- Denial is associated with abuse.
- Symptom presentation may be early, late, silent, atypical, or novel.
- Symptoms of two conditions may present concurrently, causing confusion or misinterpretation.

REFERENCES

Briggs, J.K. (Ed.). (2002). ***Telephone triage protocols for nurses.*** (2nd ed.). Philadelphia: Lippincott.

Children's Hospital of Boston. (2003). ***Facial Fractures,*** http://www.childrenshospital.org-/cfapps/A2ZtopicDisplay.cfm?Topic=Facial%20Fractures.

Lafferty, S. & Baird. M. (2001). TeleNurse: Telephone Triage Protocols. New York: Delmar.

National Institutes of Health. (2003). ***Temperomandibular Disorders (TMD).*** http://www.nidcr.nih.gov/health/pubs/tmd/text.htm.

National Institute of Neurological Disorders and Stroke. (2001). ***Bell's Palsy,*** http://www.ninds.nih.gov/health_and_medical/disorders/bells_doc.htmNINDS Bell's.

National Institute of Neurological Disorders and Stroke. (2001). ***NINDS Trigeminal Neuralgia Information Page,*** http://www.ninds.nih.gov/health_and_medical/-disorders/trigemin_doc.htm.

Schmitt, Barton. (Ed.). (1999). ***Pediatric telephone advice.*** (2nd ed.). Philadelphia: Lippincott.

Fever

FEVER

FEVER WITH ASSOCIATED SYMPTOMS

ASSESSMENT	ACUITY LEVEL	DISPOSITION/ADVICE
Key Questions	**Emergent Symptom Patterns**	**ED 0 Min - 1 Hr.**
Fever (+/- High)	+ Fever, N/V, Severe, Intractable Diarrhea, Rash, Muscle Aches, Headache, Confusion, Dizziness, Fainting? (Sepsis Syndrome)	
	+ Stiff Neck, Headache, N/V, Extreme Fatigue, +/- Pinpoint Red Purplish Spots Progressing to Purple Patches, Extremely Irritable or Unresponsive, "Toxic Child" (See Acuity Assessment)------------------------->	SA: Touch chin to chest. (Inability to perform = neck stiffness)
	+ Seizure? (Meningococcal Meningitis)	
	+ Any Age (Although 2-5 Yr Most Common): Rapid Onset High Fever > 39.5°C or 103°F, Toxic Appearing, Muffled Voice, Throat Pain, Drooling, Insp. Stridor, Difficulty Breathing/Swallowing, Sits Very Still w Jaw ExtenHfiri? fFpinlnttiti^ ------------------------>	Discourage opening mouth widely. Nothing by mouth. Do not use thermometer or give food/drink. + First Aid: Keep sitting upright and calm until you reach ED.
	+ Sore Throat, Difficulty Breathing, Nasal/Pharyngeal Infection, Throat/Neck Swelling/Pain, Difficulty Swallowing, Drooling, Neck Pain w Movement? (Retropharyngeal Abscess)	
	+ Heat/Sun Exposure or Heat Wave, +/- Extreme Exercise (*Especially* Football) + Low or No Fluid Intake, Hot, Dry Skin, Dizziness, Weakness, Headache, Confusion, Combativeness, +/- Loss of Consciousness? (Heat Stroke) (See Heat Exposure)	
	+ Possible Biological or Chemical Exposure? (Possible Biochemical Terrorism) (See Bioterrorism Information).	

Does RN feel that symptoms are severe, extreme, or emergent?

Key Questions	Urgent Symptom Patterns	ED/UCC/Office 1-8 Hr.
Fever (+/- Mod.)	+ Fatigue, Weight Loss, Swollen Lymph Node? (Occult Neoplasm/Lymphoma/HIV/TB)	
	+ Night Sweats, Fatigue, Hx of IV Drug Use/Abuse, Hx or IV Diagnostic Procedures/Central Line? (SBE)	

continues

Key Questions	Urgent Symptom Patterns	ED/UCC/Office 1-8 Hr.
Fever (+/- Mod.) (continued)	+ "Toxic" or "Very Ill Child," +/- Severe-Mod. Dehydration? (Toxicity/Dehydration) (See Toxicity/ Dehydration Assessment)--->	Come to ED Now! + SA: Pinch skin briefly and release. Describe; if skin stays pinched looking = tenting or + for dehydration.
	+ Hx of AIDS/HIV, Chemo, Splenectomy, Sickle Cell, Steroid Therapy, Transplants, All Autoimmune Disease? (> Risk of Sepsis)-->	Come to ED Now!
	+ High-Risk Groups: All Immunocompromised, AIDS/HIV, Chemo, Diabetes, Cystic Fibrosis, Asthma, Sickle Cell, Splenectomy, Steroid Therapy, Transplants, Cancer, Frail Elderly or Child? (> Risk of Sepsis)	
	+ High-Risk Groups with Diarrhea, < Intake, +/- < UA Output/8 Hr, Weak, Dizzy, Dry Mouth, Sunken Eyes, Confusion, Extreme Thirst, Frail Elderly, Bedridden, Diabetes/HIV History, > 60 Yr., > 101°F? (High-Risk Age Groups, > Risk Dehydration)	
	+ Abd./Chest/Back Pain, +/- Respirations, Difficult Breathing, Chills, Cough: +/- Productive, N/V, Fatigue? (Pneumonia) (See also Respiratory Problem)	
	+ Abd. Pain, Constant, Progresses from Periumbilical to RLQ, +/- Vomiting, +/- Anorexia, +/- Holds Abdomen, Walks Bent over? (Appendicitis) (See also Abdominal Problem)	
	+ Abdomen Pain + Vaginal Discharge: Foul Smelling, Bloody/Any Color; Chills, Walks Bent over, +/- Hx of STD Exp., +/- IUD User? (PID) (See also Abdomen Problem)	
	+ Gradual Onset: Chills, Night Sweats, Fatigue, Joint Pain, Weight Loss, Hx of IV Drug Use/Abuse, Hx of Recent Dental Work/IV Diagnostic Procedure/ Central Line? (SBE)	
	+ Facial/Sinus Pain, Prolonged URI Sx, Nasal Discharge (Any Color), Cough, +/- Periorbital Swelling, Bad Breath, Headache, Sinus Tenderness, Swollen Glands, Especially in Teen? (Sinusitis)	
	+ Breastfeeding? (Possible Mastitis)	
	+ Seizure History = Possible Upgrade? (> Risk Seizure)	
	+ Chemotherapy Hx +/- Diarrhea, Stomatitis or Respiratory Symptoms? (Possible Chemotherapy Side Effect/Complications)	

continues

continued

Key Questions	Urgent Symptom Patterns	ED/UCC/Office 1-8 Hr.
Fever (+/- Mod.) (continued)	+ N/V, Anorexia, Yellow Sclera, Fatigue, Swollen Glands, Clay Colored Stools, Dark Urine +/- Hepatitis Exposure? (Hepatitis) (See Hepatitis SI)	
	+ Fever 104-105°F in pm, normal in am, Sweating, Fatigue, Headache, Enlarged Lymph Nodes, Muscular Pain, Low Back Pain, Wildlife or Livestock Contact: Veterinarians, Farmers, Ranchers, Slaughterhouse Workers, Meat Inspectors, Lab Personnel? (Undulant Fever/Brucellosis) (See Bioterrorism Information)	
	+ Sudden Onset of Fever, Headache, Muscle Pain, +/- Red Rash? (Rocky Mountain Spotted Fever)	
Fever (+/- Mild)	+ Recent Foreign Travel? (Acute/Chronic Tropical Infection)	
	+ Temp > 72 Hr or Recurrent After 24 Hr? (Fever Unknown Origin)	
	+ New Rx or OTC Med? (Drug-Induced Fever) (See Fever SI)--->	Axiom: Drug fever often occurs 7-10 days after first dose.
Toxicity/Dehydration	+ School Age? (See Toxicity/Dehydration Assessment)	
Pain/Symptoms	+ Fever > 40°C or 104°F?--->	Come to ED Now!
Unusual Pain/Symptoms	+ Post-Op or Postprocedure? (Poss. Complications/Infection)	
Symptoms of Infection	+ Failure to Improve on Antibiotics x 48 Hr? (Ineffective Rx)	

Does RN feel that symptoms are urgent?

Key Questions	Acute/Nonacute Symptom Patterns	FA 8+ Hr. +/- HomaTx
Moderate Symptoms	+ High-Risk Patient: Extremes of Age, Communication Barrier, Emotional Distress, Hx Chronic Illness, Far from Hospital? (+/- Upgrade to Urgent)	
Minor Symptoms	+ Self-Limiting, Existing > 1 Week, Not Becoming Markedly Worse?	
	+ Failure to Improve on Home Treatment	

continued

Cross-References

Abdomen Problem
Bowel Problem
Bioterrorism Information
Breastfeeding Problem
Chest Pain
Dehydration Assessment
Ear Problem
Extremities
OB/GYN Procedures
Respiratory Problem
Skin Problem
Temperature Taking Instructions
Toxicity Assessment
Urinary Problem
Vaginal Problem
Vomiting/Nausea
And Other Protocols

Fever Supplemental Information

Quick Reference:	Dehydration	Tutorial
	Drug Side Effect (Fever)	Surgical (Postoperative Fevers)
	Fever	Oncology
	Occult Infections	

DEHYDRATION (See Rehydration Guidelines in Home Treatment Reference)

- Complication: Shock
- Prevention/Tx: Drink fluids until urine is almost clear (see Home Tx Ref Clear Liquids).

DRUG SIDE EFFECT: FEVER (CAUSED OR MADE WORSE)

- antitubercular drugs
- barbiturates
- cephalosporins
- phenytoin (Dilantin)
- erythromycin
- ibuprofen
- methyldopa (Aldomet)
- penicillin
- quinidine
- quinine
- septra, bactrim, cotrimoxazole
- streptomycin
- sulfa drugs
- sulindac (Clinoril)
- chlorpromazine (Thorazine)
- acetaminophen (Tylenol) (Paradoxical Fever)

FEVER

- Signs and symptoms: Body temperature > 37.5°C or 99.0°F. It is not dangerous unless it is > 40° C or 104° F.
- Causes: Infection by a virus or bacteria. The fever is your body's way to help fight the infection.
- Complication: Dehydration (See Dehydration above).
- HomeTx

  -Goal: Reduce fever. Increase comfort.

  -Fever: Tylenol q 4 hr

  -Fever Record: Keep a record of the fever route. Take temperature every 4 hr (how you took it, when, how high). Check temperature 1 hour after medication. It should be lower or gone.

  -Warm bath (see Home Tx Ref, Warm [Tepid] Bath)

  -Never use alcohol rub or bath to stop a fever. Fumes can be toxic (CNS depression).

-Drink 8 or more glasses of cool or iced water, juice, soda, herb tea, etc. (except patients with change in level of consciousness, abdomen pain, CV disease, renal disease, diabetes inspidus).
-Dress in single layer of clothing. Use sheet only.
-Remove heavy blankets.
-Don't overdress child or overbundle infants.
-Rest.

OCCULT INFECTIONS

- inflammatory bowel disease
- osteomyelitis
- prostatitis
- subacute bacterial endocarditis (SBE)
- sinusitis, dental abscess

TUTORIAL

Red Flags

Populations and Symptoms which increase risk (SAVED: Severe symptoms. High-risk Populations: Age, Veracity, Emotional Distress, Debilitation)
Indicators of acuity when considering Fever:

- Any high fever; or fevers of long duration
- Immunocompromised status
- Poor response to antipyretics or home treatment
- Severe associated symptoms
- Similar symptoms or illness in contacts
- Sudden onset; quickly rising fever
- "Toxic Child" or severe dehydration
- Dead tissue or blood leaked internally, i.e., heart attack, stroke, alcoholic hepatitis or pancreatitis, or blood in the belly

Rules of Thumb

Children

- Kids get sicker quicker.
- Assess all sick children for dehydration or sepsis.
- The sicker looking the child, the more serious the illness, acuity is not fever dependent.
- The younger the patient, the greater the risk for hyperthermia.
- Neonates are at increased risk for overwhelming infection due to prematurity, traumatic delivery, maternal illness, or neonatal stress.

Others

- Elderly patients have decreased or absent febrile response to infection.
- "Temperature extremes often trigger medical problems" (Clawson & Democoeur, 1998).
- Minority callers may fail to recognize acute symptoms, report fewer symptoms, or attribute them to other causes.
- Fevers normally peak in late afternoon and evening.

Red Herrings

- Remain vigilant to possible patient denial, minimization, and misinterpretation of symptoms.
- Regard with suspicion: All elderly callers and unusual sounding presentations, including symptoms that are described as "the flu," or new, sudden, or unexpected, or wakened caller from sleep.
- Patients who have been "seen recently" may still need to be seen today.
- Don't be misled by concurrent complaints or patient self-explanation.
- Don't be misled by the prospect of "normal post-op fever" or patient self-explanation.
- Symptom presentation may be early, late, silent, atypical, or novel.
- Symptoms of two conditions may present concurrently, thereby causing confusion or misinterpretation.
- Illness rarely presents as a single symptom.
- Patients often misinterpret or stereotype their symptoms.

SURGICAL: POSTOPERATIVE FEVERS

Common Sources of Post-op Fevers:

- Abscess
- Deep vein thrombosis due to restricted activity
- Phlebitis (due to IV)
- Respiratory infections: most common source of fever in first 48 hours
- Urinary tract infections
- Wound infection

ONCOLOGY

All chemotherapy patients with fevers must be evaluated within 8 hours for possible neutropenia, stomatitis, and pulmonary or cardiac toxicity, as appropriate.

REFERENCE

Clawson, J.J. & Democoeur, K.B. (1998). *Principles of emergency medical dispatch.* Salt Lake City, UT: Priority Press.

RECOMMENDED READING

Anastasia, P.J. (1997). Outpatient chemotherapy: Telephone triage for symptom management. *Oncology Nursing Forum,* 24(1), 13-22.

Centers for Disease Control. (2001). *Brucellosis.* Retrieved August 17, 2001. http://www.cdc.gov/ncidod/dbmd/diseaseinfo/brucellosis_t.htm.

Centers for Disease Control. (2000). *Rocky Mountain Spotted Fever.* Retrieved August 17, 2001. http://www.cdc.gov/ncidod/dvrd/rmsf/index.htm.

Schmitt, B.D. (1999). *Pediatric telephone advice* (2nd ed.) New York: Lippincott, 288-302.

Smith, I.M. (1996). *Solving the difficult fevers.* Virtual Hospital. Retrieved April 18, 2000 from: http://www.vh.org/patient/IHB/IntMed/ABA30/1996/FUO.html.

Head Problem

HEAD PROBLEM 1 (BIRTH-6 YR)

PAIN; LACERATION; LEVEL OF CONSCIOUSNESS CHANGE W TRAUMA

ASSOC SX/SPECIFIC/CONSIDERATIONS	DISPOSITION/ADVICE
EMERGENT SYMPTOMS	**ED IN 0 MIN-1 HOUR**
• **PENETRATING OBJECT? (Intracerebral Bleed)** ------------------------▶	• DO NOT REMOVE MISSILE/FB.
• **PAIN + TRAUMA (MAJOR): MVA, FALL, BLUNT, Witnessed or Unwitnessed** ------------------------▶ + HEADACHE ± TRAUMA (Sudden/Sharp or Gradual/Dull/Throbbing), Neck Pain/Stiffness, Resp. Changes, Progressing: Irritable/Lethargic/± Loss of Consciousness; Visual Changes, Weakness, NA/, Staggering, Slurred Speech? (Intracranial Hemorrhage/Cerebral Contusion/Subdural Hematoma) + SUSPICIOUS EXPLANATION, HIGH-PITCHED CRY, Bulging Fontanelle, Extreme Irritability, Child Will Not Look at Parent/Caretaker (Retinal Hemorrhage)? (Shaken Baby Syndrome)	• **AXIOM:** ALWAYS SUSPECT SPINE/CORD INJURY W HEAD TRAUMA. • **FIRST AID (NECK INJURY):** + DO NOT MOVE, unless absolutely necessary. Wait for help. + Keep neck still. + Place both hands on side of head to stabilize neck.
+ PAIN, TENDERNESS, SWELLING Over Injured Area, ± Blood, CSF Coming from Ear/Nose, NA/, ± Loss of Consciousness, Seizure, Sev. Weakness? (Skull Fx/Basilar Skull Fx)------------------------ «-	• **AXIOM:** Usually assoc, w other severe injuries.
• Does RN feel Sx. are severe, extreme, emergent?	
URGENT SYMPTOMS	**ED/MD/APPT. IN 1-8 HOURS**
• **LACERATION** + PERSISTENT BLEEDING, ± Hx of Bleeding Disorder, Kidney/Liver Disease, Hx of Anticoagulants? (Laceration, > Risk Hemorrhage)------------------------ ▶	• **BRING CHILD TO E.D. NOW.** • **FIRST AID:** + Lay child down. + APPLY FIRM PRESSURE W CLEAN FOLDED CLOTH. + Keep pressure on until help arrives.
• **PAIN W MOD.-MINOR TRAUMA** + SUSPICIOUS HX? (Abuse) (See ABUSE) ————▶	• **BRING CHILD TO E.D. NOW.**
+ NA/, DIZZINESS, Staggering, Confusion, Loss of Memory, ± Loss of Consciousness? (Concussion) ------------------------ ▶	• **BRING CHILD TO E.D. NOW.**
+ PERSISTENT, SEVERE, HX A-V SHUNT, Drowsiness, Vomiting, Double Vision? (Shunt Malfunction) ------------------------ ▶	• **BRING CHILD TO E.D. NOW.**
+ VISUAL CHANGES? (See EYE 1) + VOMITING > 1x ?(> Risk)	
• **AGE < 3 MO + FEVER > 38°C OR 100.4°F®? -** ————▶	• **BRING CHILD TO E.D. NOW.**
• WORSENING SX After 24-48 Hr on Home Tx? • Does RN feel Sx. are urgent?	
ACUTE SYMPTOMS	**ED/MD/APPT IN 8-24 HOURS**
• **PAIN W MOD.-MINOR TRAUMA** + Hx Trauma (Days-Months), Dizziness, Confusion, ± N/V, Sensitivity to Noise/Light? (Post-Concussive Syndrome) • Does RN feel Sx. are acute?	

continues

HEAD PROBLEM 1 (BIRTH-6 YR)

continued

ASSOC SX/SPECIFIC/CONSIDERATIONS	DISPOSITION/ADVICE
NON-ACUTE SYMPTOMS	**HOME TREATMENT W OR W/O APPT IN 24 + HOURS**
• **PAIN W MINOR TRAUMA** + Cries Immediately, Minor Headache, ± Minor Bruise/Swelling, ± Vomiting (Ix only), Quickly Returns to Baseline ADL? (New Walker, Active Child, Playground Falls) + Swelling w/o Other Sx? ("Goose Egg," Hematoma) ---------------------------------- ► • MINOR SELF-LIMITING SX EXISTING > 1 WK, NOT BECOMING MARKEDLY WORSE? • HOME TX ITEMS OR PHONE NOT AVAILABLE = POSS. UPGRADE? • Does RN feel Sx. are non-acute?	• **FIRST AID:** + Apply Ice Pack. (See HOME TX REF) + Keep head elevated. + Keep in sitting, semi-reclining position.
CROSS-REFERENCES	**STANDARD FOLLOW-UP INSTRUCTIONS**
• ABUSE • DIZZINESS • FAINTING • EYE 1; 2 • HEAD PROBLEM 2 • VOMITING/NAUSEA	PT TO CALL BACK: If symptoms become much worse or urgent or emergent symptoms arise (RN: review Protocol and advise caller). RN TO CALL BACK: If acute Sx in child AGE < 2 Years. Routinely for Abdomen pain, Respiratory problems, Fever, Diarrhea, Marked change in ADL.

HEAD PROBLEM 2 (BIRTH-6 YR)

PAIN; LEVEL OF CONSCIOUSNESS CHANGE W/O TRAUMA

ASSOC. SX/SPECIFIC CONSIDERATIONS	DISPOSITION/ADVICE
EMERGENT SYMPTOMS	**ED IN 0 MIN-1 HOUR**
• **HEADACHE W/O TRAUMA (± SUDDEN/SEVERE/PERSISTENT)** + SUDDEN/SHARP or GRADUAL/DULL/THROBBING, Neck Pain/Stiffness, Resp. Changes, Progressing: Irritable/Lethargic/ ± Loss of Consciousness; Visual Changes, Weakness, N/V, Staggering, Slurred Speech? (Intracranial Hemorrhage, Spontaneous) + FEVER, STIFF NECK, N/V, Extreme Fatigue, ± Pinpoint Red Purplish Spots Progressing to Purple Patches, Extremely Irritable or Unresponsive, ± Seizure, Infant-2 Yrs: High-Pitched Cry, Bulging/Tight Fontanelle? (Meningococcal Meningitis) + DIFFUSE, ± N/V, Confusion, ± Seizure? (Hypertensive Crisis) • Does RN feel Sx. are severe, extreme, emergent?	• **AXIOM:** Meningitis is most common in children AGE < 2 Yr and is often preceded by respiratory infection or otitis.
URGENT SYMPTOMS	**ED/MD/APPT. IN 1-8 HOURS**
• **HEADACHE (± SEV.-MOD.)** + PERSISTENT, SEVERE, Drowsiness, Vomiting, Double Vision, ± Hx A-V Shunt? (Mass, Lesion, Shunt Malfunction) ---►	• **BRING CHILD TO E.D. NOW.**
+ (SEV.-MOD.), THROBBING, ± Unilateral, N/V, Abd. Pain, > Sensitivity to Light & Noise, ± Dizziness/Staggering, ± Preceded by Aura (See HEAD PROB. INFO)? (Migraine) ---►	• **BRING CHILD TO E.D. NOW.**
+ HX OF EXP. TO STREET DRUGS/Rx, Poisonous Plant or Inhalation/Ingestion of Toxic Chemical or Pesticide? (Toxic Exposure) ---►	• **BRING CHILD TO E.D. NOW.** **CONTACT POISON CENTER.** BRING SUBSTANCE TO E.D. W YOU.
+ WEAKNESS, DIZZINESS, SOB, Drowsiness, Faintness, N/V? (Carbon Monoxide Poisoning) ---►	• **BRING CHILD TO E.D. NOW.**
+ FACIAL PAIN, PROLONGED URI SX, Nasal Discharge (Any Color), Prolonged Cough, ± Periorbital Swelling, Bad Breath, ± FEVER, ± Photophobia, Sinus Tenderness, Swollen Glands? (Sinusitis) ---►	• SA: Place head between legs. Describe results. (> Pain = +) • SA: Tap/press above eyebrows/on cheekbones. (> Pain = +)
• **AGE < 3 MO + FEVER > 38°C OR 100.4°F®?** ---►	• **BRING CHILD TO E.D. NOW.**
• FEVER > 40 °C or 104°F?	
• Does RN feel Sx. are urgent?	

continues

HEAD PROBLEM 2 (BIRTH-6 YR)

continued

ASSOC SX/SPECIFIC/CONSIDERATIONS	DISPOSITION/ADVICE
ACUTE SYMPTOMS	**ED/MD/APPT IN 8-24 HOURS**
• AGE 3 MO-6 YR + MOD. SX + (AVED) = POSS. UPGRADE? • Does RN feel Sx. are acute?	
NON-ACUTE SYMPTOMS	**HOME TREATMENT W OR W/O APPT IN 24 + HOURS**
• **HEADACHE (MOD-MILD)** + Recurrent, Generalized, AM Headache (Usually), Hx Stress/ Anxiety, w/o Aura? (Tension Headache, Depression, School Phobia) + Post-Lumbar Puncture, > When Sitting Up? (Spinal Headache) -- *■ + Generalized, > w Use of Eyes? (Refractive Error) + Hx FEVER, Muscle Aches, NA/, Diarrhea? (Viral Syndrome) (See Dehydration Assessment/Rehydration Guidelines) • MINOR SELF-LIMITING SX EXISTING > 1 WK, NOT BECOMING MARKEDLY WORSE? • HOME TX ITEMS OR PHONE NOT AVAILABLE = POSS. UPGRADE? • Does RN feel Sx. are non-acute?	• HEADACHE TX GOAL: Relieve pain. Prevent recurrence. + PAIN: Tylenol (Acetaminophen) as appropriate. + Comfort: Rest in quiet, dark room w cool damp cloth on forehead. + Relaxation techniques. • Bedrest, > fluids.
CROSS-REFERENCES	**STANDARD FOLLOW-UP INSTRUCTIONS**
• Dehydration Assessment/Rehydration Guidelines • DIZZINESS • FAINTING • HEAD PROBLEM 1 • NOSE/SINUS PROBLEM	PT TO CALL BACK: If symptoms become much worse or urgent or emergent symptoms arise (RN: review Protocol and advise caller). RN TO CALL BACK: If acute Sx in child AGE < 2 Years. Routinely for Abdomen pain, Respiratory problems, Fever, Diarrhea, Marked change in ADL.

Head Problem Supplemental Information (Birth-6 Yr)

QUICK REFERENCE: Head Injury Instructions
Hematoma ("Goose Egg")
Migraine Headache

AXIOMS

- Headache: Uncommon complaint in children age < 6 yr. The more specific the pain, the > risk of organic causes (i.e., tumor, abscess, bleed).
- Head Trauma (even mild): Can cause headache, sleepiness, and vomiting immediately following the trauma. A brief episode of staggering is very common in children following even *minor* head trauma.
- Head Trauma (Major): Most common cause of *significant* head trauma in infants/toddlers is child abuse; in preschool/school age children is playground or sports injuries; in adolescents is MVAs.
- Head Trauma Age < 2 yr: The fontanelles and sutures are open, making the skull pliable. This can lead to severe laceration of vessels, meninges, and the brain.
- Head Hematoma or Laceration: In an infant or small child, significant blood loss may occur and lead to shock.
- Hydrocephalus w Shunt in Place: *Anything* that goes wrong (trauma, headache, N/V, seizure, fever, behavior/school problems) is considered shunt malfunction and needs an immediate evaluation.

HEAD INJURY INSTRUCTIONS

- Tx Goal: Provide comfort. Observe for complications. Prevent complications.
- Tx
  - Do not leave child alone for the next 24 hr.
  - It is normal for a child to vomit right after injury, and 1-2 times in the first 8 hr. If the child doesn't vomit right away, but then starts vomiting several hours after the injury, call right away.
  - Child should be easy to awaken when sleeping.
  - Do not use any drug that could cause drowsiness x 48 hr (e.g., cough med, antihistamines).
  - Quiet play x 72 hr
  - Give child light meals: Soup, plain pasta, cereal.
- Call right away if any of following Sx occur (even within several months):
  - Vomiting: Frequent (3 or more times), persistent, sudden
  - Stiff neck
  - Fever
  - Seizures or unconsciousness
  - Blurred vision or seeing double

- Confusion, very sleepy, or very difficult to wake up
- Stumbling or other problems w arms or legs
- Ear or nose drainage in first 48 hr
- Headache that is becoming worse or more frequent

HEMATOMA ("GOOSE EGG")

- Tx
  - Swelling: Ice Packs (see Home Tx Ref)
  - Pain: Tylenol as appropriate

MIGRAINE HEADACHE

- May be preceded by aura (Aura: Visual—Flashing lights/blind spots; Motor—Weakness/staggering; Sensory—Smells/tingling).

Heat Exposure

HEAT EXPOSURE (ALL AGES)

HEAT STROKE; HEAT EXHAUSTION; HEAT CRAMPS

ASSOC SX/SPECIFIC/CONSIDERATIONS	DISPOSITION/ADVICE
EMERGENT SYMPTOMS	**ED IN 0 MIN-1 HOUR**
• **HEAT EXPOSURE ± History of > Exercise, Humidity + < or Low Fluid Intake** + RAPID ONSET: HOT, DRY SKIN, FEVER > 105°F, Marked Change in Behavior, Hallucinations, Confusion, Combativeness, ± Loss of Consciousness, Seizures? (Heat Stroke) --------------------------------- *• + CHILD: "TOXIC" or Severe Dehydration? (>Risk Toxicity/Dehydration). (see Dehydration Assessment/Toxicity Assessment) + CHILD: <AGE 3 MO + FEVER > 38°C or 100.4°F? • Does RN feel symptoms are severe, extreme, or emergent?	• **FIRST AID:** + Move to shade/cool area. + Remove clothing. + Spray, splash or sponge and fan victim. + Place covered ice packs or cold cloths: Head/neck, groin, armpits. + If victim is conscious and awake, give frequent sips of cool fluids, Gatorade or commercial sports drink. + Elevate legs. + Do not give ASA or Tylenol.
URGENT SYMPTOMS	**ED/MD/APPT IN 1-8 HOURS**
• **HEAT EXPOSURE ± History of > Exercise, Humidity + < or Low Fluid Intake** + SUSPICIOUS HISTORY? (Poss. Abuse/Neglect) (See ABUSE) ------------ ▶ + ± FEVER, THIRST, SKIN: SWEATING (May be Profuse), Cool/Clammy/Pale/ Ashen, N/V, Headache, Muscle Cramps, Dizzy, Weak, Staggering? (Heat Exhaustion) --------------------------------- ▶ + PREVIOUS MEDICAL HISTORY: Cardiac Disease, Hypertension, Thyroid Disease, DM, Cystic Fibrosis, Some Dermatologic Disorders, Obesity? (> Risk Heat Exhaustion) + MEDICATIONS: ALCOHOL/Street Drugs/or Rx: Antihypertensive, Phenothiazines, Thyroid, Amphetamines? (> Risk Heat Exhaustion) • **HEAT EXPOSURE** + HIGH-RISK AGE GROUP ------------------------- ▶ + CHILD <10 Yrs or Elderly > 65 Yrs? (>Risk) + FRAIL ELDERLY: Listless, Dizzy, No Urine Output x 8 Hr, Dry Mouth, Sunken Eyes, Bedridden? (>Risk Dehydration) • ALL AGES: FEVER >40°C OR 104°F? • Does RN feel symptoms are urgent?	• **COME TO E.D. NOW.** • **FIRST AID: See above.** • **COME TO E.D. NOW.** + SA: Pinch skin briefly and release, Describe; if skin stays pinched-looking = tenting or + for dehydration.
ACUTE SYMPTOMS	**ED/MD/APPT IN 8-24 HOURS**
• **HEAT EXPOSURE** + Dehydration (Mild)? (> Risk Dehydration) • MODERATE SYMPTOMS + RISK FACTORS (Age, Veracity, Emotional Distress, Debilitation/Distance) = POSS. UPGRADE? • FAILURE TO IMPROVE on Home Treatment x 48 Hr? • Does RN feel symptoms are acute?	
NON-ACUTE SYMPTOMS	**HOME TREATMENT W OR W/O APPT IN 24 + HOURS**
• **HEAT EXPOSURE** + Excessive Water Intake, Muscle Cramps (Legs/Abd.), Lightheadedness, Weakness, Heavy Perspiration? (Heat Cramps. Hyponatremia) • HOME TREATMENT ITEMS OR PHONE NOT AVAILABLE = POSS. UPGRADE? • Does RN feel symptoms are non-acute?	
CROSS-REFERENCES	**STANDARD FOLLOW-UP INSTRUCTIONS**
• ABUSE • BURN 2 (SKIN PROBLEMS 2) • DEHYDRATION ASSESSMENT • DIZZINESS/FAINTING • SEIZURES • TOXICITY ASSESSMENT	PT TO CALL BACK: If symptoms become much worse or urgent or emergent symptoms arise (RN: review Protocol & advise caller). RN TO CALL BACK: Routinely for Abdomen pain, Respiratory problems, Fever, Diarrhea, Marked change in ADL.

Heat Exposure Supplemental Information (All Ages)

QUICK REFERENCE High Risk Occupations & Activities
Drug Side Effect (Heat Exposure)
Prevention

COMMUNITY ALERT

- Heat waves may increase incidence of heat stroke, *even in the absence of strenuous exercise.*
- The longer (in days) and more extreme the heat wave, the higher the incidence of heat stroke.
- Predisposition to heat stroke lasts for 24+ hours. Thus, heat stroke may depend on temperature of *the previous day.*

AXIOMS

- Extremes of age add to the risk of hyperthermia. Err on the side of caution with Adults > age 60 and CHILDREN < age 10.
- Heat Extremes may aggravate other medical problems. Don't overlook other possible medical conditions that may be present.

HIGH-RISK OCCUPATIONS DUE TO INTENSE EXERTION

- Miners
- Heavy industry workers
- Military personnel

HIGH-RISK OCCUPATIONS/ACTIVITIES DUE TO IMPERMEABLE GARMENTS

- Wrestlers
- Dieters
- Firefighters
- Hazardous waste handlers

DRUG SIDE EFFECT: HEAT EXPOSURE WORSENED

- Drugs and classes of drugs that may worsen heat exposure:
  - Alcohol
  - Amphetamines
  - Anticholinergic agents
  - Antihypertensives (e.g., diuretics)
  - Beta-blockers
  - Phenothiazines (decreases diaphoresis)
    - Chlorpromazine (Thorazine)
    - Prochlorperazine (Compazine)

- Thioridazine (Mellaril)
- Trifluoperazine (Stelazine)

- Thyroid (affects heat/cold tolerance)
  - Synthroid
  - Cytomel

PREVENTION

- Drink several glasses of water before and after exercising.
- Cover head with hat, wet cloth, or scarf. Cover neck with wet scarf.
- Eat salty foods, to replace salt lost through sweating.
- Stay in shade when possible.
- Avoid overdoing exercise. Rest when possible.
- Wear loose-fitting, light-colored, lightweight cotton clothes.
- Soak your tee shirt in cool water, wring out and wear.
- If taking any medication, consult with your pharmacist regarding possible side effects related to heat.
- Remember, certain medical conditions, activities, or jobs may put you at higher risk for heat illness. (Review)
- CHILD: For infants, don't overdress in warm weather. Rule of Thumb: One more layer of clothing than adult/caretaker.

References

Auerbach, RS. (Ed.). (1995). *Wilderness medicine: Management of wilderness and environmental emergencies.* (3rd ed.). St. Louis, MO: Mosby.

Clawson, J.J., M. D,, & Democoeur, K.B. (1998). *Principles of emergency medical dispatch.* (2nd ed.). Salt Lake City, UT: Priority Press.

Goold, G.B. & Vahradian, S. (1997). *Basic first response.* Upper Saddle River, N.J.: Prentice-Hall.

Manhoff, D. (1996). *Moshv's outdoor emergency medical guide.* (1st ed.). St. Louis, MO: Mosby.

Mayo Foundation for Medical Education and Research. (1990). *Mayo Clinic family health book.* New York: William Morrow and Company.

McSwain, N.E., Paturas, J.L., & Wertz, E. (Eds.). (1990). *Pre-hospital trauma life support.* (3rd ed.). St. Louis, MO: Mosby.

Joint Problem
(Upper & Lower)

JOINT PROBLEM (UPPER AND LOWER) (BIRTH-6 YR)

PAIN W OR W/O TRAUMA; SWELLING (SHOULDER, ELBOW, WRIST, HIP, KNEE, ANKLE); LIMP

ASSOC SX/SPECIFIC/CONSIDERATIONS	DISPOSITION/ADVICE
EMERGENT SYMPTOMS	**ED IN 0 MIN-1 HOUR**
URGENT SYMPTOMS	**ED/MD/APPT IN 1-8 HOURS**
• **JOINT PAIN W TRAUMA (MOD.):**	
+ SUSPICIOUS HX? (Abuse) (See ABUSE) ----------►	• **BRING CHILD TO E.D. NOW.**
+ (ALL JOINTS), SWELLING, DEFORMITY, Skin Discoloration, < Range of Motion, Refusal to Move, Unable to Bear Weight? (Fx, Dislocation, Separation, Acute Sprain) ----------	• **FIRST AID** + Rest on pillow. Elevate above heart if possible. + Ace wrap, if available.
• **JOINT PAIN W/O TRAUMA**	
+ ± FEVER, HX OF SICKLE CELL DISEASE? (Sickle Cell Crisis)—►	• **BRING CHILD TO E.D. NOW.**
+ SWELLING/Tenderness, Hx of Hemophilia? (Hemarthrosis) ----------►	• **BRING CHILD TO E.D. NOW.**
+ (SHOULDER PAIN) REFUSAL TO USE ARM, Hx Sudden Lifting &/or Jerking of Child's Arm? (Nursemaid's Elbow)----------►	• **BRING CHILD TO E.D. NOW.**
• **LIMP/NON-USE**	
+ ± FEVER, POINT TENDERNESS, Unilateral, Non-Use, Hx of Recent Infection? (Osteomyelitis)	
+ SUDDEN ONSET, FEVER, Chills, Tenderness, Joint Swelling, Skin Warm to Touch? (Septic Arthritis, Septic Joint)	
• **AGE < 3 MO + FEVER > 38 C or 100.4 F®?** ----------►	• **BRING CHILD TO E.D. NOW.**
• FEVER >40°C or 104°F?	
• AGE < 3 MO + MOD. SX + RISK FX (AVED)?	
• FAILURE TO IMPROVE on Antibiotics x 24-48 Hr? (Ineffective Rx)	
• WORSENING SX After 24-48 Hr on Home Tx?	
• RECENT SURGERY or HOSPITALIZATION? (Poss. Complications)	
• Does RN feel Sx. are urgent?	
ACUTE SYMPTOMS	**ED/MD/APPT IN 8-24 HOURS**
• **PAIN W TRAUMA**	
+ (ANKLE/FOOT) Swelling, Discoloration, Able to Tolerate Some Weight Bearing? (Sprain, Strain)	
• **PAIN W/O TRAUMA**	
+ Hx of Tick Exp., Hx of Recent Camping? (Lyme Disease) (See TICK BITES (SKIN PROBLEM 1))	
• **LIMP**	
+ > 24 HR, ± FEVER? (Poss. Unwitnessed Accident, Infection, Neoplastic Disease)	
+ Unable to Bear Full Wt., ± Knee Pain? (Toxic Synovitis of Hip)	
• Age 3 MO-6 YR + MOD. SX + (AVED) = POSS. UPGRADE?	
• Does RN feel Sx. are acute?	

continues

JOINT PROBLEM (UPPER AND LOWER) (BIRTH-6 YR)

continued

ASSOC SX/SPECIFIC/CONSIDERATIONS	DISPOSITION/ADVICE
NON-ACUTE SYMPTOMS	**HOME TREATMENT W OR W/O APPT IN 24 + HOURS**
• **LIMP** + Gradual Onset, ± Trauma, Painful Gait? (Legg-Calv6-Perthes Disease) →	• Needs appointment in 24+ Hr.
• **JOINT PAIN (MOD.)** + Swelling, Warmth, Pain on Movement, < Range of Motion, 1 or More Joints, ± FEVER/Rash? (Juvenile Rheumatoid Arthritis) • **JOINT PAIN (MILD)** + Mild FEVER, Generalized Joint Pain, URI Sx, ± Rash? (Viral Syndrome) • MINOR SELF-LIMITING SX EXISTING > 1 WK, NOT BECOMING MARKEDLY WORSE? • HOME TX ITEMS OR PHONE NOT AVAILABLE = POSS. UPGRADE? • Does RN feel Sx. are non-acute?	
CROSS-REFERENCES	**STANDARD FOLLOW-UP INSTRUCTIONS**
• ABUSE • EXTREMITIES (UPPER); EXTREMITIES (LOWER) 1; 2 • TICK BITES (SKIN PROBLEM 1)	PT TO CALL BACK: If symptoms become much worse or urgent or emergent symptoms arise (RN: review Protocol and advise caller). RN TO CALL BACK: If acute Sx in child AGE < 2 Years. Routinely for Abdomen pain, Respiratory problems, Fever, Diarrhea, Marked change in ADL.

Joint Problem Supplemental Information (Birth-6 Yr)

QUICK REFERENCE: Ace Wrap Teaching
Dislocations (Subluxations)
Sprain
Strain

AXIOM

"RICE": Rest, Ice, Compression (Ace wrap), and Elevate above level of heart.

ACE WRAP TEACHING

- Wrap going from toes or fingers toward heart.
- Check circulation. If toes become cold, blue, numb, loosen wrap.
- The bandage will help cut down on swelling, help to reduce pain, protect the injury, and help healing.
- Remove when sleeping.

DISLOCATIONS (SUBLUXATIONS)

- Subluxed Radial Head (Nursemaid's Elbow): Usually occurs in children < 5 yr.
- Signs and Sx: Pain w movement. Child refuses to use arm.
- Causes: Injury, e.g., lifting and/or jerking child by the arm
- Dislocations Home Tx Goal: Resume use of arm; pain greatly reduced.
    - Educate parent or caretaker about cause of injuries.

SPRAIN

Injury to a joint that causes pain and disability, depending upon degree of injury to the ligaments

- Tx Goal: Prevent swelling, pain, complications.
- Assessment
    - First degree: Some fiber tear but no decreased strength, mild point tenderness, no abnormal motion, minimal swelling
    - Second degree: Partial tear w some loss of function, point tenderness, light to mod. abnormal motion, hemorrhage
    - Third degree: Complete tear w total function loss, marked abnormal motion, possible deformity
- Signs and Sx: Pain, swelling, difficult to use joint
- Causes: Trauma, wrenching or twisting of joint w partial tear of its ligaments
- Complications: Damage to adjacent muscles, blood vessels, tendons, and nerves
- Tx Goal: Prevent swelling, pain. Prevent complications.
    - Elevate the injured part to reduce swelling. Use pillows or blankets for comfort.

- Ice packs used intermittently help reduce swelling during the first 48 hr. (See Home Tx Ref, Ice Pack)
- Follow w heat to area. (See Home Tx Ref, Warm Compress)
- Tylenol as needed for discomfort.
- Limit activity until healing occurs.
- If you have an elastic bandage, don't wrap it too tight. Always take it off when you sleep.

STRAIN

Injury to muscle and tendon caused by overuse (chronic strain) or overstress (trauma)

- Assessment
  - First degree: Does not reduce strength. Local pain and tenderness increases w movement. Mild spasm and swelling may be present.
  - Second degree: Partial decrease in strength, local pain, moderate spasm, swelling, bruising
  - Third degree: Severe pain, swelling, hematoma, loss of muscle function
- Signs and Sx: Pain w/o swelling
- Causes: Overuse or overstretching of muscles around joint
- Prevention/Tx: For mild strain:
  - Rest, or don't move area.
  - Ice Pack pm for spasm and swelling. (See Home Tx Ref, Ice Pack)
  - Analgesic as appropriate

Lip Mouth

Teeth/Gums

Tongue

LIP/MOUTH; TEETH/GUMS; TONGUE (BIRTH-6 YR)

PAIN W OR W/O TRAUMA; SWELLING; LACERATION; LESIONS

ASSOC SX/SPECIFIC/CONSIDERATIONS	DISPOSITION/ADVICE
EMERGENT SYMPTOMS	**ED IN 0 MIN-1 HOUR**
• **TRAUMA (MAJOR): MVA, FALL, BLUNT** (See also FACE/JAW, HEAD PROBLEM, NECK PROBLEM) • **LIP/TONGUE SWELLING** ——→ + SOB, WHEEZING, STRIDOR, Retractions, Difficulty Swallowing, Agitation, Anxiety, Rash (Itchy, Raised, "Hive Like"), Swelling of Face, Hx of Allergies or Exp. to Allergen (Med., Drug, Food, Chemical, Substance, Bite)? (Anaphylaxis) • Does RN feel Sx. are severe, extreme, emergent?	• Benadryl (in any form) if immediately available. Dose: Age & wt. dependent.
URGENT SYMPTOMS	**ED/MD/APPT. IN 1-8 HOURS**
• **TRAUMA (MINOR-MOD.)** + SUSPICIOUS HX? (Possible Abuse) (See ABUSE)------▶	• **BRING CHILD TO E.D. NOW.**
• **BRIGHT RED MOUTH/THROAT,** Cracked Lips, Strawberry Tongue, FEVER, Red Eyes w/o Pus, Red Itchy Irregular R?*h Patches on Face/Tnjnk, Enlarged Cervical Nn- • Red/r /Tender? ——→	• **BRING CHILD TO E.D. NOW.**
• **L» -CRMTION .^- 3, TONGUE** + PERSISTEN. oi_______ OiNG, Hx of Bleeding Disorder, Ar ■ulants, Liver/Renal Disorder? (> Risk ——→	• **BRING CHILD TO E.D. NOW.** + Apply firm pressure w clean cloth until child gets to E.D. + Do not stop pressure—bleeding will get worse.
• **TOOTH PAIN** + AVULSED? (Head Injury) (See HEAD PROBLEM) ——→ + FACIAL SWELLING, FEVER? (Abscess)	• **BRING CHILD TO E.D. NOW.** + SAVE TOOTH! Place tooth in glass of milk or saline solution or in parent's mouth between gum & teeth. (See HOME TX REF, Tooth Transport)
• **AGE < 3 MO + FEVER > 38°C or 100.4°F®?**------ ——→ • FEVER >40°C or 104°F? • AGE < 3 MO + MOD. SX + RISK FX (AVED)? • FAILURE TO IMPROVE on Antibiotics x 24-48 Hr? (Ineffective Rx) • WORSENING SX After 24-48 Hr on Home Tx? • RECENT SURGERY or HOSPITALIZATION? (Poss. Complications) • Does RN feel Sx. are urgent?	• **BRING CHILD TO E.D. NOW.**

continues

ASSOC SX/SPECIFIC/CONSIDERATIONS	DISPOSITION/ADVICE
ACUTE SYMPTOMS	**ED/MD/APPT IN 8-24 HOURS**
• **TOOTH BLEEDING** (Post Op 24-48 Hr) ------------------------------ ▶ • **LESION(S)/PAIN (MOUTH/TONGUE)** + Sev. Throat Pain; Cluster of Tiny Clear Blisters, Begins w Tingling, Itching, Followed by Yellow, Crusty Crater After 1-2 Days? (Herpes, > Risk Dehydration) + Small Clusters of Blisters, Ulcers in Back of Throat, Tongue (Gums & Cheeks Are Spared); Lasts 7-10 Days? (Herpangina) + Fistula Drainage into Gum from Cheek? (Dental Root Abscess) • **RED GUMS** + Swelling, Pain, Bleeding, Bad Breath? (Gingivitis) • AGE 3 MO-6 YR + MOD. SX + (AVED) = POSS. UPGRADE? • Does RN feel Sx. are acute?	• TOOTH-BLEEDING FIRST AID: STOP BLEEDING. + Bite firmly on gauze pad x 20 Min. + Do not rinse mouth! It may remove clots & start bleeding again. + Soft Diet. (See HOME TX REF)
NON-ACUTE SYMPTOMS	**HOME TREATMENT W OR W/O APPT IN 24 + HOURS**
• **RED GUMS** + Swelling, Pain, > Irritability, Drooling? (Teething) (See BEHAVIORAL PROBLEM) • **LESION(S)/PAIN (MOUTH/TONGUE)** + Thick, White, Patchy Coating on Tongue, Sides of Mouth, ± Hx Diaper Rash, Hx of Immunosuppression, Difficulty Swallowing/Eating? (Thrush, > Risk Dehydration) • **LESIONS (ALL)** + Single Cluster of Blisters ± Pain? (Herpes) + Gum Swelling, Hx of Dilantin? (Gingival Hypertrophy) + Raised, Clear, Blister-Like Lesions on Hands/Feet/ Mouth, ± FEVER, Fatigue, > Incidence in Summer? (Hand, Foot and Mouth Disease) + Single Lesion, Painful, Red, Sore, Becoming Ulcer w Red Base, Whitish Center? (Canker Sore) • **BLACK, DAMAGED, OR DISCOLORED TEETH,** Broken, Pain, Excessive Use of Bottles, Soft, Sticky Sweets, Poor Dental Hygiene? (Dental Caries) • MINOR SELF-LIMITING SX EXISTING > 1 WK, NOT BECOMING MARKEDLY WORSE? • HOME TX ITEMS OR PHONE NOT AVAILABLE = POSS. UPGRADE? • Does RN feel Sx. are non-acute?	• TOOTH PAIN TX GOAL: Relieve pain. + PAIN: Tylenol as appropriate. + Avoid hot & cold drinks. + Ice Pack/Cold Compress to jaw area that is painful. (See HOME TX REF)
CROSS-REFERENCES	**STANDARD FOLLOW-UP INSTRUCTIONS**
• ABUSE • BEHAVIORAL PROBLEM • FACE/JAW • HEAD PROBLEM 1; 2	PT TO CALL BACK: If symptoms become much worse or urgent or emergent symptoms arise (RN: review Protocol and advise caller). RN TO CALL BACK: If acute Sx in child AGE < 2 Years. Routinely for Abdomen pain, Respiratory problems, Fever, Diarrhea, Marked change in ADL.

Lip/Mouth; Teeth/Gums; Tongue Supplemental Information (Birth-6 Yr)

QUICK REFERENCE: Canker Sore (Aphthous Ulcer)
Dental Hygiene
Hand, Foot & Mouth Syndrome
Herpes (Herpes Simplex)
Lip/Mouth/Gum Lesions
Stomatitis (Viral)

AXIOM

Do not share glasses, food, drink, utensils, kisses w person who has mouth/lip lesion. Boil nipples and pacifier if infection diagnosed.

CANKER SORE (APHTHOUS ULCER)

- Signs and Sx: Inner lip and mucous membranes only: Single lesion usually, Painful, red sore, becomes ulcer w red base and whitish center and less tender. Resolves in days—2 wk.
- Causes: Many—Hypersensitivity, physical/emotional stress, chemical/food irritants, endocrine changes
- Tx
  - Pain: Tylenol as appropriate
  - Pain: Oragel
  - Don't drink citrus juice (orange, grapefruit, lemonade).

DENTAL HYGIENE

- HomeTx
  - Brush teeth/gums at least once a day.
  - Eat hard fruits and vegetables (apple, carrot, celery, etc.).
  - New toothbrush after infection
  - No fruit roll-ups if possible

HAND, FOOT AND MOUTH SYNDROME

Throat and palms of hands and soles of feet are covered w papular/vesicular lesions. Lasts 3-10 days.

- Signs and Sx: see Protocol
- Cause: Coxsackie virus
- Tx
  - Pain and Fever: Tylenol as appropriate
  - Pain: Oragel
  - Pain: Cold drinks, popsicles (age appropriate)

HERPES (HERPES SIMPLEX) (RECURRENT OR PRIMARY)

- Signs and Sx: see Protocol
- Causes: Herpes Simplex Virus I and II
- Tx
  - Pain and Fever: Tylenol as appropriate
  - Pain: Oragel
  - Pain: Cold drinks, popsicles (age appropriate)
  - Wash hands often w warm soap and water.

LIP/MOUTH/GUM LESIONS

- Home Tx (Age Appropriate)
  - Swish and swallow antacid.
  - Oragel
    Do not let child eat or drink for 1 hr after use of "Caines" (they might choke due to numbing effect of meds).
  - Bland diet and soothing liquids (See Home Tx Refs, "BRAT" Diet, Clear Liquids)
  - No citrus juice (orange, grapefruit, lemonade)
  - Analgesics

STOMATITIS (VIRAL)

Frequent cause of throat pain. Sx should go away after a few days of home Tx. If there are lesions, white patches, severe pain, or bright red throat, the child needs to be seen.

Neck Problem

NECK PROBLEM (BIRTH-6 YR)

PAIN W OR W/O TRAUMA; SWELLING; LUMPS

ASSOC. SX/SPECIFIC CONSIDERATIONS	DISPOSITION/ADVICE
EMERGENT SYMPTOMS	**ED IN 0 MIN-1 HOUR**
• **TRAUMA (MAJOR): MVA, FALLS, ASSAULT, BLUNT** ------------------------*-	• **AXIOM:** ALWAYS CONSIDER HEAD/NECK INJURY W FACE/JAW TRAUMA. + DO NOT MOVE PATIENTI
+ ALL PENETRATING WOUNDS -- ▶	• DO NOT REMOVE PENETRATING OBJECTI + If bleeding, apply direct pressure. + Never apply pressure to both sides of the neck at the same time.
+ TROUBLE BREATHING, SEVERE PAIN or Tenderness, Crying w/o Sound, Can't Talk, Hoarseness, Coughing Up Blood, Extreme Anxiety? (Tracheal Injury/Hematoma) + WEAKNESS/NUMBNESS/TINGLING or Inability to Move 1 or More Extremities, Change in Level of Consciousness? (Cervical Spine Injury) • **PAIN** + FEVER, STIFF NECK, HEADACHE, N/V, Extreme Fatigue, ± Pinpoint Red Purplish Spots Progressing to Purple Patches, Extremely Irritable or Unresponsive, 'Toxic Child" (See Toxicity Assessment), ± Seizure, Infant-2 Yrs: High-Pitched Cry, Bulging/ Tight Fontanelle? (Meningitis) • Does RN feel Sx. are severe, extreme, emergent?	
URGENT SYMPTOMS	**ED/MD/APPT IN 1-8 HOURS**
• **TRAUMA (MINOR-MOD.)** + SUSPICIOUS HX? (Abuse) (See ABUSE)--- ▶	• **BRING CHILD TO E.D. NOW.**
• **PAIN** + TWITCHING OF NECK MUSCLES (Uncontrollable, Painful, Severe), Hx Rx, Esp. Phenothiazine OR Poss. Ingestion? (Dystonic Reaction, Ingestion) ------------------------------------- ▶	• **BRING CHILD TO E.D. NOW.**
• **AGE < 3 MO + FEVER > 38°C** or **100.4°F®?**-------------------------- ▶	• **BRING CHILD TO E.D. NOW.**
• FEVER >40°C or 104°F? • AGE < 3 MO + MOD. SX + RISK FX (AVED)? • WORSENING SX After 24-48 Hr on Home Tx? • RECENT SURGERY or HOSPITALIZATION? (Poss. Complications) • Does RN feel Sx. are urgent?	
ACUTE SYMPTOMS	**ED/MD/APPT IN 8-24 HOURS**
• **LUMP(SySWELUNG** + Redness, Tenderness, Warm to Touch, FEVER? (Cervical Adenitis) + ± Progressive > in Size, ± Non Tender, w/o Hx Recent Infection? (Cyst/Mass: Benign/Neoplastic) • AGE 3 MO-6 YR + MOD. SX + (AVED) = POSS. UPGRADE? • Does RN feel Sx. are acute?	

continues

continued

ASSOC SX/SPECIFIC/CONSIDERATIONS	DISPOSITION/ADVICE
NON-ACUTE SYMPTOMS	**HOME TREATMENT W OR W/O APPT IN 24 + HOURS**
• **LUMP(S)/SWELUNG** + Without Redness/Drainage, w Hx URI or Flu? (Lymphadenopathy) + Pain Below Ear, ± FEVER, Anorexia, Malaise, Pain on Chewing/ Swallowing Acidic Fluids, Exp. to Mumps, In Male: Scrotal Swelling? (Mumps) + Newborn? (Sternocleidomastoid Hemorrhage) • **PAIN ± TRAUMA HX:** Stiff Neck from Sleeping, Repetitive Motions, ± Hx Recent MVA? (Neck Strain, Torticollis) • MINOR SELF-LIMITING SX EXISTING > 1 WK, NOT BECOMING MARKEDLY WORSE? • HOME TX ITEMS OR PHONE NOT AVAILABLE = POSS. UPGRADE? • Does RN feel Sx. are non-acute?	
CROSS-REFERENCES	**STANDARD FOLLOW-UP INSTRUCTIONS**
• ABUSE • RESPIRATORY PROBLEM 2: THROAT	PT TO CALL BACK: If symptoms become much worse or urgent or emergent symptoms arise (RN: review Protocol and advise caller). RN TO CALL BACK: If acute Sx in child AGE < 2 Years. Routinely for Abdomen pain, Respiratory problems, Fever, Diarrhea, Marked change in ADL.

Neck Problem Supplemental Information (Birth-6 Yr)

QUICK REFERENCE: Drug Side Effect (Dystonia)
Mumps
Neck Injury Instructions

AXIOMS

- Lymph Node Swelling: Lymph nodes can double in size w minor throat or cold infections. Can take months to go down.
- Neck Trauma: Stiffness and pain are usually worst 1-2 days following injury.

DRUG SIDE EFFECT—DYSTONIA

(Possible explanation: accidental ingestion)

- Sign and Sx: Uncontrollable, painful, severe twitching of neck muscles
- Drugs and classes of drugs that may cause Dystonia:
  - fluphenazine (Prolixin)
  - haloperidol (Haldol)
  - loxapine (Loxatine)
  - molindone (Moban)
  - perphenazine (Trilafon)
  - phenothiazines:
    - chlorpromazine (Thorazine)
    - prochlorperazine (Compazine)
    - thioridazine (Mellaril)
    - trifluoperazine (Stelazine)
  - risperidone (Resperdol)
  - thiothixene (Navane)

MUMPS

See Skin Problem 5

NECK INJURY INSTRUCTIONS

- Home Tx Goal: Relieve pain. Increase movement.
- Use heat or cold (See Home Tx Ref, Warm Compress, Ice Pack) on the injured area—whichever seems to help the most. Use Warm Compress as tolerated, *never hot* (See Home Tx Ref). No heating pad.
- Pain: Tylenol as appropriate
- Rest as much as possible until child feels better.
- Don't let child do anything that causes the pain.
- Have child take a warm shower/bath; drink warm tea. Do whatever helps child to relax.
- Gentle but firm massage will relax the muscles and will help to get rid of the soreness.

Newborn Concerns
Supplemental Information

Newborn Concerns Supplemental Information (Newborn-1 Month)

(NOTE: Age > 1 mo: Regarding toddler and school age children, see Behavioral Problem.)

AXIOM

Extreme fussiness or quiet may be the first sign of a serious illness in the newborn. Always consider the possibility when asking your questions. Review Toxicity and Dehydration Assessment with caller.

APPEARANCE

- **Bones:** Your baby's legs may look bowed; the feet may also be curved inward. This is normal. His/her legs will get straighter after he or she starts to walk; the feet should straighten in a few weeks.

- **Breasts:** Newborn babies' breasts (both boys and girls) may look swollen. This is normal. It happens when the baby is in your body and is exposed to your hormones. In most babies, it will go away by six months. Never squeeze the breast. This may cause an infection. Call your doctor if a breast looks red or is very painful when you touch it.
- **Eyes**
  - **-Blocked Tear Duct:** Sometimes a baby's eye may look watery all the time. This may be a blocked tear duct. Usually the tears drain through the nose. When a tear duct is blocked, this can't happen. Most of the time, it goes away on its own by the time your baby is 1 yr.
  - **-Crossed Eyes:** Your new baby may frequently look cross-eyed. This is because your baby can't control his or her eye muscle movements very well. Eye-crossing should go away by itself in 6 mo.
  - **-Discharge:** If your baby has white, yellow, or green sticky fluid coming out of his or her eyes, she or he may have an eye infection. Often, it causes the baby's eye-lashes to stick together. Your baby needs to see an MD.
- **Genitals**
  - **-Boys:** Your baby's testicles may look big for his body. This is normal. It was caused by the mother's hormones before the baby was bom.
  - **-Girls:** The outside of your baby's vagina may look swollen. Also, you may see some clear, white, or pinkish fluid come out of her vagina. Some baby girls may have a small bloody discharge. This is normal in newborn baby girls. It was caused by the mother's hormones before the baby was bom.
- **Hair:** Sometimes new babies have fine hair all over their bodies. This is normal. It goes away in a couple of weeks.
- **Head**
  - **-Bruises:** Your baby may have some bruises or marks on his or her head. Often this happens during birth. These are caused by the birth process. Sometimes the doctor has to use special instruments that fit on the head to help pull the baby out. This can cause bruises, too (see also Abuse).
  - **-Fontanelle:** All babies have a "soft spot" on top of their heads. It is called the fontanelle. It is a place where the bone has not grown together yet. The fontanelle should be flat. If it is bulging or sunken, call your doctor right away. (Review Dehydration Assessment with caller.) It is O.K. to gently touch the soft spot on the top of your baby's head. The baby's bones will grow together over the spot by the time he or she is 1 yr.
  - **-Lumps (Hematoma):** Many babies have a bump or lump on their heads after birth. At first, it will feel soft. Then, it may get hard. It will go away in a few days to a few weeks, depending on the size. Call us right away if it starts to get bigger.
  - **-Molding:** Baby's head looks long or flat. Your baby's head was molded or shaped as it passed through your birth canal. His/her head should become more round over the next several days.
- **Mouth**
  - **-Pacifier:** Babies are comforted by sucking. Even when your baby is not hungry, he or she may still need to suck. You can give him or her a pacifier. Only give your baby a pacifier after or between feedings to help calm or soothe him or her.
  - **-Thrush:** If your baby has white patches in his or her mouth, he or she may have thrush. This is a common infection. Your baby will need to take medicine for this. If your baby is using a pacifier, do not use your mouth to wet or "clean" it. Wash all his or her pacifiers and nipple bottles in hot soap and water after a few days of giving him or her the medicine for thrush. This will prevent your baby from getting reinfected w thrush.

- **Nose**

  -Coughing, Nasal Discharge, Sneezing: It is normal for newborn babies to cough and sneeze. They often have clear drainage coming out of their noses. If the drainage is yellow or green, or if your baby has a temperature or is not eating well, he or she needs to be seen by an MD.
- **Skin—Rashes**

  -Cradle Cap (Seborrheic Dermatitis): If your baby has thick, yellow, or white crusty patches on his or her scalp, he or she may have cradle cap. You can treat this at home. Wash your baby's hair every day. After you wash his or her hair, use a soft toothbrush or your fingers to remove the crusty patches. If it does not improve or it spreads to the face, neck, or behind ears, call your MD. He or she may prescribe a medicated cream.

  -Diaper Rash: Diaper rash is very common. Your baby's skin may look red or have small bumps on the buttocks, thighs, labia, penis, or stomach. Diaper rashes are most often caused by leaving a wet or dirty diaper on too long. To help your baby's diaper rash heal: Always wash w gentle soap and water after BM or use special "wipes." Change the diaper as soon as it is wet, leave the diaper off as often as possible, and do not use plastic pants. If the rash does not get better in 4-5 days, call back.

  If you notice clusters of bumps, especially in the skin folds or near the rectum, your baby may have a *yeast infection.* If your baby already has thrush in his or her mouth, he or she may also get a yeast infection in the diaper area. He or she will need a special cream for this.

  -Eczema (Atopic Dermatitis): If your newborn has red, dry patches on his or her skin, 'he or she may have eczema. Eczema usually runs in families. To take care of your baby's skin: Bathe your baby only 2-3 x per wk. Use a mild soap. Use a skin moisturizer (Eucerin cream) frequently.

  -Erythema Toxicum: The most common rash in newborns is erythema toxicum. This rash may be anywhere on your baby's body. It has red spots with small white bumps in the middle of them. They come and go. You do not need to do anything to take care of it. It usually goes away in 2 wk.

  -Heat Rash (Miliaria, Prickly Heat): If your baby has small red bumps on the neck, upper chest, or in the skin folds, he or she may have a heat rash. It is common in very young children. Do not use ointments or cream on this rash. A warm, humid environment or excessive sweating makes it worse. Keep skin dry and clean. Avoid dressing your baby too warmly (see Care, Dressing below).

  -Milia: If your baby has tiny white bumps on his or her face (especially on the nose and cheeks), it is probably a milia rash. The bumps look like tiny pimples. You do not need to put any medicine on them. This rash usually goes away in the first 2 mo.

  -Newborn Acne (Acne Neonatorum): Some newborns have acne on their faces. You will see small red bumps on the face. It usually starts after the baby is 2 wk old and may last until 6 mo old. Do not put anything on the baby's skin.
- **Skin—Birthmarks:** About 50 percent of babies are bom with a birthmark.

  -Strawberry Hemangioma: This birthmark is usually not easy to see at birth. It slowly gets bigger over the first 6 mo. It is usually red in color and may feel rough or bumpy. The skin gets more pale when pressed with your finger.

  -Mongolian Spot: This birthmark is a blue/black or green spot, usually on the back. It may be many different sizes and shapes. Most often it is found on the baby's back or buttocks. It is very common in dark-skinned babies. Most of these go away by 5 yr old.

-**Stork Bite:** This birthmark could be pink to red in color. It is usually located on the bridge of the nose, the forehead, the eyelids, the back of the head or the neck. It is a common birthmark. Most of these go away by 2 yr old.

- **Skin—Color Change:** When your baby cries hard his or her face and lips may look blue. He or she should quickly return to his or her normal color when he or she stops crying. If the baby's hands or feet are cold he or she may look a little blue. When he or she is warm again, the skin color should be normal.
  -**Jaundice (Yellow skin):** See Skin Problem 1: Discoloration, Jaundice.

FEEDING QUESTIONS

Appetite; Adequacy of Breastfeeding/Bottle Feeding; Growth; Weight Gain

Always rule out dehydration/malnutrition and toxicity. (See Toxicity or Dehydration Assessment.) (See also Crying, below.)

- How much should I be feeding my baby? How much is enough?
  -Growth and wt. gain: A well-fed baby looks and acts satisfied after feedings, wets 6 or more diapers each day, and has 2 or more yellow to brownish stools each day.
  -Breastfeeding: He or she should be nursing at least 8-10 x/day and gradually increasing to 15 min on each breast per feeding.
  -Bottle feeding: He or she will usually eat every 3-4 hr. Most babies will drink 2-3 oz each feeding. A rule of thumb you can follow is to add 3 oz to your baby's age in months (e.g., baby age 1 mo could drink up to 4 oz each feeding).

Burping: How to; How Often

- How should I burp my baby?
  -There are different ways you can hold your baby to help him or her burp.
  -The most common way is to hold your baby up w his or her head on your shoulder. Gently rub or pat his or her back w your other hand.
  -Another way is to sit your baby on your lap. Support his or her chest and head w one hand and arm. Slightly lean him or her forward. Pat his or her back w your other hand.
- How often should I burp my baby?
  -You should stop the feeding and burp your baby if he or she becomes fussy or cranky during the feeding. He or she will only swallow more air while he or she fusses and this will just make him or her more uncomfortable.
  -You should try to burp your baby 2 x during the feeding or between breasts if you are breastfeeding. You should also try to burp him or her after each feeding. Some babies are "difficult to burp." Try burping in different positions for about 1 min after feedings.

Formula

Always rule out dehydration/malnutrition and toxicity. (See Toxicity or Dehydration Assessment.) (See also Crying, below.)

- What kind of formula should I buy?
  -Most commercially made formulas are based on cow's milk. Babies on formula should be fed formula w regular iron (not "low iron") to prevent anemia. Iron in formula does not cause constipation.

-Soy-based formulas are given to babies who may be allergic to cow milk-based formula. You should discuss w your health provider before changing your baby to a soy formula.

- How long can I save the left over formula?
  -You should throw away any left over formula after each feeding. It could have germs in it or become spoiled.
- How should I prepare formula?
  -Read labels (concentrate or ready-to-feed).
  -No need to boil water.
  -If heating by microwave, use caution—always shake well and test first.

Solids

See Behavioral Problem, Eating Problems.

Water

Always rule out dehydration and toxicity. (See also Crying, below.)

- How much water should I give my baby?
  -Your baby does not usually need water. He or she gets enough from the breast milk or formula. You should give a few oz of water during hot days or if your baby has a fever. (Review Dehydration Assessment with caller.)

Weaning

See Breastfeeding, Weaning from Breast.

BEHAVIOR

Colic

Always rule out dehydration/malnutrition and toxicity. (See Toxicity or Dehydration Assessment.)

Does *my Baby have* ***Colic?***

- Definition: Periods of intense and persistent crying or fussing. They may be brief or last for hours. Colic usually starts around age 2 wk and stops around 3-4 mo. Episodes are usually worse in the evening.
- Cause: Unknown. Possible causes are immature bowels. This may cause gassiness. Other poss. causes: Baby is sensitive to too much noise, people, activity, new places; allergy to cow's milk.
- Complication: Potential for child abuse.
- Prevention/Tx
  -Rhythmic rocking in the cradle or car ride
  -Swaddle your baby to make him or her feel snug and warm. Rock your baby from side to side.
  -Give your baby something to suck on: Bottle, breast, pacifier.
  -Warm bath and massage
  -Cuddle your baby and sing or talk to him or her soothingly.
  -Play soft, soothing music.
  -Find another person to hold your baby so you can take a break.

-Run the vacuum cleaner in the next room. Steady rhythmic sound may help him or her fall asleep.
-Lay your baby on his or her tummy on your lap. Rub your hand on his or her back.
-Take baby for walk outside.

Crying

Always rule out dehydration/malnutrition and toxicity. (See Toxicity or Dehydration Assessment.)

- **A sudden change in the quality or an abnormal sounding cry may be a sign of serious illness. Call the advice nurse if you notice a change in the baby's cry as follows:**
  -High-pitched cry (possible CNS abnormality, meningitis, Hx exposure to cocaine)
  -Hoarse or low-pitched cry (possible upper airway obstruction)
  -Marked change in pattern of sleeping and crying (possible toxicity)
  -Weak cry (possible dehydration)
  -Absence of crying when exposed to pain, cold, loud noise, etc. (possible severe illness)
- Babies age < 3 mo normally cry for 1-3 hr/day. They usually cry because they are hungry, tired, have too much gas, have a wet/dirty diaper, or are lonely. Babies will usually stop crying when their needs are met.
- If your baby cries all the time, even when he or she finishes a bottle:
  -Crying is one way your baby talks to you. It does not mean that he or she is hungry. Always check first if your baby is crying because he or she is in pain or he or she may be cold because of a wet/dirty diaper. There are different ways to cope w his or her crying. Try a different method if one does not work:
  a. Try burping.
  b. Rock your baby gently in your arms as you sway side to side or sit in a rocking chair.
  c. Lay your baby on your lap on his or her stomach and gently rub his or her back up and down w one hand.
  d. Place your baby in a sling or carrier and walk him or her.
  e. Put your baby in a stroller and take him or her for a walk outside.
  f. Swaddle your baby by wrapping him or her snugly in a baby blanket.
  g. Offer a pacifier. Babies need a lot of sucking, not just to satisfy their hunger, during the first few months. This is called nonnutritive sucking.
  h. Sing or talk to your baby in a soothing voice.
  i. Play soft music.
  j. Give your baby a warm bath.
  -If you have tried different ways and you are not able to console your baby, take his or her temperature. He or she may be sick and have a fever. Call the nurse for advice.

ELIMINATION

- **Normal bowel movement in the breastfed and bottle-fed newborn** (see also Toxicity or Dehydration Assessment.)
  -**Meconium:** Your baby's first BM is called meconium. It is thick, sticky, and will look dark green or black. After this, his or her BMs will start to change to a yellow/green color.
  -**Stools—Breastfed:** If your baby is breastfed, his or her BM will look green or yellow and be pasty, seedy, or watery. A normal breast-fed baby may have anywhere from 1 BM every time he or she feeds to 1 BM every few days.

-**Stools—Bottle-Fed:** If you feed your baby formula, his or her BM will be yellow-brown, pasty. He or she should have 1 BM at least every few days.
-**Urine Output:** Your baby may urinate as often as every hr or less often 4-6 x/day. The urine should be light yellow in color.

CARE

- **Bathing:** Babies do not need a bath every day. 2 or 3 x/wk is O.K. The most important thing is to always keep the baby's diaper area clean.
  Do not put your baby in a bath until the stump of his or her umbilical cord falls off. During the 1st wk or 2, you can sponge bathe your baby. Make sure the room is warm. Keep your baby wrapped in a towel, except for the part that you are washing. After his or her cord falls off and the belly button area is healed and dry, you may put your baby in a bath. **Be sure the water is warm, not hot.** Test the water with your elbow or wrist.
- **Circumcision care:** After a circumcision, your baby's penis may look red for about 1 wk. It may also have some yellow spots. This is normal. It should go away after 7-10 days. If it does not go away or if there is swelling or yellow crusting, there may be an infection. Call your doctor. If your baby is not circumcised, his penis should be kept clean with soap and water. Do not pull back the foreskin; it is attached to the penis tip during the first few months. You can cause irritation if you try to pull back the foreskin. (See Toxicity Assessment.)
- **Cord care:** Your baby's umbilical cord will dry out and fall off in about 2 wk. Be sure to keep the cord stump clean and dry. Clean it with a cotton-tipped swab soaked in rubbing alcohol 3 x/day. Be sure to clean around the bottom of the stump. Keep the diaper below the cord so urine does not get on it. After the cord falls off, you may see a little blood on the diaper. This is normal. If you see pus at the bottom of the stump or redness on the skin around it, call your doctor right away. This could be an infection of the cord. (See Toxicity Assessment.)
- **Dressing:** Axiom: A good rule to follow is to dress your baby w one more layer of clothing than you are wearing comfortably.
  -Outerwear/Underwear: Your baby needs several layers of clothing unless the weather is very warm. He or she may need an undershirt, diapers, and pajamas.
  -Head covering: Always put knit cap and socks on baby in cold weather.
- **Skin Care:** To help protect your baby's skin, do not use bleach and fabric softeners when you wash and dry his or her clothes. Your baby does not need lotion, oil, or powder.

CROSS-REFERENCES:

- For additional problems, consult Texts for Supplementary Advice (see Bibliography).
- For the older infant's problems and concerns, see Infant/Child Protocols in the table of contents for additional information.

Nose/Sinus Problems

NOSE/SINUS PROBLEM (BIRTH-6 YR)

PAIN W OR W/O TRAUMA; FB; BLEEDING; DISCHARGE; CONGESTION

ASSOC SX/SPECIFIC/CONSIDERATIONS	DISPOSITION/ADVICE
EMERGENT SYMPTOMS	**ED IN 0 MIN-1 HOUR**
• **TRAUMA (MAJOR): MVA, FALLS, ASSAULT BLUNT** + ALL HEAD TRAUMA? (See HEAD PROBLEM 1) • Does RN feel Sx. are severe, extreme, emergent?	
URGENT SYMPTOMS	**ED/MD/APPT. IN 1-8 HOURS**
• **PAIN W TRAUMA (MINOR-MOD.)**	
+ SUSPICIOUS HX? (Abuse) (See ABUSE)------------------------------►	• **BRING CHILD TO E.D. NOW.**
+ OBVIOUS DEFORMITY, Blocked Breathing (Unilateral)? (Septal Hematoma, Nasal Fx)	
• **BLEEDING ± TRAUMA**	
+ UNCONTROLLED w Home Tx X 20 Min, ± Hx Anticoagulants, Bleeding Disorder, Renal/Liver Disease, w/o Sx Shock? (Epistaxis, > Risk Hemorrhage) (See NOSE/SINUS SUPPLEMENTAL INFORMATION) ------------------------------►	• **BRING CHILD TO E.D. NOW.**
• **PAIN W/O TRAUMA**	
+ FACIAL, PROLONGED URI SX, Nasal Discharge (Any Color), Prolonged Cough, ± Periorbital Swelling, Bad Breath, Headache, ± FEVER, ± Photophobia, Sinus Tenderness, Swollen Glands? (Sinusitis) ------------------------------*-	• SA: Place head between legs. Describe results. (> Pain = +) • SA: Tap/press above eyebrows/on cheekbones. (> Pain = +)
• **AGE < 3 MO + FEVER > 38°C or 100.4°F®?**------------------------------►	• **BRING CHILD TO E.D. NOW.**
• FEVER >40°C or 104°F? • AGE < 3 MO + MOD. SX + RISK FX (AVED)? • FAILURE TO IMPROVE on Antibiotics X 24-48 Hr? (Ineffective Rx) • WORSENING SX After 24-48 Hr on Home Tx? • RECENT SURGERY or HOSPITALIZATION? (Poss. Complications) • Does RN feel Sx. are urgent?	
ACUTE SYMPTOMS	**ED/MD/APPT IN 8-24 HOURS**
• **DISCHARGE** + (UNILATERAL), PERSISTENT, PURULENT, Foul-Smelling, Obstruction? (Foreign Body) • AGE 3 MO-6 YR + MOD. SX + (AVED) = POSS. UPGRADE? • Does RN feel Sx. are acute?	

continues

continued

ASSOC SXS/SPECIFIC CONSIDERATIONS	DISPOSITION/ADVICE
NON-ACUTE SYMPTOMS	**HOME TREATMENT W OR W/O APPT IN 24 + HOURS**
• **NASAL CONGESTION/DISCHARGE** + AGE < 1 MO, Chronic, Afebrile, Relief w Nasal Suction? ------------------------------ ▶ + AGE > 6 MO, Nighttime & Early AM Cough X1 Wk w/o Fever, w Clear Discharge? (Post Nasal Drip ± Secondary to Asthma) + WATERY DISCHARGE, Itchy, Teary Eyes, "Allergic Shiners," Sneezing, Fatigue, Pollen Season? (Allergies) + CLEAR/WHITE MUCUS < 7 Days; Cough, Sputum; Achy Joints, Hoarseness; Swollen Glands < 7 Days, Sore Throat? (URI) (See RESPIRATORY PROBLEM 2: COUGH/CONGESTION)	• NASAL CONGESTION TX GOAL: Relieve congestion, increase comfort, increase ability to feed. + Saline Nose Drops 3-4 X /day; *gently* remove mucus w bulb syringe. (See HOME TX REF)
• **BLEEDING W/O TRAUMA** + (MILD) ± Nose Picking, Recurrent, Brief? (Simple Epistaxis)-------------------------- ▶	• Humidify air. Lubricate nostrils. (See NOSE/ SINUS SUPPLEMENTAL INFORMATION, Nosebleed)
• MINOR SELF-LIMITING SX EXISTING > 1 WK, NOT BECOMING MARKEDLY WORSE? • HOME TX ITEMS OR PHONE NOT AVAILABLE = POSS. UPGRADE? • Does RN feel Sx. are non-acute?	
CROSS-REFERENCES	**STANDARD FOLLOW-UP INSTRUCTIONS**
• ABUSE • EYE 2 • FACE/JAW • HEAD 1;2 • RESPIRATORY PROBLEM 1; 2	PT TO CALL BACK: If symptoms become much worse or urgent or emergent symptoms arise (RN: review Protocol and advise caller). RN TO CALL BACK: If acute Sx in child AGE < 2 years. Routinely for Abdomen pain, Respiratory problems, Fever, Diarrhea, Marked change in ADL.

Nose/Sinus Problem Supplemental Information (Birth-6 Yr)

QUICK REFERENCE: Allergies
Nasal Suction
Nosebleed
Sinus Infection

GENERAL GUIDELINES

- Second-Hand Smoke Exposure: Increases risk for URI and ear infections
- Blowing nose too hard may lead to earache, nosebleeds.
- When child has a cold, give more clear liquids. (See Home Tx Ref)

ALLERGIES

- Tx Goal: Relieve Sx. Prevent > exposure to allergen.
  - Don't go outdoors on hot, windy days in pollen season.
  - No indoor flowers, feather pillows, pets
  - Vacuum and dust house often.
  - Drink 2-3 extra glasses water, juice, soda, daily.
  - Nasal Congestion: Saline nose drops (See Home Tx Ref)
  - Congestion: No OTC nasal sprays
  - Steam treatment (See Home Tx Ref)

NASAL SUCTION

- Tx: Suction with saline nose drops before feedings and bedtime/nap time (See Home Tx Ref). Don't overdo it!

NOSEBLEED

- Tx Goal: Stop nosebleed. Prevent more nosebleeds.
  - Sit up, lean forward.
  - Don't swallow blood, spit it out.
  - Pinch soft part of nose x 10 min; if bleeding continues, call back.
  - Apply cold compress to bridge of nose. (See Home Tx Ref)
- Prevention
  - No hot beverages x 24 hr after nosebleed (may start bleeding)
  - No heavy lifting, straining x 24 hr
  - No ASA, Motrin, Ibuprofen, Naprosyn, Advil (> bleeding)
  - Child may throw up from swallowing blood. It will look like coffee grounds.
  - After nosebleed stops, do not blow nose. It can cause bleeding to start again.
  - Always blow nose gently.

- In allergy season, or w rhinorrhea, put 1 gtt. K-Y Jelly just inside opening of nose every 12 hr.
- Steam treatment (See Home Tx Ref)

SINUS INFECTION

There are four sinuses in the head. They help to warm and moisturize the air.

- Cause: Viral URI or hay fever
- Complication: Untreated, could lead to brain abscess
- Prevention/Tx
  - Swimming allowed, avoid jumping in water feet first.
  - Warm washcloth over face, nose, TID
  - Sinus infection may be serious if untreated.
  - Needs antibiotics

Penile/Scrotal/Testicle Problem

PENILE/SCROTAL/TESTICLE PROBLEM (BIRTH-6 YR)

TRAUMA; FB; PAIN; DISCHARGE; LUMPS; LESIONS

ASSOC SX/SPECIFIC/CONSIDERATIONS	DISPOSITION/ADVICE
EMERGENT SYMPTOMS	**ED IN 0 MIN-1 HOUR**
• **TRAUMA (MAJOR): FALL, MVA, BLUNT,** LACERATION/BLEEDING, Severe Hemorrhage, Refusal to Urinate? (Urethral Rupture/Poss. Pelvic Fx) • Does RN feel Sx. are severe, extreme, emergent?	
URGENT SYMPTOMS	**ED/MD/APPT IN 1-8 HOURS**
• **DISCHARGE/LESION/ULCERATION (ALL)?** (Abuse) (See ABUSE)- →	• **BRING CHILD TO E.D. NOW.** • **AXIOM:** GENITAL/RECTAL TRAUMA (pain, bruising, laceration, bleeding) and abnormal discharge or lesions in a child *may* be an indication of abuse. Use a sensitive approach. Immediate evaluation is necessary. DO NOT be accusatory, arouse suspicion, or unduly alarm parent/caretaker. (See ABUSE)
• **TRAUMA (MINOR-MOD.)**	
+ SUSPICIOUS HX, Foreign Body? (Abuse) (See ABUSE) →	• **BRING CHILD TO E.D. NOW.** (See AXIOM above)
+ STRADDLE INJURY w or w/o Bleeding at Meatus, Swelling? (Urethral Injury)	
+ ZIPPER INJURY w Gians or Foreskin Imbedded in Zipper? ------------------------------*■	• Do not attempt to unzip.
+ SCROTUM PAIN/Swelling? (Hematocele)	
• **PAIN (SCROTAL/TESTICLE)**	
+ (SUDDEN, SEVERE, UNILATERAL) SWELLING, N/V? (Testicular Torsion) ------------------------------*-	• **BRING CHILD TO E.D. NOW. KEEP NPO.**
+ BULGE AT GROIN/Scrotum, Tender, N/V, Uncomfortable/ Inconsolable? (Incarcerated Hernia) (See ABDOMEN PROBLEM)—►	• **BRING CHILD TO E.D. NOW. KEEP NPO.** + SA: Touch: Tense or hard = +
• **PAIN (PENILE)**	
+ SWOLLEN GLANS w Uncircumcised Foreskin Stuck in Retraction at Base of Gians? (Paraphimosis)------------------------------►	• **BRING CHILD TO E.D. NOW.** **+ FIRST AID:** Put Cold Compress on penis to < swelling. (See HOME TX REF)
+ UNCIRCUMCISED W BALLOONING OF FORESKIN w Urination, ± Pain? (Obstructive Phimosis)	
+ CONTINUOUS ERECTION > 1 HR, Hx Sickle Cell Disease/Leukemia? (Priapism) ------------------------------►	• **BRING CHILD TO E.D. NOW.**
+ RECENT CIRCUMCISION, RED SKIN ± STREAKING, Swollen, Tender, Hot; ± Discharge, Often w FEVER, Swollen Nodes, Hx of Infection? (Cellulitis)	
+ RECENT CIRCUMCISION, BLEEDING CONTINUOUS? (> Risk Hemorrhage) ------------------------------*-	• **BRING CHILD TO E.D. NOW.**
• **AGE > 2 YR, ALL FB (PENILE),** BLOODY DISCHARGE? (FB)	
• **AGE < 3 MO + FEVER > 38°C or 100.4°F®?**------------------------------→	• **BRING CHILD TO E.D. NOW.**
• FEVER >40°C or 104°F? • AGE < 3 MO + MOD. SX + RISK FX (AVED)? • WORSENING SX After 24-48 Hr on Home Tx? • RECENT SURGERY or HOSPITALIZATION? (Poss. Complications) • Does RN feel Sx. are urgent?	

continues

PENILE/SCROTAL/TESTICLE PROBLEM (BIRTH-6 YR)

continued

ASSOC SX/SPECIFIC/CONSIDERATIONS	DISPOSITION/ADVICE
ACUTE SYMPTOMS	**ED/MD/APPT IN 8-24 HOURS**
• **SCROTAL SWELLING** + Bulge at Groin/Scrotum, Tender, No *UN* & Comfortable? (Inguinal Hernia) (See ABDOMEN PROBLEM) • **IRRITATION (PENILE)** + Redness, Irritation Around Opening to Urinary Tract, Circumcised w Agg. Diaper Rash? (Meatitis) (See PENILE PROBLEM SUPPLEMENTAL INFORMATION) • AGE 3 MO-6 YR + MOD. SX + (AVED) = POSS. UPGRADE? • Does RN feel Sx. are acute?	
NON-ACUTE SYMPTOMS	**HOME TREATMENT W OR W/O APPT IN 24 + HOURS**
> **IRRITATION (PENILE)** + Cheesy Material, Circumcised Penis Head Edge? (Smegma) + Uncircumcised or Incompletely Circumcised? (Adhesions) (See PENILE PROBLEM SUPPLEMENTAL INFORMATION) + Lump, Firm/Curved/Non-Tender at Head Edge? (Boil/Inclusion Cyst) (See SKIN PROBLEM 5) + Pinpoint Spraying or Unusual Direction of Urinary Stream, Hx of Meatitis, Circumcised? (Meatal Stenosis) + Hx Circumcision, Questions? (See NEWBORN CONCERNS: Circumcision Care) • **SWELLING (SCROTAL)** + Pain/Swelling below Jaw/Ear Fever, Headache, Anorexia, Fatigue, Pain on chewing/swallowing Acidic fluid, Exp. to Mumps? (Mumps) + Unilateral, > Size w Crying? (Hydrocele) • **NEWBORN (SCROTAL SWELLING)?** (See NEWBORN CONCERNS) • MINOR SELF-LIMITING SX EXISTING > 1 WK, NOT BECOMING MARKEDLY WORSE? • HOME TX ITEMS OR PHONE NOT AVAILABLE = POSS. UPGRADE? • Does RN feel Sx. are non-acute?	
CROSS-REFERENCES	**STANDARD FOLLOW-UP INSTRUCTIONS**
• ABDOMEN PROBLEM • ABUSE • NEWBORN CONCERNS • SKIN PROBLEM 5: LESION/LUMP/SWELLING	PT TO CALL BACK: If symptoms become much worse or urgent or emergent symptoms arise (RN: review Protocol and advise caller). RN TO CALL BACK: If acute Sx in child AGE < 2 years. Routinely for Abdomen pain, Respiratory problems, Fever, Diarrhea, Marked change in ADL.

Penile/Scrotal/Testicle Problem Supplemental Information (Birth-6 Yr)

QUICK REFERENCE: Adhesions
Circumcision
Meatitis
Mumps
Penile Hygiene
Smegma
Undescended Testicle

GENERAL AXIOM

Parents may overreact to problems related to genitalia because of the taboo nature of sexual organs. Fears and anxiety of parents/caretakers may call for problem upgrade.

ADHESIONS

- Definition: Scar tissue, contracted tissue stuck to infection/trauma site/surface
- Causes: Infection, trauma, previous surgery, chronic manipulation of tissue
- Complications: Inability to retract tissue w > amount of adhesions (i.e., foreskin)
- Prevention/Tx: Sitz Bath (See Home Tx Ref) to release adhesions to widen opening/tissue ROM. Only pull foreskin if it pulls back easily. *Never force it back!* Clean w soap and water.

CIRCUMCISION

- Definition: Surgical removal of the foreskin (prepuce) from the penis
- Causes: Surgery is done for cultural or religious reasons, or because parents want it done.
- Complications: Hemorrhage, infection
- Prevention/Tx: Cover glans after procedure w sterile gauze and petroleum jelly to prevent infection and irritation from diaper. Change dressing w diaper change. Watch for signs and Sx of bleeding, infection, urine output. Heals within 3-4 days.

MEATITIS

- Definition: Inflammation/infection of urethra at end of penis
- Causes: Mild phimosis, hypospadias, trauma, diaper rash
- Complications: UTI, meatal ulcerations, meatal stenosis, septicemia
- Prevention/Tx
  - Penile hygiene if uncircumcised; Sitz Bath. (See Home Tx Ref) Age > 4 yr: Only pull foreskin if it pulls back easily. *Never force it back!* Clean w soap and water.
  - Systemic antibiotic therapy
  - Change diaper frequently when rash; use ointment/cream on diaper rash.

MUMPS

See Skin Problem 5

PENILE HYGIENE

- Prevention/Tx: Sitz Bath. (See Home Tx Ref) Age>4yr: Only pull foreskin if it pulls back easily. *Never force it back!* Clean w soap and water.

SMEGMA

- Definition: Cheesy material in or around foreskin of penis; may smell bad
- Cause: Normal discharge
- Prevention/Tx: Sitz Bath. (See Home Tx Ref) Age > 4 yr: Only pull foreskin if it pulls back easily. *Never force it back!* Clean w soap and water.

UNDESCENDED TESTICLE

- Definition: Lack of one or both testicles in scrotum
- Causes: Hernias, adhesions, narrow inguinal canal, endocrine problems, delayed descent
- Complications: Damage to testes, infertility, or sterility if not brought down by age 4 yr.
- Prevention/Tx: 80 percent of all undescended testes will be in scrotum during first few months of life. Differentiate between undescended and retractile by "milking down" from inguinal or groin area to scrotum. Warm hands to "milk." See M.D. for evaluation, treatment (i.e., hormone Tx) or surgery.

Rectal Problems

RECTAL PROBLEM (BIRTH-6 YR)

PAIN W OR W/O TRAUMA; FB; BLEEDING; ITCHING; DISCHARGE; LESION

ASSOC SX/SPECIFIC/CONSIDERATIONS	DISPOSITION/ADVICE
EMERGENT SYMPTOMS	**ED IN 0 MIN-1 HOUR**
URGENT SYMPTOMS	**ED/MD/APPT. IN 1-8 HOURS**
• **TRAUMA (MINOR-MOD.)** + SUSPICIOUS HX? (Abuse) **(See ABUSE)** → + FOREIGN BODY, Suspicious Explanation? (Abuse) (See ABUSE)	• **BRING CHILD TO E.D. NOW.**
• **DISCHARGE/LESIONS** → + PURULENT, ITCHING, Burning, Painful BM, Throbbing (Severe), Swelling, FEVER? (Perirectal Abscess/GC, Abuse) (See ABUSE)	• **BRING CHILD TO E.D. NOW.** • **AXIOM:** GENITAL/RECTAL TRAUMA (pain, bruising, laceration, bleeding) and abnormal discharge or lesions in a child *may* be an indication of abuse. Use a sensitive approach. Immediate evaluation is necessary. DO NOT be accusatory, arouse suspicion, or unduly alarm parent/caretaker. (See ABUSE)
• **AGE < 3 MO + FEVER > 38°C or 100.4°F®?** → • FEVER > 40°C or 104°F? • AGE < 3 MO + MOD. SX + RISK FX (AVED)? • FAILURE TO IMPROVE on Antibiotics x 24-48 Hr? (Ineffective Rx) • WORSENING SX After 24-48 Hr on Home Tx? • Does RN feel Sx. are urgent?	• **BRING CHILD TO E.D. NOW.**
ACUTE SYMPTOMS	**ED/MD/APPT IN 8-24 HOURS**
• **PAINLESS PROTRUSION** + AGE 1-3 YR: Pink, Rectal Tissue Visible? (Rectal Prolapse) • **ITCHING** + Beefy Red, Worse Around Anus/Creases/Folds, Blister-Like Lesions, ± Hx Oral Thrush? (Candidiasis, Strep) • AGE 3 MO-6 YR + MOD. SX + (AVED) = POSS. UPGRADE? • Does RN feel Sx. are acute?	

continues

continued

ASSOC SX/SPECIFIC/CONSIDERATIONS	DISPOSITION/ADVICE
NON-ACUTE SYMPTOMS	**HOME TREATMENT W OR W/O APPT IN 24 + HOURS**
• **BLEEDING (W MILD PAIN OR W/O PAIN)** + Small Amount, Bright Red, on Outside of BM or Toilet Tissue or Toilet Bowl? (Hemorrhoids, Fissure, Polyps) • **PAIN** + Hx of Constipation x 5 Days, Anorexia, Malaise, Abd. Fullness (Lower)? (Fecal Impaction) (See BOWEL PROBLEM 2) • **ITCHING** + Hx of Pinworm Infestation in Household/Daycare? (Pinworms) + Excessive Scratching? (Contact Dermatitis) (See SKIN PROBLEM 6: RASHES; CHILDHOOD RASHES) • **RASH,** Red, Generalized, Bum-Like Appearance Under Diaper Area or Near Anus? (Diaper Rash) • MINOR SELF-LIMITING SX EXISTING > 1 WK, NOT BECOMING MARKEDLY WORSE? • HOME TX ITEMS OR PHONE NOT AVAILABLE = POSS. UPGRADE? • Does RN feel Sx. are non-acute?	• PINWORM HOME TX: (See SUPPLEMENTAL INFORMATION)
CROSS-REFERENCES	**STANDARD FOLLOW-UP INSTRUCTIONS**
• ABUSE • ABDOMEN PROBLEM • BOWEL PROBLEM 1; 2 • SKIN PROBLEM 6: RASHES; CHILDHOOD RASHES	PT TO CALL BACK: If symptoms become much worse or urgent or emergent symptoms arise (RN: review Protocol and advise caller). RN TO CALL BACK: If acute Sx in child AGE < 2 years. Routinely for Abdomen pain, Respiratory problems, Fever, Diarrhea, Marked change in ADL.

Rectal Problem Supplemental Information (Birth-6 Yr)

QUICK REFERENCES: Constipation
Fissures
Pinworms

CONSTIPATION

See Bowel Problem.

FISSURES

- Defmition/Cause: Cracks in rectal area caused by stretching and tearing of skin
- Complication: Constipation
- Prevention/Tx
  - Sitz Baths (see Home Tx Ref)

PINWORMS

- Definition: A common parasite, 90 percent found in children.
- Identification: Apply sticky side of Scotch tape to anus after awakening and before bath. Look >r tiny white worms. Can sometimes be seen in stool.
- cause: Carried by touching rectum, then mouth, easily spread.
- Complications: Itching; irritation of skin from scratching; constipation
- Previ ition/Tx
  - Handwashing
  - Rx of entire family w medication

Respiratory Problem

RESPIRATORY PROBLEM 1: BREATHING PROBLEM/COUGH (BIRTH-6 YR)

RESPIRATORY DISTRESS; CHOKING; SOB; STRIDOR; W OR W/O TRAUMA

ASSOC. SX/SPECIFIC/CONSIDERATIONS	DISPOSITION/ADVICE
EMERGENT SYMPTOMS	**ED IN 0 MIN-1 HOUR**
• **SEVERE CHOKING EPISODE W ANXIETY/AGITATION** + ASSOC. W SOLID FOOD/FB W COLOR CHANGE, Wheeze, Unable to Breathe/Talk/Cry, ± Loss of Consciousness? (FB Aspiration)	**AXIOM:** Meninigitis is most common in children AGE < 2 years and is often preceded by respiratory infection or otitis.
• **STRIDOR** + ANY AGE (2-5 Yr Most Common): RAPID ONSET HIGH FEVER > 39.5°C or 103°F, Toxic Appearing Child, Muffled Voice, Throat Pain, Drooling, Insp. Stridor, Difficulty Breathing/Swallowing, Sits Very Still w Jaw Extended? (Epiglottitis) ----------*-	• DISCOURAGE OPENING MOUTH WIDELY. NOTHING BY MOUTH. Do not use thermometer or give food/drink. + First Aid: Keep child sitting upright & calm until you reach E.D.
+ SOB, WHEEZING, STRIDOR, Retractions, Difficulty Swallowing, Agitation, Anxiety, Rash (Itchy, Raised, "Hive-Like"), Swelling of Face/ Tongue, Hx of Allergies or Exp. to Allergen (Med, Drug, Food, Chemical, Substance, Bite)? (Anaphylaxis) ----------►	• Benadryl (in any form) if immediately available. Dose: Age & wt. dependent.
• **SOB** (± **SEVERE)** + ± TRAUMA (MAJOR): MVA, FALL, BLUNT, SHARP, SEV. CHEST PAIN Referred to Shoulder/Abd., Dry Hacking Cough, Hx of TB, Cystic Fibrosis, Pneumonia? (Pneumothorax: Spontaneous/Traumatic) + KNOWN ASTHMATIC W FAILURE TO RESPOND to 2-3 Doses of Rx Inhaled 1 Nebulized Bronchodilator; Resp. Distress: Labored/Rapid, Wheezing; Nasal Flaring; Substemal/Intercostal Retractions; Cyanosis; Diaphoresis; Agitation, Confusion, Lethargy? (Status Asthmaticus)	
+ STEAM, SMOKE, OR TOXIC INHALANT: Ammonia, Fertilizers, Chem. Fumes? (Chemical/Thermal Bum)----------►	• **CONTACT POISON CENTER.** BRING SUBSTANCE TO E.D. W YOU.
• **DECREASED/SHALLOW RESPIRATIONS** + CONFUSION, LETHARGY, BLUE LIPS, ± OD or Ingestion? (Respiratory Failure) + Does RN feel Sx. are severe, extreme, emergent?	

continues

RESPIRATORY PROBLEM 1: BREATHING PROBLEM/COUGH (BIRTH-6 YR)

continued

ASSOC SX/SPECIFIC/CONSIDERATIONS	DISPOSITION/ADVICE
URGENT SYMPTOMS	**ED/MD/APPT. IN 1-8 HOURS**
• **APNEIC EPISODE** > 10-15 SEC IN PREEMIE/NEWBORN INFANT? (Apnea) ----«-	• **BRING CHILD TO E.D. NOW.**
• **COUGH W FEVER**	
+ AGE 2-6 MO (Typically): HX URI, Breathing More Rapid, Nasal Flaring, Retraction, Grunting Respiration, High-Pitched Whistling Sound (Wheeze), Irritable, Feeding Poorly, ± Blue Tint Around Mouth/ Fingertips? (Bronchiolitis) ----►	• **BRING CHILD TO E.D. NOW.**
+ SHAKING, CHILLS, Substemal/Intercostal Retractions, Nasal Flaring, ± Wheezing, Rapid/Shallow Resp., ± Abd. Pain, Anorexia, Fatigue? (Pneumonia: Bacterial, Viral, Aspiration) ----►	• **BRING CHILD TO E.D. NOW.**
+ AGE: 6 MO-3 YR (Most Common): PRECEDED BY URI, Abrupt Onset: Barking, Seal-Like Cough, Worse at Night/Early AM, Usually FEBRILE, Hoarse Voice, ± Insp./Expir. Stridor? (Croup)	
• **COUGH ± SOB**	
+ TRAUMA (ALL) + SUSPICIOUS HX? (Abuse) (See ABUSE)----►	• **BRING CHILD TO E.D. NOW.**
+ SUDDEN OR GRADUAL SOB, CHEST TIGHTNESS, Wheezing, ± Retractions, Nasal Flaring? (Asthma) ----*•	• **BRING CHILD TO E.D. NOW.** + SA: Remove shirt, look at chest. Can see ribs when breathing = + retractions.
+ HX OF URI, Worsening After 2 Wk, Bursts of Rapid Cough w Insp., w "Whoop" at End, Cyanosis, Exhaustion, No Immz? (Pertussis/ Whooping Cough)	
+ (CHRONIC) W KNOWN FOREIGN BODY, ± Chest Pain, w/o SOB or Color Change, ± Wheezing? (FB)----►	• **BRING CHILD TO E.D. NOW.**
• **AGE < 3 MO + FEVER > 38°C or 100.4°F®?** ----►	• **BRING CHILD TO E.D. NOW.**
• FEVER >40°C or 104°F? • AGE < 3 MO + MOD. SX + RISK FX (AVED)? • FAILURE TO IMPROVE on Antibiotics X 24-48 Hr? (Ineffective Rx) • WORSENING SX After 24-48 Hr on Home Tx? • RECENT SURGERY or HOSPITALIZATION? (Poss. Complications) • Does RN feel Sx. are urgent?	
ACUTE SYMPTOMS	**ED/MD/APPT IN 8-24 HOURS**
• **COUGH (GRADUAL ONSET)** + X 2 Wk, w/o Other Sx? (FB, TB, Asthma, CF, GE Reflux) + Made Worse by Exercise or Cold Air, ± Hx of Asthma? (Exercise-Induced Asthma) • AGE 3 MO-6 YR + MOD. SX + (AVED) = POSS. UPGRADE? • Does RN feel Sx. are acute?	
NON-ACUTE SYMPTOMS	**HOME TREATMENT W OR W/O APPT IN 24 + HOURS**
• **COUGH/CONGESTION** + ± Productive, Runny Nose, ± FEVER? (URI) + Chronic W Clearing, > AM, Seasonal Rhinitis + Hx of Allergy? (Allergy, Post-Nasal Drip) • MINOR SELF-LIMITING SX EXISTING > 1 WK, NOT BECOMING MARKEDLY WORSE? • HOME TX ITEMS OR PHONE NOT AVAILABLE = POSS. UPGRADE? • Does RN feel Sx. are non-acute?	• COUGH TX GOAL: Relieve coughing. Prevent complications. + Cough Suppressant or Rx from M.D. + Steam Tx. (See HOME TX REF)
CROSS-REFERENCES	**STANDARD FOLLOW-UP INSTRUCTIONS**
• ABUSE • CHEST PROBLEM • RESPIRATORY PROBLEM 2: THROAT	PT TO CALL BACK: If symptoms become much worse or urgent or emergent symptoms arise (RN: review Protocol and advise caller). RN TO CALL BACK: If acute Sx in child AGE < 2 Years. Routinely for Abdomen pain, Respiratory problems, Fever, Diarrhea, Marked change in ADL.

RESPIRATORY PROBLEM 2: THROAT (BIRTH-6 YR)

CHOKING; FB/TRAUMA; PAIN; BURN: CHEMICAL/THERMAL

ASSOC SX/SPECIFIC/CONSIDERATIONS	DISPOSITION/ADVICE
EMERGENT SYMPTOMS	**ED IN 0 MIN-1 HOUR**
• **SEVERE CHOKING EPISODE W ANXIETY/AGITATION** + ASSOC. W SOLID FOOD/FB W COLOR CHANGE, Wheeze, Unable to Breathe/Talk/Cry, ± Loss of Consciousness? (FB ASPIRATION)	**AXIOM:** Meningitis is most common in children AGE < 2 years and is often preceded by respiratory infection or otitis.
• **TRAUMA (MAJOR): MVA, FALL, BLUNT** + PENETRATING Object? (Laceration/Hemorrhage) ---------- ▶	• DO NOT REMOVE IMPALED OBJECT!
+ RESPIRATORY DISTRESS? (Tracheal Injury/Hematoma)	
• **PAIN** + ANY AGE (2-5 Yr Most Common): RAPID ONSET HIGH FEVER > 39.5°C or 103°F, Toxic Appearing Child, Muffled Voice, Throat Pain, Drooling, Insp. Stridor, Difficulty Breathing/Swallowing, Sits Very Still w Jaw Extended? (Epiglottitis/Peritonsillar Abscess) ---------- ▶	• DISCOURAGE OPENING MOUTH. WIDELY. NOTHING BY MOUTH. Do not use thermometer or give food/drink. **+ FIRST AID:** Keep child sitting upright & calm until you reach E.D.
+ HX OF INGESTION or Inhalation of Caustic Substance, Steam, Smoke or Toxic Inhalant: Chemical/Fertilizer/Ammonia? (Chemical/Thermal Burn) ---------- ▶	• **CONTACT POISON CENTER.** BRING SUBSTANCE TO E.D. W YOU.
+ THROAT/NECK SWELLING, FEVER, Difficulty Swallowing, Drooling, Hx of OM, Nasal/Pharyngeal Infection, Stiff Neck, Neck Pain w Movement? (Retropharyngeal Abscess)	
+ SOB, WHEEZING, STRIDOR, Retractions, Difficulty Swallowing, Agitation, Anxiety, Rash (Itchy, Raised, "Hive-Like"), Swelling of Face/Tongue, Hx of Allergies or Exp. to Allergen (Med, Drug, Food, Chemical, Substance, Bite)? (Anaphylaxis) ---------- ▶	• Benadryl (in any form) if immediately available. Dose: Age & wt. dependent.
• Does RN Feel Sx. are severe, extreme, emergent?	
URGENT SYMPTOMS	**ED/MD/APPT. IN 1-8 HOURS**
• **TRAUMA (MINOR-MOD.)** + SUSPICIOUS HX? (Abuse) (See ABUSE) ---------- ▶	• **BRING CHILD TO E.D. NOW.**
• **AGE < 3 MO, NEWBORN/INFANT STRIDOR (ALL)** + > STRIDOR (Insp. & Expir.), > RR, Color Changes w Feeding, < PO Intake? (Tracheal Stenosis, Tracheomalacia) ---------- ▶	• **BRING CHILD TO E.D. NOW.**
• **AGE < 3 MO + FEVER > 38°C OR 100.4°F®?** ---------- ▶	• **BRING CHILD TO E.D. NOW.**
• FEVER >40°C or 104°F?	
• AGE < 3 MO + MOD. SX + RISK FX (AVED)?	
• FAILURE TO IMPROVE on Antibiotics x 24-48 Hr? (Ineffective Rx)	
• WORSENING SX After 24-^48 Hr on Home Tx?	
• RECENT SURGERY or HOSPITALIZATION? (Poss. Complications)	
• Does RN Feel Sx. are urgent?	

continues

continued

ASSOC SX/SPECIFIC/CONSIDERATIONS	DISPOSITION/ADVICE
ACUTE SYMPTOMS	**ED/MD/APPT IN 8-24 HOURS**
• **PAIN (SEVERE)** + THROAT PAIN, Difficulty Swallowing, Headache, FEVER > 38.5°C or 101.3°F, Chills, Pus, Foul Taste, White Patches in Throat, ± Abd. Pain, Vomiting, Swollen Lymph Nodes, ± Hx Strep/Impetigo Exp.? (Strep Pharyngitis/Tonsillitis) • AGE 3 MO-6 YR + MOD. SX + (AVED) = POSS. UPGRADE? • Does RN feel Sx. are acute?	
NON-ACUTE SYMPTOMS	**HOME TREATMENT W OR W/O APPT IN 24 + HOURS**
• **PAIN (MOD.-MILD) W/O RESPIRATORY DISTRESS** + Loud Snoring? (Enlarged Tonsils) + Hx Allergies? (Allergic Rhinitis) (See NOSE/SINUS PROBLEM) + Runny Nose, Hoarseness, Cough, Minor Aches & Pains, ± FEVER, Strep Unlikely? (URI) • MINOR SELF-LIMITING SX EXISTING > 1 WK, NOT BECOMING MARKEDLY WORSE? • HOME TX ITEMS OR PHONE NOT AVAILABLE = POSS. UPGRADE? • Does RN feel Sx. are non-acute?	
CROSS-REFERENCES	**STANDARD FOLLOW-UP INSTRUCTIONS**
• ABUSE • NOSE/SINUS PROBLEM • RESPIRATORY PROBLEM 1: BREATHING PROBLEM/COUGH	PT TO CALL BACK: If symptoms become much worse or urgent or emergent symptoms arise (RN: review Protocol and advise caller). RN TO CALL BACK: If acute Sx in child AGE < 2 Years. Routinely for Abdomen pain, Respiratory problems, Fever, Diarrhea, Marked change in ADL.

Respiratory Problem Supplementary Information (Birth-6 Yr)

QUICK REFERENCE: Asthma
Bronchiolitis
Croup
Epiglottitis
Pneumonia
Pneumothorax
Retractions (Intercostal)
SIDS
Sore Throat (Pharyngitis)
Strep Pharyngitis
Tuberculosis
URI

GENERAL GUIDELINES

Throw away unused or old antibiotics! Never use another person's Rx!

ASTHMA

Chronic disease of lung

- Signs and Sx: see Protocol
- Cause: Anxiety, allergies, and stress may be triggers.
- Complications: Severe, life-threatening asthma attack; death
- Prevention/Tx
  - Take Rx.
  - Avoid triggers: Exposure to cigarette smoke, pollen, dust, pets, sulfites, exercise, food allergies, strong fumes
  - Avoid sudden change in temperature, altitude, humidity.
  - Avoid ASA, possible ASA-induced asthma.

BRONCHIOLITIS

Viral infection of part of lung in children under age 2 yr

- Signs and Sx: see Protocol
- Cause: Viral, mucous buildup, edema, bronchospasm. Over 50 percent of cases are caused by RSV.
- Complications: Pneumonia, collapse of lung
- Prevention/Tx
  - Happens most in winter. Peak age of child: 4-6 mo During winter months, don't send child to day care; avoid crowds when possible.
  - Review w parent/caretaker: Color changes, > wheezing, poor fluid intake, "Toxic" or "Very 111 Child." (See Toxicity Assessment.)
  - Reassurance and review emergent Sx with parent/caretaker.
  - Use cool mist vaporizer.

CROUP

- Signs and Sx: see Protocol
- Cause: Virus/infection
- Complications: Usually none
- Prevention
  - Steam Treatment. Sit in steamy bathroom w child until coughing stops. (See Home Tx Ref.)
  - > Clear liquids intake. Drink 2-3 extra glasses of water every day.
  - Monitor for "Toxic Child" and fever. (See Toxicity Assessment.)
  - Use cool mist vaporizer.
  - Expose to night air.

EPIGLOTTITIS

- Signs and Sx: see Protocol
- Cause: Bacterial infection
- Complications: Swelling blocks throat.
- Prevention
  - Paramedic transport
  - Immunization
- Tx
  - Antibiotics
  - Hospitalization

PNEUMONIA

Serious infection of lung; contagious

- Signs and Sx: see Protocol
- Cause: Bacteria, vims, or chemical; aspiration
- Complications: Lungs can be permanently damaged; death
- Prevention/Tx
  - Take all antibiotics. Follow M.D. orders.
  - Pneumovax vaccine for: Splenectomy, Sickle Cell, all immunocompromised patients. (See Appendix E, Recommended Childhood Immunization Schedule.)

PNEUMOTHORAX

Collapsed lung due to break in lung or break in chest wall (trauma)

- Signs and Sx: see Protocol
- Cause: Injury or disease such as trauma, TB
- Complications: Shock, tension pneumothorax

RETRACTIONS (INTERCOSTAL)

Skin between ribs being pulled back, w ea. expiration. "Marked" vs. "mild." Marked: Extends throughout upper and lower rib cage. Mild: Extends to upper rib cage only.

- Signs and Sx: Labored breathing, "can see ribs" when breathing. May be accompanied by nasal flaring, SOB.
- Causes: Poor air exchange due to infection/trauma
- Complications: > Oxygen in blood
- Tx Goal: Change breathing pattern. If fever, give Tylenol; if asthma, suggest bronchodilatation.

SUDDEN INFANT DEATH SYNDROME (SIDS)

- Definition: Sudden death of an infant under 1 year of age that remains unexplained even after an autopsy
- Incidence: 1-2 in 1000 live births
  - Leading cause of death in infants between 1 mo and 1 yr of age
  - Peak incidence 2-3 mo of age
  - Rare before 1 mo and after 9 mo
- Risk Factors
  - Sleeping on stomach; always put child on ***side,*** firmly propped w pillows, or on back
  - Babies with a family of SIDS
  - Premature infants
  - Mothers who smoke
  - Acute life-threatening events (apneic episode)
- Support: National Sudden Infant Death Syndrome Foundation
  Two Metro Plaza, Suite 104
  8200 Professional Plaza
  Landover, MD 20785
  1-800-221-SIDS

SORE THROAT (PHARYNGITIS)

- Signs and Sx: Pain, difficulty swallowing
- Causes: Virus
- Complication: Tonsillitis
- Prevention/Tx
  - Rest. Drink 2-3 extra glasses of clear liquids—makes mucus easier to cough up.
  - Steam treatment or humidifier at bedtime/nap time. (See Home Tx Ref)
  - Throat Pain: Tylenol as appropriate. Lozenges, Life Savers, popsicles, saline gargles. (Age appropriate; See Home Tx Ref)
  - Soft diet x 2 days (bland, cooked, non-spicy foods)
  - Don't eat ice cream, cheese, yogurt, milk (makes mucus thicker).

- Stop smoking in house—reduces throat irritation.
- Avoid overheated rooms, esp. at night—reduces drying of throat.
- Most sore throats are caused by a virus. Antibiotics don't work. (Home treatment as above.)

STREP PHARYNGITIS

Serious, contagious infection of throat, acute in onset and lasts 3-4 days

- Signs and Sx: see Protocol
- Cause: Caused by bacteria, streptococcal
- Complications: Rheumatic fever, kidney disease, acute post-strep glomerulonephritis
- Prevention/Tx
  - Wash hands with soap frequently, esp. before meals.
  - Do not share food, drinks, kisses.
  - Do not go to work or school until p 24 hr on antibiotics.
- Always take all Rx! Call back if no improvements within 48 hr.
  - Throat Pain: Tylenol as appropriate. Lozenges, Life Savers, popsicles, saline gargles (Age appropriate; See Home Tx Ref)
  - Soft diet x 2 days (bland, cooked, non-spicy foods)
  - Don't eat ice cream, cheese, yogurt, milk (makes mucus thicker).
  - Stop smoking in house—reduces throat irritation.
  - Avoid overheated rooms, esp. at night—reduces drying of throat.

TUBERCULOSIS

Highly contagious lung infection

- Signs and Sx: see Protocol
- Cause: Bacteria
- Complications: May come back again and again. May affect bones, heart, kidneys.
- Prevention
  - Always take all of your medicine. If you stop, the infection may come back stronger than before and may not respond to the medicine again.
  - Family members and other contacts should have TB skin test.

URI

Upper respiratory infection of throat, nose—"Cold."

- Cause: Virus
- Complications: Bacterial infections; pneumonia; sinusitis
- Prevention
  - Avoid spreading germs by washing hands with soap + water frequently.
  - Avoid kissing and sharing food.
  - Antibiotics do not work on viruses, only bacteria.

- Tx
  - Comfort: Relieve cough; liquefy secretions; < fever.
  - Rest.
  - Drink 2-3 extra glasses of clear liquids every day.
  - Saline nose drops (See Home Tx Ref)
  - Steam treatment (See Home Tx Ref)
  - Pain/Fever: Tylenol as appropriate
  - Cough: Robitussin—DM (trade name)
  - Congestion: Sudafed

Seizures

SEIZURES (BIRTH-6 YR)

W OR W/O TRAUMA

ASSOC SX/SPECIFIC/CONSIDERATIONS	DISPOSITION/ADVICE
EMERGENT SYMPTOMS	**ED IN 0 MIN-1 HOUR**
• **SEIZURE (ALL)** (Sudden Falling, Pale, Loss of Consciousness, Twitching, Jerking, Stiffening, Incontinence, Eyes Roll Upward) + MOST OFTEN GRAND MAL Type; Continuous Seizure Activity Lasting > 5-10 Min; Also Recurrent Seizures (> 2) w/o Regaining Consciousness Between Seizures? (Status Epilepticus) →	• **AXIOM: ALL FIRST-TIME SEIZURES MUST COME IN.** ■ KTIDOT AIR + Do not pry jaw open. Do not put anything in mouth 1 + If vomiting, turn on side. + Protect child from injury (e.g., move furniture or objects). + Do not restrain child but be ready to protect head and clear out mouth if child vomits. + Child may sleep after seizure. You don't have to keep child awake.
[Listed Below Are POSSIBLE CAUSES of SEIZURES]	
• **HYPERPYREXIC** + FEBRILE, Heat Stroke? →	• DO NOT BUNDLE OR OVERDRESS CHILD ON WAY TO HOSPITAL! • **FIRST AID FOR HEAT STROKE** + Move to shade/cool area. + Remove clothing. + Cool off as rapidly as possible w cool water by sponging skin: Head, groin, armpits. + If child is conscious and awake, give frequent sips of cool fluids. + Massage extremities to > peripheral blood flow. + Do not give ASA or Tylenol.
• **CNS INFECTION:** + Meningitis, Encephalitis, Abscess, Post-DPT Immunization?	
• **TRAUMA/SUSPICIOUS EXPLANATION:** + Skull Fx, Shaken Baby Syndrome, Abuse?	
• **TOXIC EXPOSURE:** + Hx of Exp. to Street Drugs/Rx, Poisonous Plant or Inhalation/ Ingestion of Toxic Chemical or Pesticide? →	• **CONTACT POISON CENTER.** BRING SUBSTANCE TO E.D. W YOU.
• **METABOLIC:** + Hypoglycemia, Liver Failure, Inborn Errors of Metabolism?	
• **A-V SHUNT:** + Shunt Infection, Blockage?	
• **BRAIN LESIONS:** + Hematoma, Tumor?	
URGENT SYMPTOMS	**ED/MD/APPT IN 1-8 HOURS**
• **SEIZURE,** Single Episode < 5-10 Min (See description above), Followed by Deep Sleep, Memory Loss, Confusion + HX SEIZURE DISORDER? (Subtherapeutic Anticonvulsant Level: Noncompliance, LowBreo oeizure i nresnoiu Due 10 iiiness; → + BRIEF LAPSES IN AWARENESS, w/o Loss of Consciousness, ± Rhythmic Blinking, Staring, Nodding? (Petit-Mal Seizure)	• DM. Are you laKing your meoiciner (INO — noncompliance) + May need to come in for blood test.
ACUTE SYMPTOMS	**ED/MD/APPT IN 8-24 HOURS**
NON-ACUTE SYMPTOMS	**HOME TREATMENT W OR W/O APPT IN 24 + HOURS**
CROSS-REFERENCES	**STANDARD FOLLOW-UP INSTRUCTIONS**
• ABUSE	

Shock

SHOCK (ALL AGES)

DISTRIBUTIVE; CARDIOGENIC; HYPOVOLEMIC

ASSOC SX/SPECIFIC/CONSIDERATIONS	DISPOSITION/ADVICE
EMERGENT SYMPTOMS	**ED IN 0 MIN-1 HOUR**
• SHOCK ----------▶ + PROGRESSIVELY: Anxious, Weak, Dizzy, Thirsty, N/V, SKIN: Pale, Blotchy/Discolored/Cool or Cold, Sweaty, LIPS/NAILBED: Blue, PULSE: Weak/Fast, BREATHING: Rapid/Shallow, Unresponsive, Loss of Consciousness? (Shock)	• **CALL 911.** • **FIRST AID** (GOAL: Prevent worsening shock.) + Keep victim CALM, WARM and QUIET. + Cover w blanket, if cold. + Make sure victim can breathe easily. + IF NO BACK OR NECK TRAUMA (see below): + Lie patient flat. Raise feet 8-12 inches. + Loosen clothing, tight belts, collar. + Do not give food or drink. + Stay w victim; watch carefully for signs of worsening shock.
+ MAJOR TRAUMA HISTORY: MVA, Fall, Possible Head/Spine Injury/ Paraplegia? (Neurogenic) ----------▶	• SA: SPINAL INJURY (IF YES, DONT MOVE UNLESS IN DANGER) + Loss of feeling? + Unable to move hands, legs, feet? + Numbness, tingling of hands/feet? + Sore spine?
+ SOB, WHEEZING, STRIDOR, Difficulty Swallowing, NA/, Abdomen Pain, Agitation/Anxiety, Rash (Itching, Raised, "Hive-Like"), Swelling of Face/Tongue, Allergy History or within minutes of exposure to Allergen (Med., Drug, Food, Chemical, Substance, Bite)? (Anaphylaxis)----------▶ + HEADACHE, NECK PAIN, Photophobia, FEVER/Chills, NA/, ± Confusion, Restlessness, Somnolence, ± History of HIV? (Sepsis, Meningitis) + CHILD/INFANT-2 Yrs: FEVER, Stiff Neck, Headache, NA/, Extreme Fatigue, ± Pinpoint Red/Purplish Spots Progressing To Purple Patches, Extremely Irritable or Unresponsive, High-Pitched Cry, Bulging/Tight Fontanelle, ± Seizure? (Sepsis, Meningitis) + CHEST PAIN: ± Exertion (Dull Ache, Pressure, Squeezing, Crushing, Radiates to Neck/Jaw/Arms), SOB, Sweating, Dizziness, Lightheaded, N/V, Pale, Anxiety, Sense of Impending Doom? (MI/Angina, Cardiogenic) + DRUG INGESTION: ACCIDENTAL/PURPOSEFUL, Street Drugs/Rx/ Barbiturates, Poisonous Plant, Toxic Chemical or Pesticide? (Toxic Exposure/Ingestion) ----------▶	• Epi Kit as appropriate. + Benadryl in any available form. + Dose: Age and weight dependent. • **CONTACT POISON CENTER.** BRING SUBSTANCE TO E.D. W YOU.
+ PELVIC PAIN, Sharp, Progressive, Unilateral, ± Radiates to Shoulder, Pale, Lightheaded, Fainting, History of STD, PID, Tubal/Any Abdominal Surgery, Prior IUD Use, Missed Period x 3-6 Wks, Spotting, Painful Intercourse? (Ectopic Pregnancy) + Nausea/Vomiting, FEVER, Severe Intractable Diarrhea, Rash, Muscle Aches, Headache, Confusion, Dizziness, Fainting? (Sepsis Syndrome) « UICTADV nc cm i rwA/iKin- ----------▶ + Heat Exposure? (See HEAT EXPOSURE) + Cold Exposure? (See COLD EXPOSURE)	• **FIRST AID (AS APPROPRIATE)**
+ Electric Shock? ----------▶ + Severe Burn? (See BURN 1) + Severe Dehydration, Dizziness, Weakness, Diarrhea, Hyperthermia? + Severe Trauma to Lower Extremity? (Femur Fracture, 2 or More Long-Bone Fracture) + Abdominal Trauma, Abdominal Pain, Left Shoulder Pain? (Liver/Spleen Rupture)	• **DO NOT ADVISE ANY FIRST AID UNLESS RESCUER CAN BE SURE IT IS SAFE TO APPROACH VICTIM.**
+ Severe Bleeding/Hemorrhage/Laceration? ----------▶ • Does RN feel symptoms are severe, extreme, emergent?	• **FIRST AID (see above)** + Direct pressure to control bleeding. (See SUPPLEMENTAL INFORMATION)
URGENT SYMPTOMS	**ED/MD/APPT IN 1-8 HOURS**
ACUTE SYMPTOMS	**ED/MD/APPT IN 8-24 HOURS**

continues

ASSOC SX/SPECIFIC/CONSIDERATIONS	DISPOSITION/ADVICE
NONACUTE SYMPTOMS	HOME TREATMENT W OR W/O APPT IN 24 + HOURS
CROSS-REFERENCES	STANDARD FOLLOW-UP INSTRUCTIONS

Shock Supplemental Information (All Ages)

QUICK REFERENCE Aggravating Factors
First Aid for Bleeding

AXIOM

- Any accident or illness can lead to shock.

AGGRAVATING FACTORS

- Pain
- Temperature Extremes: Heat/Cold Exposure.
- Exhaustion due to extreme physical exertion; lack of food intake or dehydration.
- Chronic Illness: Chronic disease like heart disease or diabetes.
- Individual response to injury, pain, or emotional stress.
- Improper care: Rough handling; improper treatment.

FIRST AID FOR BLEEDING: PRESSURE POINTS

- Raise extremity above heart to slow the bleeding.
- Arm wound: Put pressure (firm and without stopping) to pulse inside of upper arm. Use four fingers. Put pressure firmly along bone until you can no longer feel pulse in wrist.
- Leg wound: Place victim on back. Feel for pulse in groin area—at top of leg where it bends. Put heel/palm of hand against artery and bone. Keep your arm straight and press with both hands if needed.

References

Auerbach, P. S. (Ed.). (1995). *Wilderness medicine: Management of wilderness and environmental emergencies.* (3rd ed.). St. Louis, MO: Mosby.

Clawson, J.J., M. D. & Democoeur, K.B. (1998). *Principles of emergency medical dispatch.* (2nd ed.). Salt Lake City, UT: Priority Press.

Manhoff, D. (1996). *Mosby s outdoor emergency medical guide.* (1st ed.). St. Louis, MO: Mosby.

Skin Problem

SKIN PROBLEM 5: LESION/LUMP/SWELLING

Skin Problem 5 (Lesion/Lump/Swelling) Supplemental Information

Adult

Protocol General Information

Skin Problem 5 follows the typical content and format for most Protocols. This Protocol may be used in conjunction with Rash (Skin Problem 6).

See Skin Problem 5 Supplemental Information for additional information.

Age 6-18 Yr

Protocol General Information

See Adult section above.

Age Birth-6 Yr

Protocol General Information

See Adult section above.

SKIN PROBLEM 6: RASH W OR W/O ITCHING (AGE 18+)

SKIN PROBLEM 6: RASHES; CHILDHOOD RASHES (AGE 0-6, 6-18)

Skin Problem 6 (Rash w or w/o Itching) Supplemental Information (Age 18+)

Skin Problem 6 (Rashes; Childhood Rashes) Supplemental Information (Age 0-6, 6-18)

Adult

Protocol General Information

Skin Problem 6 includes several childhood rashes, namely, measles, chicken pox, and scarlet fever. It follows the typical content and format for most Protocols. This Protocol may overlap with Lesion/Lump/Swelling (Skin Problem 5).

See Skin Problem 6 Supplemental Information for additional information.

Age 6-18 Yr

Protocol General Information

Title variation: Rashes; Childhood Rashes.

See Adult section above.

Age Birth-6 Yr

Protocol General Information

Title variation: Rashes; Childhood Rashes.

See Adult section above.

SKIN PROBLEM 3: DISCOLORATION (BIRTH-6 YR)

BRUISE; YELLOW; ALL COLOR CHANGES

ASSOC SX/SPECIFIC/CONSIDERATIONS	DISPOSITION/ADVICE
EMERGENT SYMPTOMS	**ED IN 0 MIN-1 HOUR**
• **BRUISE W TRAUMA (MAJOR): MVA, BLUNT, FALL** + WEAK, DIZZY, Cold/Mottled/or Pale Skin, Blue Lips/ Nailbeds, Rapid/Shallow Breathing, Unresponsive, Loss of Consciousness? (Shock/Intemal Hemorrhage) (See SHOCK)	
• **BRUISE W/O TRAUMA** + FEVER, STIFF NECK, HEADACHE, N/V, Extreme Fatigue, ± Pinpoint Red Purplish Spots Progressing to Purple Patches, Extremely Irritable or Unresponsive, "Toxic Child" (See Toxicity Assessment), ± Seizure, Infant-2 Yrs: High-Pitched Cry, Bulging/Tight Fontanelle? (Meningitis)	
• Does RN feel Sx. are severe, extreme, emergent?	
URGENT SYMPTOMS	**ED/MD/APPT IN 1-8 HOURS**
• **BRUISE W HX TRAUMA (MINOR-MOD.)**	
+ SUSPICIOUS HX? (Abuse) (See ABUSE)------------------------------►	• **BRING CHILD TO E.D. NOW.**
+ MOUTH + SUSPICIOUS HX? (Abuse/Sexual) (See ABUSE) + MULTIPLE, Unusual Pattern, Various Stages of Healing? (Abuse) + QUICKLY ENLARGING BRUISE, w Swelling, Unresponsive to First Aid? (Hematoma) (See SKIN PROBLEM 3 SUPPLEMENTAL INFORMATION)	• **AXIOM:** GENITAL/RECTAL TRAUMA (pain, bruising, laceration, bleeding) and abnormal discharge or lesions in a child *may* be an indication of abuse. Use a sensitive approach. Immediate evaluation is necessary. DO NOT be accusatory, arouse suspicion, or unduly alarm parent/ caretaker. (See ABUSE)
• **BRUISE (W/O TRAUMA)** + SPONTANEOUS, Hx of Anticoagulants, Bleeding Disorder, Kidney/Liver Disease? (Leukemia/ Hemorrhage) + DIFFUSE PINPOINT PURPLISH/RED RASH, Recent Viral Illness? (Idiopathic Thrombocytopenic Purpura)	
• **YELLOW SKIN** + NEWBORN: 'TOXIC CHILD" (See Toxicity Assessment), FEVER or Subnormal Temp., Jaundiced Palms/Soles? (Sepsis) ------------------------------►	• **BRING CHILD TO E.D. NOW.**
+ NEWBORN (FIRST WEEK): All Jaundice? (Physiologic Jaundice)	
• **AGE** < **3 MO** + **FEVER** > **38°C** or 1**00.4°F®?**------------------------►	• **BRING CHILD TO E.D. NOW.**
• FEVER >40°C or 104°F? • AGE < 3 MO + MOD. SX + RISK FX (AVED)? • WORSENING SX After 24-48 Hr on Home Tx? • RECENT SURGERY or HOSPITALIZATION? (Poss. Complications) • Does RN feel Sx. are urgent?	

continues

SKIN PROBLEM 3: DISCOLORATION (BIRTH-6 YR)

continued

ASSOC SX/SPECIFIC/CONSIDERATIONS	DISPOSITION/ADVICE
ACUTE SYMPTOMS	**ED/MD/APPT IN 8-24 HOURS**
• **YELLOW SKIN** + FEVER, N/V, Anorexia, Yellow Sclera, Fatigue, Swollen Glands, Clay-Colored Stools, Dark Urine, ± Exp. to Hepatitis? (Hepatitis) (See APPENDIX A) • AGE 3 MO-6 YR + MOD. SX + (AVED) = POSS. UPGRADE? • Does RN feel Sx. are acute?	
NON-ACUTE SYMPTOMS	**HOME TREATMENT W OR W/O APPT IN 24 + HOURS**
• **SKIN COLOR CHANGE** (See also SKIN PROBLEM 3 SUPPLEMENTAL INFORMATION) + White Patches of Skin, Hx of Eczema, Any Hx of Skin Problem? (Vitiligo, Pityriasis Alba, Tinea Versicolor, Hypopigmentation) + Yellow/Orange Color, Esp. Palms & Soles of Feet? (Carotenemia) (See SKIN PROBLEM 3 SUPPLEMENTAL INFORMATION) + Hx Rx/Food Causing Color Change? (Drug/Food Side Effect) • MINOR SELF-LIMITING SX EXISTING > 1 WK, NOT BECOMING MARKEDLY WORSE? • HOME TX ITEMS OR PHONE NOT AVAILABLE = POSS. UPGRADE? • Does RN feel Sx. are non-acute?	
CROSS-REFERENCES	**STANDARD FOLLOW-UP INSTRUCTIONS**
• ABUSE • HEPATITIS • SKIN PROBLEM 5: LESION/LUMP/SWELLING • SKIN PROBLEM 6: RASHES, CHILDHOOD RASHES	PT TO CALL BACK: If symptoms become much worse or urgent or emergent symptoms arise (RN: review Protocol and advise caller). RN TO CALL BACK: If acute Sx in child AGE < 2 years. Routinely for Abdomen pain, Respiratory problems, Fever, Diarrhea, Marked change in ADL.

Skin Problem 3 (Discoloration) Supplemental Information (Birth-6 Yr)

QUICK REFERENCE:
- Disease Side Effect (Discoloration)
- Drug Side Effect (Color Change)
- Food Side Effect (Carotenemia)
- Hematoma
- Jaundice
- Petechiae
- Purpura

DISEASE SIDE EFFECT (DISCOLORATION)

- Causes
  - Blood disorders (pale)
  - Liver (yellow)
  - Vitiligo (white patches)

DRUG SIDE EFFECT (COLOR CHANGE)

- Cause: Anti-malarials

FOOD SIDE EFFECT (CAROTENEMIA)

- Causes
  - Beets
  - Carrots
  - Squash

HEMATOMA

- Hematoma Tx Goal: Reduce swelling, pain; provide comfort.
- First Aid
  - Ice pack QID x 48 Hr (See Home Tx Ref, Ice Pack)
  - Raise injured part up above heart level.
  - Rest the part that was bruised.
  - Do not rub or massage area.
  - Mark the border of the bruise w pen.
  - Watch to see if the bruise gets bigger.
  - If it gets bigger, you will need to come in w/in 2 hr.
  - Warm, moist compress QID after 48 hr.
  - Watch for: > Size, change in sensation, temperature of limb, Sx of shock
  - Bruise will change color and reabsorb over time. It may move down arm or leg.

JAUNDICE

- Signs and Sx: Yellow skin and whites of the eyes
- Causes: Possible liver, gallbladder, blood problem, or newborn jaundice; breast milk jaundice (See Newborn Concerns.)
- Complications: Could become a serious health problem if the cause is infectious.

PETECHIAE

- Signs and Sx: Multiple, pinpoint, purplish red spots
- Cause: Bleeding under the skin caused by bacterial infection
- Complications: Serious Sx of infection (meningitis, blood infection, coagulation disorder)

PURPURA

- Signs and Sx: Large, purplish-red areas that look like flat bruises
- Cause: Bleeding under the skin caused by bacterial infection
- Complications: Serious Sx of infection (meningitis, blood infection, coagulation disorder)

SKIN PROBLEM 4: LACERATION/WOUND (BIRTH-6 YR)

AMPUTATIONS; MAJOR & MINOR LACERATIONS; ABRASIONS; PUNCTURE WOUNDS

ASSOC. SX/SPECIFIC/CONSIDERATIONS	DISPOSITION/ADVICE
EMERGENT SYMPTOMS	**ED IN 0 MIN-1 HOUR**
• **PENETRATING WOUND** (HEAD/CHEST/ABDOMEN/THROAT)? -▶	• NEVER REMOVE IMPALED OBJECT! (Unless it is penetrating the trachea.)
• **AMPUTATIONS (ALL)?**---------▶	• CONTROL BLEEDING, APPLY FIRM PRESSURE. Save body part, wrap in clean cloth. (Place in plastic bag on top of ice.)
• **LACERATION/STAB WOUND (TRUNK, NECK, GROIN)** ---------▶	• **AXIOM:** STAB WOUNDS OF CHEST/ ABDOMEN may be worse than they first appear!
+ FORCEFUL, SPURTING, Uncontrolled by Direct Pressure, Bright Red Bleeding? (> Risk Hemorrhage, Shock) ---------▶ + BLUE, COLD, Pale Extremity, Numbness Distal to Wound? (> Risk of Loss of Limb) • **WOUND (ALL)** + NEWBORN W INFECTED UMBILICAL STUMP, "Toxic Child" (See Toxicity Assessment)? (Neonatal Tetanus) • Does RN feel Sx. are severe, extreme, emergent?	• **FIRST AID:** + Lay child down. + APPLY FIRM PRESSURE W CLEAN FOLDED CLOTH. (See Supplemental Information.) + Keep pressure on until help arrives. + Elevate extremity above heart if possible.
URGENT SYMPTOMS	**ED/MD/APPT IN 1-8 HOURS**
• **LACERATION(S) (MINOR-MOD.)** + SUSPICIOUS HX? (Abuse) (See ABUSE)---------▶	• **BRING CHILD TO E.D. NOW.**
+ PERSISTENT BLEEDING, Hx of Bleeding Disorder, Kidney/Liver Disease, Hx of Anticoagulants? (> Risk Hemorrhage) ---------*	• Apply pressure. (See Supplemental Information)
+ ABLE TO SEE FAT WHEN SEPARATED SLIGHTLY, or Large Cut, Facial or Hand Cut? (Needs Sutures) ---------▶ • **IMBEDDED OBJECT(S) (ALL):** Nail, Glass, etc.? (Foreign Body) • **LACERATION HX** + (ALL SKIN) RED, ± STREAKING, Swollen, Tender, Hot; ± Discharge, Often w FEVER, Swollen Nodes, Hx of Trauma/Bite/ Local Infection? (Cellulitis) • **PUNCTURE WOUND**	• **FIRST AID:** + Cover w clean, dry dressing. + If blood saturates, reinforce w another dressing. DO NOT REMOVE!
+ RUSTY, DIRTY NAIL, Gardening Wounds, Through Rubber Footwear? (> Risk Infection) ---------▶	• **FIRST AID:** Scrub X 5 Min., soak in soapy water X 15 Min.
• **AGE < 3 MO + FEVER > 38°C or 100.4°F?**---------▶ • FEVER >40°C or 104°F? • AGE < 3 MO + MOD. SX + RISK FX (AVED)? • FAILURE TO IMPROVE on Antibiotics X 24-48 Hr? (Ineffective Rx) • WORSENING SX After 24-48 Hr on Home Tx? • Does RN feel Sx. are urgent?	• **BRING CHILD TO E.D. NOW.**
ACUTE SYMPTOMS	**ED/MD/APPT IN 8-24 HOURS**
• **LACERATION(S) (MINOR)** + Immunizations Not Up-to-Date? (Immz) + Dirty, Puncture Wound, Last Tetanus > 5 Yr? (Immz) • AGE 3 MO-6 YR + MOD. SX + (AVED) = POSS. UPGRADE? • Does RN feel Sx. are acute?	• CARETAKER CALL BACK: IF SX BECOME MUCH WORSE OR EMERG/URG SX ARISE (Review pertinent emergent & urgent Sx)

continues

SKIN PROBLEM 4: LACERATION/WOUND (BIRTH-6 YR)

continued

ASSOC SX/SPECIFIC/CONSIDERATIONS	DISPOSITION/ADVICE
NON-ACUTE SYMPTOMS	**HOME TREATMENT W OR W/O APPT IN 24 + HOURS**
• **ABRASION (SEVERE)** + "Road Burn," Heavily Encrusted w Dirt/Foreign Body, Parent/ Caretaker Able to Carry Out First Aid? **(> Infection Risk)** → • **LACERATION(S) (MINOR),** Abrasion, Splinter, Puncture Wound? (Superficial Wound) • **SUTURE REMOVAL QUESTIONS?** • MINOR SELF-LIMITING SX EXISTING > 1 WK, NOT BECOMING MARKEDLY WORSE? • HOME TX ITEMS OR PHONE NOT AVAILABLE = POSS. UPGRADE? • Does RN feel Sx. are non-acute?	• LACERATION/WOUND TX GOAL: Prevent infection. Promote healing. (See SKIN PROBLEM 4 SUPPLEMENTAL INFORMATION) • **FIRST AID:** + Pain: Tylenol (Acetaminophen) as appropriate 1 Hr prior to Tx. + Flush/scrub w washcloth to area w water x 5 Min. + Use tweezers to remove large particles. + Warm Soapy Soak. (See HOME TX REF)
CROSS-REFERENCES	**STANDARD FOLLOW-UP INSTRUCTIONS**
• ABUSE • BITES (SKIN PROBLEM 1) (As Appropriate) • NEWBORN CONCERNS	PT TO CALL BACK: If symptoms become much worse or urgent or emergent symptoms arise (RN: review Protocol and advise caller). RN TO CALL BACK: If acute Sx in child AGE < 2 years. Routinely for Abdomen pain, Respiratory problems, Fever, Diarrhea, Marked change in ADL.

Skin Problem 4 (Laceration/Wound) Supplemental Information (Birth-6 Yr)

QUICK REFERENCE: Abrasion/Scrapes
Laceration & Wound Care
Pressure Points
Puncture
Suture Removal
Tetanus

ABRASION/SCRAPES

- Causes: Scraping of skin or mucous membranes
- Complications: Infection
- Prevention/Tx
  - Check tetanus status.
  - Wash area w warm, soapy water 3 x /day. Cover w dry, sterile dressing.

LACERATION AND WOUND CARE (CUTS, ABRASIONS, BURNS, ETC.)

- Check tetanus status.
- Tetanus must be given within 72 hr.
- Wash w warm soapy water. Remove all dirt. Cover w sterile dressing. (See Home Tx Ref, Warm Soapy Soak)
- If there is dirt in wound, remove all dirt by scrubbing gently.
- Keep cut clean and dry.
- Elevate the wound to help relieve soreness and speed wound healing.
- Watch for signs and Sx of infection.
- Despite the greatest care, any cut can become infected. Return if any of the following develop:
  - Increasing pain or tenderness after the first 24 hr
  - Pus
  - Red streaks
  - Increasing swelling
  - Fever

PRESSURE POINTS

- Raise extremity above heart to < bleeding.
- Arm Wound: Apply pressure (firm and continuous) to pulse point inside the upper arm. Use four fingers. Apply pressure firmly against bone until you can no longer feel pulse.

- Leg Wound: Place victim on back and feel for pulse in groin area—at top of leg where leg bends. Use the heel/palm of hand, keep arm straight, press artery against bone. If you need to, use both hands.

PUNCTURE

Small cut or wound made by sharp, thin object (nail, needle)

- Axiom: **Puncture wounds w rubber footwear always need antibiotics.**
- Signs and Sx: Skin pierced w pointed object or instrument
- Causes: Penetration or piercing of skin w pointed object or instrument
- Complications: Infection, bleeding, tetanus
- Prevention/Tx
  - Wear shoes outside.
  - Wear gloves when gardening.

SUTURE REMOVAL SCHEDULE (MODIFY AS APPROPRIATE)

Area	*Days*
Face	3-4
Neck	5
Scalp	7
Chest, Abdomen	7
Arms	7
Legs	10
Back	12
Palms, Soles, Over Joints	14

TETANUS

- Definition: A serious, life-threatening bacterial infection
- Signs and Sx: Pain at wound site, muscle spasms, stiff jaw and neck, difficulty swallowing or opening mouth, irritability, convulsions
- Cause: A germ enters the skin through a wound. The germ is often found in the soil or on sharp pieces of metal.
- Complication: The death rate is very high.
- Prevention
  - Tetanus is completely preventable by immunization. Get an immunization booster every 10 yr.
  - Adults who have never been immunized require 2 doses of tetanus toxoid 1 mo apart, w booster dose 6-12 mo later, and booster every 10 yr thereafter.
- Tx
  - Anyone who has been immunized but has not had a booster within the past 5 yr and who has a puncture wound, dirty wound, bum, or frostbite should receive a tetanus booster.

- Any non-immunized person w a puncture wound, dirty wound, bum, or frostbite should receive tetanus immune globulin I.M. (passive immunity) and antibiotics.
- Careful washing of cut w soap and water (See Laceration and Wound Care above.)
- Dirty wounds—Get booster every 5 yr.

SKIN PROBLEM 5: LESION/LUMP/SWELLING (BIRTH-6 YR)

W OR W/O TRAUMA

ASSOC SX/SPECIFIC/CONSIDERATIONS	DISPOSITION/ADVICE
EMERGENT SYMPTOMS	**ED IN 0 MIN-1 HOUR**
URGENT SYMPTOMS	**ED/MD/APPT IN 1-8 HOURS**
• **SWELLING W TRAUMA (MILD-MOD.)** [illegible] ——→	• **BRING CHILD TO E.D. NOW**
+ Quickly Enlarging, ± Bruise/Discoloration Unresponsive to First Aid? (Hematoma)	
• **SWELLING W/O TRAUMA** + (ALL AREAS), SWOLLEN NODES, RED ± STREAKING, Swollen, Tender, Hot; ± Discharge, Often w FEVER, Bite/Local Infection? (Cellulitis)	
• **LESION(S)/WARTS** + ON RECTUM OR GENITALIA? (STD, Abuse) (See VAGINAL, PENILE, or RECTAL PROBLEM)--------→	• **BRING CHILD TO E.D. NOW** • **AXIOM:** Abnormal discharge or lesions in a child *may* be an indication of abuse. Use a sensitive approach. Immediate evaluation is necessary. DO NOT be accusatory, arouse suspicion, or unduly alarm parent/caretaker. (See ABUSE)
• **LESION(S)** + NEWBORN: ± FEVER, Sm. Blisters w Red Base, Near Umbilical Cord Stump, &/or Groin? (Staph Pustulosis Impetigo)	
• **AGE < 3 MO + FEVER > 38°C or 100.4°F®?** ——→	• **BRING CHILD TO E.D. NOW.**
• FEVER >40°C or 104°F? • AGE < 3 MO + MOD. SX + RISK FX (AVED)? • FAILURE TO IMPROVE on Antibiotics x 24-48 Hr? (Ineffective Rx) • WORSENING SX After 24-48 Hr on Home Tx? • RECENT SURGERY or HOSPITALIZATION? (Poss. Complications) • Does RN feel Sx. are urgent?	•
ACUTE SYMPTOMS	**ED/MD/APPT IN 8-24 HOURS**
• LUMP/SWELLING + (NECK), Redness, Tenderness, Warm to Touch, FEVER? (Cervical Adenitis) • **LESION(S)** + Cluster of Tiny Clear Blisters, Begins w Tingling, itching, Pain, Followed by Yellow, Crusty Crater After 1-2 Days; First Time; Near Eye; w Severe Throat Pain ± Sev.-Mod. Dehydration? (Herpes) + Itchy, Honey Colored Crusted? (Impetigo) (See SKIN PROBLEM 5) + Redness, Swelling, Blisters, Broken Skin Over Pressure Points, Mentally Challenged, Cerebral Palsy, or Muscular Dystrophy? (Pressure Sore/Decubitus Ulcer/Neglect) + Facial, Red, Hot, Painful, Thickened Tissue; ± FEVER; Pea- to Walnut-Sized, 3 or More, Soft & Mushy, > 7 Days? (Abscess) + NEWBORN: Umbilical Stump, Redness, Swelling, ± FEVER? (Omphalitis) • AGE 3 MO-6 YR + MOD. SX + (AVED) = POSS. UPGRADE? • Does RN feel Sx. are acute?	

continues

SKIN PROBLEM 5: LESION/LUMP/SWELLING (BIRTH-6 YR)

continued

ASSOC SX/SPECIFIC/CONSIDERATIONS	DISPOSITION/ADVICE
NON-ACUTE SYMPTOMS	**HOME TREATMENT W OR W/O APPT IN 24 + HOURS**
• **LESION(S)** + NEWBORN: Papules, Pustules, Face/Back/Chest? (Acne) (See NEWBORN CONCERNS) + Patches of Cracked Skin, Dry, Scaly, Flaky, Itchy Areas, Face, Trunk, Inner Arm, ± Hx Allergies? (Atopic Dermatitis) + Plaques, Irregular, Greasy Surface, Sun-Exposed Area, Yellow, Dark, Tan, Defined Edge? (Seborrhea Dermatitis) + Linear/Painful, Follows the Path of Nerve, Unilateral, Begins as Cluster of Bumps, Becomes Blisters, Then Dry Crust, ± Sev. Itching? (Herpes Zoster) + Raised, Clear, Blister-Like Lesions on Hands/Feet/Mouth, ± FEVER, Fatigue, > Incidence in Summer? (Hand, Foot and Mouth Disease) • **LESION(S)/WARTS** + Small Skin-Colored Bumps w Rough Surfaces? (Warts) • **SWELLING/LUMP** • Small, Not Warm to Touch, w/o Fever or Tenderness, May Be Felt in Neck, Behind Ears, Axilla, Groin, Base of Skull? (Lymphadenopathy) • MINOR SELF-LIMITING SX EXISTING > 1 WK, NOT BECOMING MARKEDLY WORSE? • HOME TX ITEMS OR PHONE NOT AVAILABLE = POSS. UPGRADE? • Does RN feel Sx. are non-acute?	
CROSS-REFERENCES	**STANDARD FOLLOW-UP INSTRUCTIONS**
• ABUSE • LIP/MOUTH; TEETH/GUMS; TONGUE • NEWBORN CONCERNS • SKIN PROBLEM 6: RASHES; CHILDHOOD RASHES	PT TO CALL BACK: If symptoms become much worse or urgent or emergent symptoms arise (RN: review Protocol and advise caller). RN TO CALL BACK: If acute Sx in child AGE < 2 years. Routinely for Abdomen pain, Respiratory problems, Fever, Diarrhea, Marked change in ADL.

Skin Problem 5 (Lesion/Lump/Swelling) Supplemental Information (Birth-6 Yr)

QUICK REFERENCE: Boil
Cellulitis
Herpes Simplex (Cold Sore, Fever Blister)
Impetigo
Mumps

BOIL

- Definition: see Protocol
- Causes: Infection caused by staph germs.
- Complications: May come back for months or years.
- Prevention/Tx: Handle very gently.
  - Warm, moist soaks 4 x /day or more
  - Clean w soap often.
  - Don't squeeze boil. Wait for it to "pop" and infection will come out.

CELLULITIS

- Signs and Sx: see Protocol
- Causes: Bacterial infection w streptococci, staphylococci, or other organisms
- Complications: Infection in blood and skin; potentially dangerous, esp. around face—can spread to brain.
- Prevention/Tx
  - Keep skin clean.
  - Clean wounds immediately.

HERPES SIMPLEX (COLD SORE, FEVER BLISTER)

May appear anywhere on skin—Lips, eye, genitals, thumb (thumb suckers).

- Signs and Sx: see Protocol
- Causes: Contagious virus
- Complications: Usually heal by themselves in 1-2 wk.
- Prevention/Tx
- Oral (Herpes Simplex 1)
  - OTC ointment, e.g., glyoxide
  - Cool compresses (See Home Tx Ref)
  - No kissing.
- Genital (Herpes Simplex 2)
  - May need prescription.
  - Keep sores clean and dry.
  - Pain: Tylenol as appropriate
  - Sitz baths (See Home Tx Ref)

IMPETIGO

- Signs and Sx: see Protocol
- Causes: Bacterial infection, Group A strep and staphylococcus species; highly contagious
- Complications: Severe infection; kidney problems; can be fatal to newborns
- Prevention/Tx
  - Wash w soap and water.
  - Keep open to air so it will dry out and heal.
  - Don't scratch. Isolation—Don't touch sores and pus. Wash hands after touching.
  - Needs antibiotics.

MUMPS

- Signs and Sx: see Protocol
- Causes: Virus; contagious childhood infection
- Complications: May cause meningitis, encephalitis, pancreatitis, or inflammation of testicles and ovaries. Usually does not affect fertility. Male family members of childbearing age who have not been immunized may be at increased risk of infertility if they get the mumps.
- Tx: Soft Diet (See Home Tx Ref); isolation. No acidic drinks.
- Prevention: MMR immunization at age 15 mo and booster (5-10 yr)

TETANUS

(See Skin Problem 4, Laceration/Wound.)

SKIN PROBLEM 6: RASHES; CHILDHOOD RASHES (BIRTH-6 YR)

W OR W/O ITCHING

ASSOC SX/SPECIFIC CONSIDERATIONS	DISPOSITION/ADVICE
EMERGENT SYMPTOMS	**ED IN 0 MIN-1 HOUR**
• **RASH** ——————————————————— *■ + "HIVE-LIKE," ITCHY, RAISED; SOB, Wheezing, Stridor, Retractions, Difficulty Swallowing, Agitation, Anxiety, Swelling of Face/Tongue, Hx of Allergies or Exp. to Allergen (Med, Drug, Food, Chemical, Substance, Bite)? (Anaphylaxis) + ± PINPOINT RED PURPLISH SPOTS PROGRESSING TO PURPLE PATCHES, FEVER, Stiff Neck, Headache, N/V, Extreme Fatigue, Extremely Irritable or Unresponsive, 'Toxic Child" (See Toxicity Assessment), ± Seizure, Infant-2 Yrs: High-Pitched Cry, Bulging/Tight Fontanelle? (Meningitis) • Does RN feel Sx. are severe, extreme, emergent?	• FOR ALL APPOINTMENTS, REVIEW ISOLATION PROCEDURE. • Benadryl (in any form) if immediately available. Dose: Age & wt. dependent.
URGENT SYMPTOMS	**ED/MD/APPT IN 1-8 HOURS**
• **RASH WITCHING** + RED ITCHY IRREGULAR RASH PATCHES ON FACE/TRUNK, Bright Red Mouth/Throat, Cracked Lips, Strawberry Tongue, FEVER, Red Eyes w/o Pus, Enlarged Cervical Nodes, Hands/Feet: Red/Swollen/ Shiny/Tender? (Kawasaki Disease) ——————— *- + SEVERE ITCHING, w Red, Weepy, Oozing Blisters? (Poison Oak, > Risk Infection)	• **BRING CHILD TO E.D. NOW.**
• **RASH W/O ITCHING** + PRECEDED BY COUGH, ± FEVER, Pink > Red, Flat, Face to Trunk & Extremities, Red Eyes, "Toxic Child" (See Toxicity Assessment)? (Measles) ———————	• **AXIOM:** Measles vaccine is 90-95% effective. • **BRING CHILD TO E.D. NOW.**
+ STARTS W CRUSTED INFECTION, Scarlet Tender Areas Appear Nearby in 24 Hr, Progressing to Large Blisters, Fatigue, Chills/FEVER? (Staph Scalded Skin Syndrome) ——————— ▶ + DIAPER AREA, REDNESS, SWELLING, Blisters or Pustules, Oozing, ± FEVER? (Infected Diaper Rash) + SANDPAPER-LIKE RASH (Most Intense on Neck, Axilla, Groin, Behind Knees, May Cover Entire Body), Lasts 7 Days Then Peels; ± Hx of Sore Throat/FEVER? (Scarlet Fever)	• **BRING CHILD TO E.D. NOW.**
• **AGE** < **3 MO** + **FEVER** > **38°C** or **100.4°F®?** ——————— ▶ • FEVER >40°C or 104°F? • AGE < 3 MO + MOD. SX + RISK FX (AVED)? • FAILURE TO IMPROVE on Antibiotics x 24-48 Hr? (Ineffective Rx) • WORSENING SX After 24-48 Hr on Home Tx? • Does RN feel Sx. are urgent?	• **BRING CHILD TO E.D. NOW.**

continues

SKIN PROBLEM 6: RASHES; CHILDHOOD RASHES (BIRTH-6 YR)

continued

ASSOC SX/SPECIFIC/CONSIDERATIONS	DISPOSITION/ADVICE
ACUTE SYMPTOMS	**ED/MD/APPT IN 8-24 HOURS**
• **RASH W ITCHING** + Intense Itching at Night, Tiny Blisters in 'Tracks," Fingers, Webs of Fingers, Toes, Heels, Wrists, Elbows, Armpits, Breast, Crease of Buttocks, ± Hx of Contact? (Scabies) + Cluster of Red Bumps, Becomes Blisters, Painful, Follows Nerve, One Sided, Then Dry Crust, ± Burning/Itching in Young Child? (Herpes Zoster/Shingles) • AGE 3 MO-6 YR + MOD. SX + (AVED) = POSS. UPGRADE? • Does RN feel Sx. are acute?	
NON-ACUTE SYMPTOMS	**HOME TREATMENT W OR W/O APPT IN 24 + HOURS**
• **RASH W ITCHING** + Redness, Swelling on Area of Skin in Contact w Irritants (e.g., Plants, Chem., Fabric Softener, Soaps, Cosmetic)? (Contact Dermatitis) + Red, Dry, Scaly, Excoriated, Extreme Itching? (Eczema) + Skin Breakdown, Eyelids/Scalp, Gray White Lice Eggs Attached to Eyelashes, Eyebrows, or Hair Shaft, Hx of Contact? (Head/Body Lice) + FEVER, Red Rash (Dewdrop on Rose Petal Appearance), Starts on Trunk/Face, Intensely Itchy, Turns to Crusts When Blisters Break? (Chicken Pox) + ± Itching, Hx Rx or OTC Drug Within Past 2 Wk? (Drug Allergy) ----------►	• Call for new Rx as appropriate.
+ Circular Pattern, Raised Border, Itchy, Scaly Center? (Ringworm) • **RASH W/O ITCHING W FEVER** + Red Rash, Slightly Raised or Flat, Face to Trunk/Extremities, Swollen Glands Behind Ears/Neck, No MMR Hx, Not Very Sick? (German Measles/Rubella) ----------►	• Avoid contact w pregnant women.
+ Pink Rash, Flat, Occasional Bumps, Preceded by FEVER (High), on Trunk Then Arms & Neck, < on Face or Legs? (Roseola) + Raised, Clear, Blister-Like Lesions on Hands/Feet/Mouth, ± FEVER, Fatigue, > Incidence in Summer? (Hand-Foot and Mouth Disease) • **RASH W/O ITCHING OR FEVER** + Red Rash, Flat/Lacey, "Slapped Cheek" Appearance, Comes & Goes, Face Then Arms, Legs & Rest of Body? (Fifth Disease) + (DIAPER AREA) Beefy Red, Worse Around Anus/Folds/Creases, Blister-Like Lesions, ± Hx Oral Thrush? (Candidiasis) + (DIAPER AREA) Red, Generalized, Bum-Like Appearance? (Diaper Rash) • **NEWBORN RASHES (ALL)?** (See NEWBORN CONCERNS) • MINOR SELF-LIMITING SX EXISTING > 1 WK, NOT BECOMING MARKEDLY WORSE? • HOME TX ITEMS OR PHONE NOT AVAILABLE = POSS. UPGRADE? • Does RN feel Sx. are non-acute?	
CROSS-REFERENCES	**STANDARD FOLLOW-UP INSTRUCTIONS**
• LIP/MOUTH; TEETH/GUMS; TONGUE • NEWBORN CONCERNS • SKIN PROBLEM 3: DISCOLORATION • SKIN PROBLEM 5: LESION/LUMP/SWELLING	PT TO CALL BACK: If symptoms become much worse or urgent or emergent symptoms arise (RN: review Protocol and advise caller). RN TO CALL BACK: If acute Sx in child AGE < 2 years. Routinely for Abdomen pain, Respiratory problems, Fever, Diarrhea, Marked change in ADL.

Skin Problem 6 (Rashes; Childhood Rashes) Supplemental Information (Birth-6 Yr)

QUICK REFERENCE: *Childhood Rashes*

Isolation Procedures At Home	Red or 7-Day Measles (Rubeola)
Chicken Pox	Roseola
Fifth Disease	Scarlet Fever
German Measles (Rubella)	

Other Rashes

Contact Dermatitis	Lice (Head & Body)
Drug Side Effect (Rash)	Poison Oak
Eczema	Scabies
Hives	Tinea (Ringworm)

Childhood Rashes

AXIOM

Treat all rashes as contagious until proven differently.

- Isolation procedure when coming to clinic or hospital
  - Avoid contact with people who are pregnant, have been on cancer drugs, or who have AIDS. They are very susceptible to contagious infections.
  - If you follow these instructions, you will not expose others to infection.

ISOLATION PROCEDURE AT HOME

- Child should stay home, not go outside, or play w other children or high-risk groups. (See Axiom above.)
- Wash hands in warm soapy water every time you eat.
- Prevent infection of rashes by washing hands with soap and water at least four times a day.
- Do not share food, spoons, forks, towels, handkerchiefs, bath, or kisses with child.

CHICKEN POX

- Cause: Virus—Antibiotics will not work.
  - Exp. to Chicken Pox, Measles, Hx splenectomy, or immune compromised person (see above)? (> Risk)
- Treatment/Course: Chicken pox lasts about 10-14 days. Chicken pox should be treated at home unless the child becomes very sick. Complications are rare.

- For Itching
  - Cut fingernails and try not to scratch.
  - Baking soda baths (See Home Tx Ref.)
  - Benadryl (Dose: Age and wt. dependent)
- Sores in Mouth
  - Pain: Tylenol as appropriate. Cold non-acid drinks.
- Prevention: Chicken pox is very contagious, spread by coughing, sneezing, kissing, or sharing food. It is contagious from one day before the rash appears to 6 days after the rash appears. Most brothers and sisters of children who have it will get it too. Once someone has had chicken pox, they rarely ever get it again. But sometimes people who have had chicken pox get shingles later on.

FIFTH DISEASE

- Cause/Course: Possibly a virus. Rash lasts 3-7 days. Not serious but contagious. There is rarely a fever.
- Treatment: No treatment; watch and wait. Check for fever.

GERMAN MEASLES (RUBELLA)

- Cause/Course: Mild virus. Antibiotics will not work. It is not as contagious as measles or chicken pox. Spread by coughing, sneezing, kissing, sharing food. The rash lasts for 2-4 days.
- Prevention: German measles is very dangerous to pregnant women who have not had their vaccination (MMR). If it happens in the first 3 months of pregnancy, the child may be bom deaf, have serious eye or heart problems, or brain damage. Do not let child have contact with or go near anyone who could possibly be pregnant.
- Treatment: Treat at home.
  - Fever: Tylenol as appropriate

RED OR SEVEN-DAY MEASLES (RUBEOLA)

- Cause/Course: Highly contagious viral illness. No antibiotics are needed. The red measles last 4-7 days.
- Prevention: Spread through the air or by coughing, sneezing, kissing, sharing food, or contact w used tissue. Not contagious after the rash is gone. All children who have had contact with the child with measles should come in immediately to get their immunizations (MMR).
- Treatment: Do not let other children visit.
  - Fever: Tylenol as appropriate
  - Cough: Vaporizer
  - Eye sensitivity to light: Darken the room; sunglasses when outside

ROSEOLA

- Cause/Course: Vims. Antibiotics won't work. Rash lasts 1-2 days. Usually found in children under the age of 3 yr but may occur at any age.

- Prevention/Tx
  - Do not let other children visit. Watch for complications.
  - Should not last more than 4-5 days.
  - Fever: Tylenol as appropriate

SCARLET FEVER

- Cause/Course: Streptococcus bacteria. Needs antibiotics. Rash lasts 5-7 days.
- Treatment
  - Fever: Tylenol as appropriate
  - Sore throat: Cold clear liquids (See Home Tx Ref, Clear Liquids)

Other Rashes

CONTACT DERMATITIS

- Causes: Exposure to things your body is extra sensitive to, like metal
- Complications: Itching, discomfort
- Prevention/Tx
  - Wash exposed area well. Also wash contaminated clothing with soap and water.
  - Avoid exposure in future by wearing protective clothing, gloves, etc.
  - Always wash hands after contact with any skin rash.
  - Avoid scratching (will spread if contagious).
  - Avoid sun exposure; keep as cool as possible.
  - Avoid powders/comstarch: They can cake in skin folds and increase irritation.

DRUG SIDE EFFECT—RASH

(Possible explanation: accidental ingestion)

Axiom: All drugs have the potential to cause a rash at any time. The drags and classes of drags below are related to a serious drag reaction, Toxic Epidermal Necrolysis.

- antibiotics (many)
- allopurinol (Zyloprim)
- barbiturates
- nonsteroidal anti-inflammatory drags
  - Aleve
  - Advil
  - Ibuprofen
  - Midol 200
  - Motrin
  - Nuprin
- penicillin
- phenytoin (Dilantin)
- sulfas

ECZEMA

- Cause: Skin sensitivity
- Complication: Infection
- Prevention/Tx
  - Avoid rough clothing, wool, overheating.
  - Use Lowilla soap, Cetaphil, Keri, Nivea Lotion. Use after bath and 4-6 x /day.
  - Hydrocortisone cream 0.5% to itching areas
  - Bathe 3 x /wk.

HIVES

- Signs and Sx: Itching, raised, pink rash. Hives may come and go for 3-4 days, then disappear.
- Causes: Your body reacts in a bad way to something that you come into contact with. Too much cold, heat, stress, tension, or allergies to Rx, food, plant, chemical, or insect bite/sting.
- Complications: Itching, swelling, discomfort
- Prevention/Tx
  - Take medicine for itching. Don't wait for hives to disappear. Continue until hives are gone x 24 hr.
  - Cool baking soda bath (See Home Tx Ref)
  - Stay out of sun—makes itching worse.
  - Stop whichever Rx caused rash. Talk w M.D. immediately.
  - Be careful about eating foods such as shellfish, nuts, etc.
  - Benadryl-Chlortrimaton (Dose: Age and wt. dependent)
  - Calamine lotion (*not* Calydryl)
  - Try to discover and avoid what makes you itch or causes hives/rash.

LICE (HEAD AND BODY)

- Signs and Sx: Itching; tiny white lumps on hair strands
- Causes: Parasites. Lice may be spread by linens, toilet seats, and sexual contact.
- Complications: Discomfort; spreading lice to others
- Prevention: Do not share combs, brushes, hats, clothing.
- Tx Goal: Remove parasites. Prevent others from getting them. Prevent them from coming back.
  - RID: Follow directions on medication package.
  - Wash all clothes/bedding.
  - You may put bedding in plastic bags for 10-14 days instead of sending them to the dry cleaners.
  - It is important to treat everyone in the family and clean everything the same day. Otherwise the lice may come back.
  - Med for lice is not recommended for pregnant women or very young children.

POISON OAK (3-LEAF LOW-GROWING SHRUB)

- Signs and Sx: Severe itching rash, red swelling, weeping, oozing blisters
- Causes: Oil from plant forms an invisible coating on the skin. Smoke from burning bush can also cause rash or severe allergic reaction.
- Complications: Rash may spread to eyes. Infection could develop.
- Prevention/Tx
  - Shower and wash well w strong soap (Dial) as soon as possible after touching plant. Wash clothes. Do not put them back on until they have been washed with soap and water.
  - If it becomes worse, or fever develops, see M.D.
  - Avoid exposure in future.
  - Avoid sun exposure; keep as cool as possible.
  - Avoid r vvders/comstarch: They can cake in skin folds and increase irritation.

_ jt'-t

t_____& wt. dependent)

Dress cooi, bathe cool, sleep cool.

C 's every 2 hr (See Home Tx Ref)

■_,c_ ..dKing . d Aveeno Baths (Vfe cup baking soda/tub) (See Home Tx Ref, Baking Soda Batn,

Calamine lotion *(not* Caladryl)

Hydrocortisone 1%

Tylenol as appropriate

SCABIES

- Signs and Sx: see Protocol
- Cause: Parasites lay eggs under skin.
- Prevention/Tx
  - Needs appt. and Tx with prescription med.
  - Scabies is highly contagious. All family members and close contacts need to be notified and treated. Incubation period is 2-6 wk. Bedding needs to be washed in HOT, soapy water. Dry in dryer x 20 min or more; or put in double plastic bag x 7 days.

TINEA (ATHLETE'S FOOT, RINGWORM)

Contagious fungal infections.

- Athlete's Foot
  - Signs and Sx: Most common fungal infection, often persistent. Redness, scaling between toes, cracks/small blisters; itching.

- Complication: Infection
- Prevention/Tx

    Clean feet carefully w soap and water. Dry carefully.
    Wear shoes that are made of canvas, or sandals.
    Wear cotton socks, change often if possible.
    Lotrimin

■ Ringworm

- Signs and Sx: see Protocol
- Cause: Fungus living on dead skin
- Complication: Secondary infection
- Prevention/Tx: Use topical antifungal cream 2-3 x/day. If it doesn't clear up in 3 days, make an appt.

    Lotrimin
    Tinactin

Urinary Problem

URINARY PROBLEM (BIRTH-6 YR)

PAIN W OR W/O TRAUMA; FREQUENCY; URGENCY; DISCHARGE; CHANGE IN OUTPUT/COLOR; BLOODY URINE

ASSOC SX/SPECIFIC/CONSIDERATIONS	DISPOSITION/ADVICE
EMERGENT SYMPTOMS	**ED IN 0 MIN-1 HOUR**
• **TRAUMA (MAJOR): MVA, FALL, BLUNT (URETHRAL/FLANK/ RIBS REGION)** + WEAK, DIZZY, Cold/Mottled/or Pale Skin, Blue Lips/Nailbeds, Rapid/Shallow Breathing, Unresponsive, Loss of Consciousness, + Bloody Urine, Bruise on Flank? (Hemorrhage, Shock) (See SHOCK) • Does RN feel Sx. are severe, extreme, emergent?	
URGENT SYMPTOMS	**ED/MD/APPT. IN 1-8 HOURS**
• **TRAUMA (MINOR-MOD.)** + (FLANK/BACK), BLOODY URINE, ± N/V, ± Abd. Pain? (Renal Contusion)----------►	• **BRING CHILD TO E.D. NOW.**
+ SUSPICIOUS EXPLANATION? (Abuse) (See ABUSE) ----------►	• **BRING CHILD TO E.D. NOW.**
• **DISCHARGE (ALL)?** (Poss. Abuse) (See AXIOM; See ABUSE) • **PAIN/BURNING ON URINATION** + PAIN (SEV.-MOD.), RADIATING FROM ABD./FLANK/BACK TO GROIN, Colicky Then Constant & Severe, FEVER/Chills, N/V, Dysuria, ± Hematuria, Frequency/Urgency? (Pyelonephritis) + HX OF SPINA BIFIDA w Intermittent Catheterization, < or No Urine Output? (Neurogenic Bladder w Urinary Retention) • **BLOODY URINE** + BLOODY STOOLS, ± Abd. Pain, Hx Runny Nose, Cough, N/V? (Hemolytic Uremic Syndrome) + ABD. MASS, ± AbdVFlank Pain, ± FEVER? (Wilm's Tumor) • **DIFFICULT URINATION** + LOWER ABD. PAIN, < Urine Output, Anesthesia? (Urinary Retention)	• **AXIOM:** GENITAL/RECTAL TRAUMA (pain, bruising, laceration, bleeding) and abnormal discharge or lesions in a child maybe an indication of abuse. Use a sensitive approach. Immediate evaluation is necessary. DO NOT be accusatory, arouse suspicion, or unduly alarm parent/caretaker. (See ABUSE)
• **AGE** < **3 MO** + **FEVER** > **38°C** or **100.4°F®?**----------*-	• **BRING CHILD TO E.D. NOW.**
• FEVER >40°C or 104°F? • AGE < 3 MO + MOD. SX + RISK FX (AVED)? • FAILURE TO IMPROVE on Antibiotics x 24-48 Hr? (Ineffective Rx) • WORSENING SX After 24-48 Hr on Home Tx? • RECENT SURGERY or HOSPITALIZATION? (Poss. Complications) • Does RN feel Sx. are urgent?	

continues

URINARY PROBLEM (BIRTH-6 YR)

continued

ASSOC SX/SPECIFIC/CONSIDERATIONS	DISPOSITION/ADVICE
ACUTE SYMPTOMS	**ED/MD/APPT IN 8-24 HOURS**
• **DIFFICULT URINATION** + Mild Pain, Redness Around Urethra, Hx of Mild Pain, Masturbation, Bubble Bath, Mild Trauma? (Urethritis) • **PAIN/BURNING ON URINATION** + Frequency, Urgency, ± Blood-Tinged Urine, ± Nocturia, ± Cloudy, Foul or Strong Smelling Urine, ± FEVER? (UTI) • **OUTPUT CHANGE** + Decreased (Progressive), Generalized Edema, < Stream? (Acute Renal Failure) + Decreased, Hx New Rx? (Drug Side Effect) + Increased (Extreme), Dilute Urine, ± Trauma? (Diabetes Insipidus) + Increased, Weight Loss, Thirst, > Hunger? (Diabetes Mellitus) + Incontinence, Hx New Rx? (Drug Side Effect) • **Color Change** + Dark Urine, FEVER, N/V, Anorexia, Yellow Skin, Yellow Sclera, Fatigue, Swollen Glands, Clay-Colored Stools, ± Exp. to Hepatitis? (Hepatitis) (See APPENDIX A) + Bloody Urine, Dysuria, ± < Urine Output, ± *UN,* ± FEVER? (Hemorrhagic Cystitis) + ± Bloody Urine + Hx New Rx? (Drug Side Effect) • AGE 3 MO-6 YR + MOD. SX + (AVED) = POSS. UPGRADE? • Does RN feel Sx. are acute?	
NON-ACUTE SYMPTOMS	**HOME TREATMENT W OR W/O APPT IN 24 + HOURS**
• **UNUSUAL COLOR** OF URINE > 24 HR? (See URINARY PROBLEM SUPPLEMENTAL INFORMATION) • MINOR SELF-LIMITING SX EXISTING > 1 WK, NOT BECOMING MARKEDLY WORSE? • HOME TX ITEMS OR PHONE NOT AVAILABLE = POSS. UPGRADE? • Does RN feel Sx are non-acute?	
CROSS-REFERENCES	**STANDARD FOLLOW-UP INSTRUCTIONS**
• ABDOMEN PROBLEM • ABUSE • HEPATITIS	PT TO CALL BACK: If symptoms become much worse or urgent or emergent symptoms arise (RN: review Protocol and advise caller). RN TO CALL BACK: If acute Sx in child AGE < 2 years. Routinely for Abdomen pain, Respiratory problems, Fever, Diarrhea, Marked change in ADL.

Urinary Problem Supplemental Information (Birth-6 Yr)

QUICK REFERENCE: Bladder Infection
Drug Side Effect (Urinary Color Change)
Drug Side Effect (Urine, Bloody)
Drug Side Effect (Urinary Retention)
Food Side Effect (Urinary Color Change)

AXIOMS

- Major changes in urine output (greater or less than usual) = needs appt.
- Age < 3 mo: UTIs are more common in boys.
- Age > 3 mo: UTIs are more common in girls.

BLADDER INFECTION

- Axiom: Signs and Sx may be nonspecific for this age group.
- Definition: Having a lot of germs in any part of bladder or kidneys
- Signs and Sx
  - Age < 2 yr: May present w generalized Sx, i.e., fever, irritability, < appetite, diarrhea, vomiting
  - Age > 2 yr: Frequency, urgency, painful urination, blood in urine w pressure, leaking, fever
- Complications: Sepsis, kidney infection Sx: Flank/side pain, severe shaking, chills and fever, kidney failure
- Prevention
  - Goal: Comfort. Prevent Infection.
  - Drink 2-3 extra glasses of water and/or cranberry juice/day, esp. in warm weather.
  - Don't let child put off going to bathroom. Should go when he/she feels the need to urinate.
  - Take all antibiotics as prescribed. Call if no improvement in 24-48 hr or 8 doses.
  - Avoid ASA, Advil, Motrin, antihistamines, decongestants—may cause constriction of ureters.
  - Travel: Drink water often. Go to bathroom often.
  - Prevent constipation.
  - Females

    Always wipe from front to back to avoid bacteria from rectum.

    Avoid bubble bath: Irritates skin in genital area.

    Advise urination following baths.

    Wear cotton underwear.

DRUG SIDE EFFECT—URINARY COLOR CHANGE

(Possible explanation: accidental ingestion)

Drugs and classes of drugs that may cause urinary color change

- metronidazole (Flagyl): yellow
- nitrofurantoin (Furadantin, Macrodantin): yellow, brown or darker
- phenazopyridine (Pyridium): orange/red
- rifampin (Rifadin): red/orange
- sulfonamides: yellow
- vitamins: orange/yellow
- vitamin B-complex: green

DRUG SIDE EFFECT—URINE, BLOODY

(Possible explanation: accidental ingestion)

Drugs and classes of drugs that may cause hematuria

- anticoagulants
- aspirin
- methenamine (Azo-mandelamine)
- methotrexate (Folex, Mexate)
- sulfonamides

DRUG SIDE EFFECT—URINARY RETENTION

(Possible explanation: accidental ingestion)

Drugs and classes of drugs that may cause retention

- alpha-adrenergic agents
- anticholinergics
    - atropine
    - belladonna
    - scopolamine
- ephedrine
- pseudoephedrine (Actifed, Chlortrimeton, Pediacare, Sudafed)
- phenylpropanolamine (Acutrim, Allerest, Contac, Dexatrim, Dimetapp, Omade, Tri-aminic)

FOOD SIDE EFFECT—URINARY COLOR CHANGE

Foods that may cause color change

- beets (red)
- rhubarb (brown)
- blackberry (red)

Vaginal Bleeding

VAGINAL BLEEDING (BIRTH-6 YR)

ABNORMAL BLEEDING; TRAUMA; FB

ASSOC SX/SPECIFIC/CONSIDERATIONS	DISPOSITION/ADVICE
EMERGENT SYMPTOMS	**ED IN 0 MIN-1 HOUR**
URGENT SYMPTOMS	**ED/MD/APPT IN 1-6 HOURS**
• **BLEEDING + TRAUMA (MINOR-MOD.)** + SUSPICIOUS EXPLANATION, FOREIGN BODY? (Abuse) (See ABUSE)---	• **BRING CHILD TO E.D. NOW.** • **AXIOM:** GENITAL/RECTAL TRAUMA (pain, bruising, laceration, bleeding) and abnormal discharge or lesions in a child maybe an indication of abuse. Use a sensitive approach. Immediate evaluation is necessary. DO NOT be accusatory, arouse suspicion, or unduly alarm parent/caretaker. (See ABUSE)
+ SEVERE LACERATION/BLEEDING w/o Sx of Shock + SEVERE PAIN? (> Risk Hemorrhage)--*-	• **BRING CHILD TO E.D. NOW.** • **FIRST AID:** + Lay child down. + APPLY FIRM PRESSURE W CLEAN CLOTH. + Keep pressure on until help arrives. + See AXIOM above.
+ KNOWN BLEEDING DISORDER, Bleeding/Bruising Elsewhere? (> Risk Hemorrhage) ——————►	« BRING CHILD TO E.D.NOW + See AXIOM above.
+ WITNESSED STRADDLE INJURY, Bruising, Pain, Swelling, Unable to Urinate? (Urethral Injury)---►	• **BRING CHILD TO E.D. NOW.** + See AXIOM above.
• Does RN feel Sx. are urgent?	
ACUTE SYMPTOMS	**ED/MD/APPT IN 8-24 HOURS**
• Does RN feel Sx. are Acute?	
NON-ACUTE SYMPTOMS	**HOME TREATMENT W OR W/O APPT IN 24 + HOURS**
• **BLEEDING** + NEWBORN: Sm. Amt. Blood Appears 5-10 Days After Birth? (Withdrawal of Maternal Estrogens) + Witnessed or Unwitnessed Straddle Injury, Minimal Bleeding w or w/o Pain? (Minor Straddle Injury) • Does RN feel Sx. are non-acute?	
CROSS-REFERENCES	**STANDARD FOLLOW-UP INSTRUCTIONS**
• ABUSE • NEWBORN CONCERNS • SKIN PROBLEM 4: LACERATION/WOUND • VAGINAL PROBLEM	PT TO CALL BACK: If symptoms become much worse or urgent or emergent symptoms arise (RN: review Protocol and advise caller). RN TO CALL BACK: If acute Sx in child AGE < 2 years. Routinely for Abdomen pain, Respiratory problems, Fever, Diarrhea, Marked change in ADL.

Vomiting/Nausea

VOMITING/NAUSEA (BIRTH-6 YR)

W OR W/O DIARRHEA; HEADACHE; ABDOMINAL PAIN

ASSOC SX/SPECIFIC/CONSIDERATIONS	DISPOSITION/ADVICE
EMERGENT SYMPTOMS	**ED IN 0 MIN-1 HOUR**
• **NAUSEA/VOMITING** + VOMITING, ± PROJECTILE, IRRITABLE, LETHARGIC, ± Loss of Consciousness, Recent Head Trauma? (> Intracranial Pressure) + BRIGHT RED BLOOD/COFFEE GROUND, ± Abd. Pain? (Upper G.I. Bleed) + HX OF EXP. TO STREET DRUGS/Rx, Poisonous Plant or Inhalation/Ingestion of Toxic Chemical or Pesticide? (Toxic Exposure)------------------------------► + CONTINUOUS VOMITING, FEVER, 'Toxic Child"/ Severe Dehydration (See Toxicity/Dehydration Assessment)? (Severe Toxicity/Dehydration) + FEVER, STIFF NECK, Extreme Fatigue, ± Pinpoint Red Purplish Spots Progressing to Purple Patches, Extremely Irritable or Unresponsive, 'Toxic Child" (See Toxicity Assessment), ± Seizure, Infant-2 Yrs: High-Pitched Cry, Bulging/Tight Fontanelle? (Meningitis) • Does RN feel Sx. are severe, extreme, emergent?	• **KEEP NPO.** • **CONTACT POISON CENTER.** BRING SUBSTANCE TO E.D. W/YOU.

continues

continued

ASSOC SX/SPECIFIC/CONSIDERATIONS	DISPOSITION/ADVICE
URGENT SYMPTOMS	**ED/MD/APPT IN 1-8 HOURS**
• **NAUSEA/VOMITING W/O DIARRHEA**	
+ LOWER ABD. PAIN, SUDDEN ONSET, CRAMPY, ± Vomiting Thick, Bright Green, Bitter Tasting Fluid? (Volvulus) ----------*	• **BRING CHILD TO E.D. NOW. KEEP NPO.**
+ W FIRM/TENDER BULGE AT GROIN/Scrotum, Groin Pain? (Incarcerated Hernia) ----------»	• **BRING CHILD TO E.D. NOW. KEEP NPO.**
+ PAIN (SEVERE) RADIATING FROM ABD./FLANK/ BACK TO GROIN, Colicky Then Constant & Severe, FEVER/Chills, Dysuria, ± Hematuria, Frequency/ Urgency? (Pyelonephritis)	
+ AGE < 5 MO: W FEEDING, ± PROJECTILE, ± Vomiting Thick, Bright Green, Bitter Tasting Fluid, ± Dehydration (See Dehydration Assessment)? (Pyloric Stenosis)	
• **NAUSEA/VOMITING W DIARRHEA**	
+ COLICKY, Abd. Distention, Hx of Major Change in Bowel Habits? (Bowel Obstruction) ----------▶	• **BRING CHILD TO E.D. NOW. KEEP NPO.**
+ AGE < 2 YR (USUALLY): ABD. PAIN, SUDDEN ONSET, RECURRENT, COLICKY, SHARP, ± Vomiting Thick, Bright Green, Bitter Tasting Fluid, ± Bloody Mucous Stool (Currant Jelly Stool), "Toxic Child" ± Sev. Dehydration? (Intussusception) ----------▶	• **BRING CHILD TO E.D. NOW. KEEP NPO.**
+ CRAMPY ABD. PAIN; Watery Stools ± Blood/Mucous/ Pus, Alternating W Normal Stools, ± N/V, FEVER, Recent Immigration, Hx of Foreign Travel, Exp. to Contaminated Water, Undercooked Meat/Seafood/ Poultry/Improperly Stored Food? (Infectious Diarrhea, "Food Poisoning" (See V/N SUPPLEMENTAL INFORMATION)----------▶	• **BRING CHILD TO E.D. NOW. KEEP NPO.**
+ "VERY ILL CHILD" (See Acuity Assessment) + Moderate Dehydration (See Dehydration Assessment)? (Dehydration, Mod.) ----------▶	• **BRING CHILD TO E.D. NOW.**
• **NAUSEA/VOMITING W HEADACHE/DIZZINESS**	
+ DIZZINESS/STAGGERING (SUDDEN ONSET), Jerky Eye Movement, ± Hx URI, ± Hearing Loss? (Labyrinthitis, Vestibular Neuronitis)----------*■	• **BRING CHILD TO E.D. NOW.**
+ HEADACHE (SEV.-MOD.), Throbbing, ± Unilateral, Abd. Pain, > Sensitivity to Light & Noise, ± Dizziness/ Staggering, ± Preceded by Aura (See HEAD PROBLEM)? (Migraine) (See HEAD PROBLEM 2)	
• **AGE < 3 MO + FEVER > 38°C or 100.4°F®?----------▶**	• **BRING CHILD TO E.D. NOW.**
• FEVER >40°C or 104°F?	
• AGE < 3 MO + MOD. SX + RISK FX (AVED)?	
• FAILURE TO IMPROVE on Antibiotics x 24-48 Hr? (Ineffective Rx)	
• WORSENING SX After 24-48 Hr on Home Tx?	
• RECENT SURGERY or HOSPITALIZATION? (Poss. Complications)	
• Does RN feel Sx. are urgent?	

continues

VOMITING/NAUSEA (BIRTH-6 YR)

continued

ASSOC SX/SPECIFIC/CONSIDERATIONS	DISPOSITION/ADVICE
ACUTE SYMPTOMS	**ED/MD/APPT IN 8-24 HOURS**
• **NAUSEA/VOMITING** + FEVER, Anorexia, Yellow Skin, Yellow Sclera, Fatigue, Swollen Glands, Clay-Colored Stools, Dark Urine, ± Exp. to Hepatitis? (Hepatitis) + "Sick Child", ± Mild Dehydration (See Toxicity/ Dehydration Assessment)? (Toxicity or Mild-Mod Dehydration) + Hx Effortless Vomiting w/o Pain Following Meal, ± Hx Poor Feeding? (Gastroesophageal Reflux) + Following Antibiotics? (Drug Reaction) + Following Meds for Chronic Condition (i.e., Seizure Med)? (> Risk Seizures or Disease) • AGE 3 MO-6 YR + MOD. SX + (AVED) = POSS. UPGRADE? • Does RN feel Sx. are acute?	
NON-ACUTE SYMPTOMS	**HOME TREATMENT W OR W/O APPT IN 24 + HOURS**
• **NAUSEA/VOMITING** + Crampy Abd. Pain w/o Dehydration Sx: Diarrhea, ± FEVER ± Headache? (Gastroenteritis) + Coughing Spasm Leading to Vomiting, Worse at Night? (Paroxysmal Coughing) + NEWBORN: Spitting Up in Happy, Contented New Baby? (Spitting Up) (See NEWBORN CONCERNS) • HOME TX ITEMS OR PHONE NOT AVAILABLE = POSS. UPGRADE? • Does RN feel Sx. are non-acute?	
CROSS-REFERENCES	**STANDARD FOLLOW-UP INSTRUCTIONS**
• ABDOMEN PROBLEM • DEHYDRATION/ASSESSMENT/REHYDRATION GUIDELINES • DIZZINESS • HEAD PROBLEM 1; 2 • NEWBORN CONCERNS • TOXICITY ASSESSMENT • URINARY PROBLEM	PT TO CALL BACK: If symptoms become much worse or urgent or emergent symptoms arise (RN: review Protocol and advise caller). RN TO CALL BACK: If acute Sx in child AGE < 2 years. Routinely for Abdomen pain, Respiratory problems, Fever, Diarrhea, Marked change in ADL.

Vomiting/Nausea Supplemental Information (Birth-6 Yr)

DRUG SIDE EFFECT—VOMITING/NAUSEA

(Possible explanation: accidental ingestion)

Drugs and classes of drugs that may cause nausea and vomiting

- antibiotics (many)
- antihypertensives
- codeine
- cytotoxic drugs
- digoxin (Lanoxin)
- iron preparations
- nicotine and nicotine gum
  - Nicoderm
  - Habitrol
  - Nicorette
- nonsteroidal anti-inflammatory drugs
  - Advil
  - Aleve
  - Ibuprofen
  - Midol 200
  - Motrin
  - Nuprin
- quinidine
- salicylates
  - aspirin
  - bismuth subsalicylate (Pepto Bismol)
- xanthine bronchodilators (Theophylline, Aminophylline)
- Prevention
  - Take med w 1 full glass of water and/or food, if possible, to prevent GI upset.

INFECTIOUS DIARRHEA ("FOOD POISONING")

- Signs and Sx: see Protocol
- Cause: Bacteria
- Complications: Shock, dehydration; rare fatalities in very young and the elderly or those w chronic illness
- Prevention
  - Never eat home-preserved meat, fish, poultry, or milk products that have been unrefrigerated or left in sun for any length of time.
  - Wash hands before preparing foods.
  - Cover and refrigerate foods quickly.
  - Boil home canned foods 30 min.
- TX
  - Bedrest
  - Convenient access to a bathroom
  - See Dehydration Assessment/Rehydration Guidelines.

MOTION SICKNESS

- Signs and Sx: Pale, cold, sweating, fast breathing, nausea and vomiting
- Causes: > Activity of the middle ear caused by > motion
- Prevention
  - Don't eat large meals before traveling by car, boat, air.
  - In airplane: Sit by window near wing.
  - In car: Sit in front seat near window. Leave window open.
  - Don't read while in motion, it will make it worse.
- Tx
  - < The problem by being where least motion in airplanes, on ships
  - Take Rx 1 hr before going on the ship, driving, or flying.

NAUSEA/VOMITING

- Tx Goal: Keep clear liquids down. Drink more water, juice to prevent dehydration.
- Causes: Illness, obstruction, trauma, food poisoning, medications, poison ingestion, motion
- Complication: Dehydration
- Prevention/Tx: See Dehydration Assessment/Rehydration Guidelines.

PROJECTILE VOMITING

- Signs and Sx: Sudden forceful expulsion of stomach contents through nose or mouth
- Causes: Bowel obstruction; pyloric stenosis, head injuries

APPPENDIX TABLE OF CONTENTS

APPENDIX A

Home Treatment Supplemental Information

Listed below are common home remedies that must be approved in-house by medical staff.

Standards for home treatments: All home treatments must be approved foods, drinks, activities done at home by patient or caretaker.

1. Effective: Provide some relief from symptoms.
2. Harmless: No ill effect can come from using it as directed.
3. Accessible: Low cost, easily available to most clients.

Directory

Baking Soda Bath	Hot Pack	Rehydration Guidelines
Baking Soda Paste	Hot Soapy Soak	"RICE"
"BRAT " Diet	Ice Collar	Rice Water
Breast Cold Pack	Ice Massage	Saline Gargle/Mouthwash
Clear Liquids	Ice Pack	Saline Nose Drops
Clove Remedy	Increase Fluids	Sitz Bath
Cold/Cool Compress	Jell-0 Water	Soft Diet
Cold Pack	Mint Tea	Steam Treatment
Cornstarch Bath	Motion Sickness Remedies	Tooth Transport
Cornstarch Paste	Nausea Remedies	Vinegar Douche
Elevate	Night Air	Warm Compress
Eyewash	Nose Pinch	Warm Soapy Soak
Gatorade	Oatmeal Bath	Warm (Tepid) Bath
Ginger Tea	Popsicle	
Honey-Lemon Mix	Pressure Points	

Home Treatment	Formula	Purpose
Baking Soda Bath	Add 7, cup baking soda to tub of warm water	Itching; skin irritation
Baking Soda Paste	A smooth paste of baking soda and water	Pain/itching; bee sting; insect bites; chickenpox lesions
"BRAT" Diet	Bananas (ripe), rice (white), applesauce, toast (white), and other foods easily digested	GI upset, diarrhea
Breast Cold Pack	Baggie of frozen vegetables, wrapped in thin dry cloth or pillowcase, placed on breasts after feedings for 10 minutes or less; cool cabbage leaves are effective as well	Breast engorgement
Clear Liquids	Drinks you can see through: water, soda, clear fruit juice, Gatorade, herb tea, chicken broth, boullion,)ell-0	GI upset, diarrhea
Clove Remedy	Place whole clove between gum and painful tooth	Toothache
Cold/Cool Compress	Cold, damp cloths, wrung out; change every 10 min	Swelling; discomfort
Cold Pack	Bags of frozen peas, corn, lima beans, wrapped in pillowcase, dish towel or soft cloth use cold pack for 10-20 minutes every 2-4 hr for 24 hr	Reduce swelling, muscle spasms and pain

(continued)

Home Treatment	Formula	Purpose
Cornstarch Bath	One handful of cornstarch added to tub of tepid water soak for about 15 min	Itching
Cornstarch Paste	A smooth paste made from cornstarch and water	Itching
Elevate	Raise above the level of the heart	Swell ing/bleeding
Eyewash	Hold eye open put head under gentle lukewarm kitchen tap; or have someone pour lukewarm water gently in steady stream into eye X 20-30 min. Fill bowl w water, open eyes and put face into bowl x 5 min or gently flood eye w water for 15 min by the clock. Bring chemical to hospital for MD to see	Eye irritation; chemical/ toxic burn
Gatorade	Drink Gatorade or similar drink drink slowly but frequently until urine becomes light, clear yellow	Dehydration, electrolyte replacement
Ginger Tea	Make a tea with ginger drink small amounts slowly until upset disappears	Nausea
Honey-Lemon Mix	Two parts honey to one part lemon juice; one part alcohol (brandy, rum, vodka, etc.) may be added if desired (check for Hx alcohol abuse) The honey soothes the throat and helps to bring up mucus; lemon juice helps to make mucus more watery and easier to cough up; alcohol reduces cough This Rx may be taken by teaspoon as needed for cough	Cough
Hot Pack	Put cloths soaked in hot water and wrung out in plastic bag; place on swelling for 20 min on and off Don't place directly on skin (use with caution for children under 18 yr or elderly, or use warm compress)	Swelling; muscle spasm
Hot Soapy Soak	Fill tub or bucket w hot water and enough liquid hand soap or liquid dish soap to make bubbles. Soak for 10-15 min 3 x per day in the morning, afternoon, and before you go to bed at night For hands/fmgers, wash dishes in hot soapy water 3 x a day the infection should get better after three soaks. (Use with caution for children under 18 yr or elderly, or use warm soapy soak)	Minor infections
Ice Collar	Put crushed ice in plastic bag, cover w towel, and drape across patient's neck. Wet dishtowel frozen around a large cylinder (e g , can) also good Reduces discomfort	Sore throat; swollen glands
Ice Massage	Wrap a cloth around a frozen juice can or put frozen juice can in a sock and roll the can over the muscle in spasm. Cold and massage help relieve muscle spasm	Muscle spasm
Ice Pack	Fill a Ziploc bag w crushed ice; wrap the bag in pillowcase, dishtowel, or soft cloth. Use the ice pack for 10-20 minutes every 2-4 hr for 24 hr	Swelling; muscle spasm, and pain (See also Cold Pack)

(continued)

Home Treatment	Formula	Purpose
Increase Fluids	Drink one glass of water each hr while awake, up to 6-8 glasses. Elderly patients or those w heart disease should drink one glass every 2 hr while awake	Dehydration/constipation
Jell-0 Water	Mix hot water w Jell-0 to taste	Sore throat, cough
Mint Tea	Mint herbal tea; drink small amounts slowly until upset disappears	Nausea
Motion Sickness Remedies	Keep your head still. Avoid bad odors—engine Himes, cigarette smoke, and strong smelling foods. Avoid smoking. Avoid others who are getting sick. Travel at night. Sit in the front seat of the car or drive the car. Get fresh air—in car, open the window; on a plane, turn on overhead vent. Avoid alcohol. Avoid fatigue—it increases the chance of motion sickness. Always get enough sleep. Try acupressure wristbands (See also Nausea and Rehydration Guidelines)	Relieve nausea, prevent vomiting
Nausea Remedies	Rest in a quiet, cool room. Take ice chips or drink in small amounts: room temperature Jell-0 or clear juice; e g., soft drinks, 7-Up, ginger ale—fizzy or flat, whichever works best. Try warm, clear liquids like ginger, peppermint, or chamomile tea Try small amounts of soda crackers, white toast, plain pasta, or rice avoid spicy, greasy foods, caffeine (cola and coffee) (See also Rehydration Guidelines)	Relieve nausea
Night Air	Damp, cool night air	Croup cough, wheezing
Nose Pinch	Pinch soft part of nose x 5 min by the clock	Nosebleed
Oatmeal Bath	Fill thin cloth or toe of old nylon stocking w uncooked oatmeal (about 1 cup); tie it closed; allow it to float in bathtub of w arm w ater. Bag of oatmeal can be cooked for 7, hr, then squeeze the bag in warm bath water to extract the gelatinous starch. Be careful, the tub may be slippery. Place bath towel in bottom of tub	Skin irritation, itching
Popsicle	Give popsicle to cut down on bleeding, pain, and act as a distraction	Cut lip
Pressure Points	Raise extremity above heart to < bleeding; Arm Wound: Apply pressure (firm and continuous) to pulse point inside the upper arm; use four fingers; Apply pressure firmly against bone until you can no longer feel pulse Leg Wound Place victim on back and feel for pulse in groin area—at top of leg or where leg bends. Use the heel/palm of hand, keep arm straight, press artery against bone. If you need to, use both hands	To decrease bleeding

(*continued*)

Home Treatment	Formula	Purpose
Rehydration Guidelines	First 24 hr Slowly give small amounts of the following: + Water, ice chips, popsicles, Gatorade, soda, diluted clear fruit juice + */2 to 1 cup every 30-60 min + Give more if person is able to hold it down. Slowly give larger amounts and more often as long as the person does not throw up. If the person vomits, allow to rest for 30 min and try again. When the person has not vomited x 8 hr, start "BRAT" and soft diet (See "BRAT" Diet; Soft Diet) After 24 hr w/o vomiting, begin solids. Do not take any dairy products (milk, cheese, ice cream, yogurt) for 24 hr. Use the " BRAT" diet x 24 hr (See "BRAT" diet) After 24 hours on above diet After 2 days, begin slowly giving solids. If not tolerated, person needs to be evaluated	To prevent dehydration
"RICE" (Rest, Ice, Compression, Elevation)	Using several pillows, large blankets, or bolsters, raise arm or leg above the level of the heart. Remove any jewelry. Using RICE x 24 hr will reduce swelling and avoid further injury. Do not use the injured part or walk on it (See also Cold Pack; Ice Pack)	Reduce swelling/pain/injury of extremities
Rice Water	Boil white rice in water, drain off before absorbed	Diarrhea
Saline Gargle/ Mouthwash	Use '/4 teaspoon salt to one cup of water, warm or cool, whichever feels better	Sore throat
Saline Nose Drops	Use 7, teaspoon salt to one cup of warm water; use w' a dropper prn nasal congestion; put in 3 gtts w nose dropper; wait 3 min and blow nose	Nasal congestion
Sitz Bath	A shallow, warm tub bath, 3 x or more per day x 20 min	Rectal irrigation; hemorrhoid, vaginal irrigation; vaginal lesion or boil
Soft Diet	Don't eat or drink anything that is very hot or very cold. First 12-24 hr clear liquids (See Clear Liquids). After diarrhea stops x 2 days: white toast, crackers, nonsweetened cereals of rice or corn, bread (not whole grain), white rice, macaroni, potatoes, cooked yellow vegetables (squash or carrots), light-colored fruits (applesauce or bananas), and meats; soft-boiled/poached eggs, boiled chicken. For 3-4 days, avoid the following: milk, cheese, ice cream, yogurt, alcohol, coffee, caffeine drinks, diet soda, raw fruits and vegetables, fatty/very sweet/spicy foods	Diarrhea
Steam Treatment	Run hot shower w doors and windows closed; breathe steam for 20 min 3 x a day	Respiratory congestion or croup, cough, wheezing

(continued)

Home Treatment	Formula	Purpose
Tooth Transport	Hold tooth in mouth between gum and cheek during transport to MD. or place in glass of milk	Avulsed tooth
Vinegar Douche	Use 1 tbsp. of white vinegar to 1 qt. of tepid water in a douche bag	Yeast infection
Warm Compress	Soak cloths in warm water, wring out, and place on skin for 20 min on and off	Swelling; muscle spasm
Warm Soapy Soak	Fill tub or bucket w warm water and enough liquid hand soap or liquid dish soap to make bubbles. Soak for 10-15 min 3 x per day: in the morning, afternoon, and before you go to bed at night. For hands/fingers, wash dishes in warm soapy water 3 x a day; the infection should get better after three soaks	Minor infections
Warm (Tepid) Bath	Warm (not hot) water deep enough to cover patient's legs. Splash water on trunk. Get head wet. Do not submerge in water. Keep pt. in tub 20-30 min. The water will draw heat from body as it cools. Try not to make water so cool as to start pt. shivering. Make it comfortably warm	Fever

APPENDIX B

Policy Statements

Position Statement of the Emergency Nurses Association

Access to Quality Healthcare

Description

The Affordable Care Act (ACA) constitutes the broadest change to American healthcare since the institution of Medicare in 1965.[1] The ACA has had the greatest impact on families and adults aged 18-64, while Medicare primarily (although not exclusively) affects adults 65 years old and older. As a result of the ACA, between January 2012 and March 2016, the number of uninsured American adults is estimated to have declined by between 43% and 48%.[2] As of February 2016, however, there were still between 20.8 and 26.5 million non-elderly uninsured adults, and 19 states had chosen not to expand Medicaid, the vehicle by which the ACA offers health insurance to the poor.[2,3,4]

Although the ACA has increased the number of individuals who have insurance, increased access to insurance does not necessarily correlate with increased access to quality healthcare. Many people continue to have high-deductible health plans (HDHPs) and limited networks from which to choose a primary care provider (PCP).[5] By April 2014, 85% of patients who had obtained private health insurance through the ACA marketplace had HDHPs, defined in 2015 as a minimum annual deductible of $1,300 for individuals and $2,600 for families (in 2016, out of pocket expenses were capped at $6,850 per person and $13,700 per family, per year).[6-8] Deductibles for employer-sponsored insurance rose three times faster than premiums, and seven times faster than wages and inflation combined, between 2010 and 2015,[10] and a 2015 survey found that 75% of insured patients who had problems paying their medical bills stated that it was because they could not afford copays, deductibles, or coinsurance.[11] Others have plans that include up to 50% coinsurance.[9] Medicare-insured patients also face difficulties paying for needed services and medications, whether because of fixed incomes (half of which were less than $23,500 in 2013), annual increases in premiums and deductibles, or difficulty affording medications.[59]

The consolidation of health insurance companies has contributed to this problem. Often touted as good for the consumer because increased market share means increased buying power and lower healthcare costs, consolidation has instead resulted in increased premiums and deductibles.[60] Furthermore, increased competition within the healthcare insurance industry has been associated with decreased costs for patients, but consolidation has resulted in exclusive, non-overlapping market territories and increased barriers to entry for smaller companies.[60] In 2014, private insurance premiums averaged $16,834 per family, and out of pocket spending averaged $800 per individual; the four largest insurance companies commanded approximately 83% of the market share (up from 74% in 2006), and the largest of them recorded $5.6 billion in profits.[60,6*]

This problem of unaffordable healthcare is especially prevalent among those with chronic health conditions[12] and is often compounded by a lack of patient knowledge of helpful resources: 47% of those patients who had problems paying their medical bills were unaware of hospital-fee-reduction programs[13] and 37% of patients in another survey did not know that their insurance plan fully covered preventive care services.[14]

Access to quality hospital-based healthcare is impeded by emergency department (ED) overcrowding, which is associated with increased patient mortality, length of stay, cost, and an overall decreased access to timely treatment, regardless of insurance type.[15-17] EDs are a major gateway for hospital admissions and by law must provide care to all patients regardless of citizenship, legal status, or ability to pay.[2,18,19] As a result, EDs have become the healthcare system's safety net, treating the non-emergent and primary care needs of those who cannot access a PCP, while also being reimbursed poorly or not at all by Medicaid-insured and uninsured patients. The problem of overcrowded EDs is exacerbated by a shortage of PCPs[20,21] and a dearth of healthcare workers specifically trained to treat those patients with behavioral health problems who comprise 12.5% of ED visits, spend almost 3 times longer in the ED, and are 2.5 times more likely to be admitted than other patients.[22]

The greater the number of barriers to primary care access, the greater the ED utilization,[23] and Medicaid-insured patients continue to have more barriers and receive lower quality healthcare than privately insured patients. Contributing factors include:

1. Limited physician willingness to accept Medicaid insurance[23-25]
2. Discrimination against and stigmatization of Medicaid-insured patients by healthcare providers[26]
3. Medical and non-medical hurdles associated with lower socio-economic status[26]
4. Barriers to access to primary care and other outpatient services[23,27,49]
5. Significant mental and physical disease burden[26,49]
6. Other barriers specific to the Medicaid population[28]

The ACA has achieved much-needed reform of the U.S. healthcare system,[29] but more is needed. The current state of the U.S. national healthcare system, particularly the EDs, is not robust enough to meet the future needs of an aging population, growing racial and ethnic diversity, a mounting income gap, and increasing chronic health problems.

ENA Position

It is the position of the Emergency Nurses Association that:

1. All people, regardless of geographical locale or socio-economic status, need equal access to comprehensive healthcare services for critical, acute, and chronic medical conditions, including mental health and substance use disorders.

2 The definition of comprehensive healthcare includes preventive healthcare, wellness promotion, palliative and end-of-life care, and illness and injury prevention.

3 There is compelling evidence that gender, race, ethnicity, and socio-economic class are correlated with persistent and often increasing health disparities that impact and are impacted by diminished access to healthcare.

4 ED staff be knowledgeable about fee reduction programs offered by their facility so that they can refer their patients to support staff and resources that will help them to navigate payment for their care.

5 The use of EDs for primary care and for non-urgent needs can be decreased by expanding primary, preventive, and community healthcare services through a variety of proven strategies, including those listed at the end of this document.

6 Access to primary, preventive, and community healthcare services can be increased by allowing Advanced Practice Registered Nurses (APRNs) to practice to the full extent of their educational preparation, in addition to allowing them equitable reimbursement for services provided.

7 Primary care and non-urgent ED return visits can be reduced through the use of nurse navigators, case managers, and clinical social workers in the ED who assist patients in accessing preventative, primary care, and follow-up resources.

8 Emergency departments and hospital systems can implement evidence-based approaches that increase throughput and reduce patient wait times along with their associated adverse events.

9 Public education and social media initiatives can be implemented to increase public awareness of preventive, community, and primary care resources in an effort to reduce the impact of non-urgent needs on EDs.

10 Our understanding of the ACA's impact on access to quality healthcare is still evolving; therefore, a commitment to ongoing research and review of the ACA's impact on access is critical for the future of the healthcare system.

11 Health insurance companies, by virtue of the human object of their business, have an obligation to responsibly balance commercial profit with the thoughtful and innovative provision of affordable healthcare plans that promote wellness, prevention, and the management of chronic conditions.

Background

Over the past half century the utilization of EDs in the U.S. healthcare system has shifted from treating patients with emergent conditions to one of primarily providing care for non-emergent needs. The rate of ED visits over the past 15 years has outpaced population growth, increasing at double the expected rate between 1997 and 2007.[30-32] In addition, a retrospective study of more than 241,000 ED visits from 1997-2009 concluded that 70% were for primary-care-treatable conditions,[33] and the most recent data from the CDC's National Hospital Ambulatory Medical Care Survey found that 86% of ED visits in 2011 were triage levels 3, 4, or 5 (i.e., urgent, semi-urgent, or non-urgent).34 Patients without insurance accounted for more than 21 million of those visits, and only 11.9% of the total visits resulted in admission.[35]

These problems are worse in non-metropolitan areas, where there are lower odds that seriousness of the medical problem will be the reason for an ED visit. Indeed, non-metropolitan ED patients are almost twice as likely as metropolitan ED patients to indicate that the reason for their visit is that their doctor's office was not open.49 Perhaps unsurprisingly, multiple studies have found decreased rates of hospital admission from ED visits in rural and non-metropolitan areas, as compared to hospitals in metropolitan areas.34,53 These problems are often magnified by the budget and staffing challenges that many rural and community hospitals face, which impede the implementation of technological and specialized solutions.

The ACA was anticipated to provide solutions to these problems by increasing the number of patients with healthcare insurance, thereby allowing patients to have their non-emergent healthcare needs met by PCPs, while at the same time also providing insurance payment for those patients who still utilize the ED. However, many studies predicted that the ACA would likely cause a slight long-term decrease in ED visits, but would increase ED visits by up to 21% among some patient populations in the first three years after its implementation.7,41 A nationwide survey of emergency physicians concluded that ED visits were still on the rise as of March 2015.40

The majority of patients receiving new healthcare insurance under the ACA did so under Medicaid, and although multiple studies have shown an increased use of preventive care among Medicaid recipients,36,37 early studies also revealed that Medicaid patients visited EDs up to 46% more frequently than patients with other types of insurance or with no insurance at all.33,38,39 The most recent data from the CDC's National Health Interview Study, which looked at ED visits in 2013-2014, found that adults with Medicaid had the highest prevalence of both a single ED visit and multiple ED visits in the previous 12 months, when compared with patients with private insurance and patients without insurance, and almost four times the odds of having one or more ED visits in the previous 12 months when compared with privately insured adults.49

One of the ways that the ACA pays for itself is by offering tiered plans that trade lowered monthly premiums for cost-sharing approaches to payment.43 Such health plans and their high out-of-pocket costs are a burden for households with incomes between 100% and 250% of the Federal Poverty Limit (FPL), 80% of which do not have the assets to meet the high deductibles required by their healthcare plans.42 They are also a burden for households with incomes between 250% and 400% of the FPL, which do not benefit from the ACA's provisions for subsidized insurance.42 HDHPs are particularly prevalent in the private healthcare market, in part because this cost-sharing approach allows employers to reduce their portion of their employees' coverage. In 2013, 58% of companies with fewer than 200 workers offered insurance that had an average annual deductible of at least $1,000.43 Some studies have found that the ACA's elimination of out-of-pocket costs for preventative services has improved screening among patients with HDHPs;44 however, HDHPs also force patients to stop essential treatment,45 decrease the dosage of or cease taking prescribed medications to reduce costs,46 and schedule expensive diagnostic procedures late in the calendar year in order to minimize out-of-pocket costs.47 Many are simply unable to pay their medical bills.46

As mentioned above, the problem is compounded by insurance companies' established track record of decreasing competition through consolidation and driving down healthcare costs through the power of volume bargaining, while at the same time increasing premiums and deductibles rather than passing those savings on to the patient.60 The degree of consolidation within the healthcare industry can be appreciated by comparing it with the airline industry. In 2014 the market share of the top four insurance companies was 83%, while the market share of the top four airlines was only 62%.60 The consequences of HDHPs and insurance company consolidation for hospitals and providers include decreased reimbursement from insured patients who are nevertheless unable to pay their portion and increased acuity and number of comorbidities in patients who have avoided treatment to cut costs.

Some of the changes brought about by the ACA improved benefits to Medicare patients (e.g., closing the gap in Part D prescription drug coverage by 2020), but many patients with Medicare still struggle to pay for needed services and medications. In 2016, Part B premiums and deductibles for 16 million Americans rose by 16% and 13%, respectively, and both premiums and deductibles are projected to rise by up to 8% per year between 2016-2024.56,57 Perhaps more problematic, the Medicare system can be incredibly complex and difficult to navigate, and an inability to understand it can lead to poor decisions and lost healthcare access.58 The potential for insolvency of the program, increased eligibility age, and increasing numbers of eligible Americans constitute future potential barriers to access to quality healthcare that are yet to be solved.

The use of EDs for primary care and non-urgent needs can be decreased by expanding primary, preventive, and community healthcare services through a variety of proven strategies, including:

- Increasing access to local community health centers, neighborhood and specialty chronic disease clinics, and nurse-managed health clinics
- Expanding evidence-based community prevention and wellness programs
- Increasing the use of mobile integrated health and community paramedicine programs
- Increasing the use of advanced practice nurses and allowing them full practice authority in all states

- Eliminating barriers that prevent triaging of patients from the ED to primary care health facilities
- Collaborating with community-based programs to build and maintain a coordinated system of services that advance a continuum of quality care for patients with mental illnesses and substance use disorders
- Increasing the use of case managers and clinical social workers in the ED who can help patients access non-ED resources whenever possible[52,53]

EDs can also help combat the problem of overcrowding by adopting practices that more efficiently treat all patients, including those requiring specialized care,22 thereby improving ED patient flow.[43].

Resources

Claxton, G., Cox, C., & Rae, M. (2015, February 1). *The cost of care with marketplace coverage.* The Henry J. Kaiser Family Foundation.

Emergency Nurses Association. (2013). *White paper: Care of the psychiatric patient in the emergency department.*

Emergency Nurses Association. (2014). *Topic brief: Care of behavioral health patients in the emergency department.*

Emergency Nurses Association. (2014). *Topic brief: Collaborative care of the older adult.*

Emergency Nurses Association. (2015). *Position statement: Emergency nursing interface with mobile integrated health (MIH) and community paramedicine (CP) programs.*

Gindi, R. M., Black, L. I., & Cohen, R. A. (2016). Reasons for emergency room use among U. S. adults aged 18-64: National Health Interview Study, 2013 and 2014. *National Health Statistics Reports,* 90, 1-15.

Health Insurance Industry Consolidation: What Do We Know From the Past, Is It Relevant in Light of the ACA, and What Should We Ask?: Hearings before the Committee on the Judiciary, Senate, 114th Cong. 1 (2015) (Testimony of Leemore S. Dafny).

Heisler, E. J., & Tyler, N. L. (2014). *Hospital-based emergency departments: Background and policy considerations.* Washington, DC: Congressional Research Service.

Medford-Davis, L. N., Eswaran, V., Shah, R. M., & Dark, C. (2015). The Patient Protection and Affordable Care Act's effect on emergency medicine: A synthesis of the data. *Annals of Emergency Medicine,* 66(5), 496-506. doi: 10.1016/j.annemergmed.2015.04.007

Shenkin, B. N., & the American Academy of Pediatrics Committee on Child Health Financing, 2013-2014. (2014). Policy Statement: High-Deductible Health Plans. *Pediatrics 133(5),* e1461-1470.

U.S. Department of Health and Human Services, Centers for Disease Control and Prevention. (2016). *National Center for Health Statistics.*

U.S. Department of Health and Human Services, Centers for Disease Control and Prevention, National Center for Health Statistics. (2015). *Health insurance and access to care.*

References

1 The Affordable Care Act is made up of the Patient Protection and Affordable Care Act of 2010 (Pub. L. No. 111-148) and the Health Care and Education Reconciliation Act of 2010 (Pub. L. 111-152), retrieved from https://www.gpo.gov/fdsys/pkg/PLAW-111publ152/pdf/PLAW-111publ152.pdf and https://www.gpo.gov/fdsys/pkg/PLAW-111 publ148/pdf/PLAW-111 publ148.pdf

2 Uberoi, N., Finegold, K, & Gee, E. (2016, March 3). *ASPE issue brief: Health insurance coverage and the Affordable Care Act, 2010-2016.* Washington, DC: U. S. Department of Health and Human Services Office of the Assistant Secretary for Planning and Evaluation, Figure 4, p. 6. Retrieved from https://aspe.hhs.gov/sites/default/files/pdf/187551/ACA2010-2016.pdf

3 The Henry J. Kaiser Family Foundation. (2016, March 14). *Status of state action on the Medicaid expansion decision.* Retrieved from http://kff.org/health-reform/state-indicator/state-activity-around-expanding-medicaid-under-the-affordable-care-act/

4 Garfield, R., & Damico, A. (2016, January 21). *The coverage gap: Uninsured poor adults in states that do not expand Medicaid - An update.* Retrieved from the Henry J. Kaiser Family Foundation website: http://kff.org/health-reform/issue-brief/the-coverage-gap-uninsured-poor-adults-in-states-that-do-not-expand-medicaid-an-update/

5 Wharam, J. F., Zhang, F., Landon, B. E., Soumerai, S. B., & Ross-Degnan, D. (2013). Low-socioeconomic-status enrollees in high-deductible plans reduced high-severity emergency care. *Health Affairs,* 32(8), 1398-1406. doi: 10.1377/hlthaff.2012.1426

6 Internal Revenue Service. (2015). *Publication 969.* Washington, DC: Author. Retrieved from https://www.irs.gov/publications/p969/ar02.html

7 Medford-Davis, L. N., Eswaran, V., Shah, R. M., & Dark, C. (2015). The Patient Protection and Affordable Care Act's effect on emergency medicine: A synthesis of the data. *Annals of Emergency Medicine,* 66(5), 496-506. doi: 10.1016/j.annemergmed.2015.04.007

8 Department of Labor, Employee Benefits Security Administration. (2015). *FAQs about Affordable Care Act implementation (part XXVII).* Retrieved from http://www.dol.gov/ebsa/pdf/faq-aca27.pdf

9 Claxton, G., Cox, C., & Rae, M. (2015, February 11). *The cost of care with marketplace coverage.* Retrieved from The Henry J. Kaiser Family Foundation website: http://kff.org/health-costs/issue-brief/the-cost-of-care-with-marketplace-coverage/

10 Claxton, G., Rae, M., Long, M., Panchal, N., Damico, A., Kenward, K., & Whitmore, H. (2015). *Employer health benefits: 2015 annual survey.* Chicago, IL: The Henry J. Kaiser Family Foundation & the Health Research & Educational Trust. Retrieved from http://files.kff.org/attachment/report-2015-employer-health-benefits-survey

11 Hamel, L., Norton, M., Pollitz, K., Levitt, L., Claxton, G., & Brodie, M. (2016, January 5). *The burden of medical debt: Results from the Henry J. Kaiser Family Foundation/New York Times Medical Bills Survey. Section 2: The role of health insurance.* Retrieved from The Henry J. Kaiser Family Foundation website: http://kff.org/report-section/the-burden-of-medical-debt-section-2-the-role-of-health-insurance

12 Galbraith, A. A., Ross-Degnan, D., Soumerai, S. B., Rosenthal, M. B., Gay, C., & Lieu, T. A. (2011). Nearly half of families in high-deductible health plans whose members have chronic conditions face substantial financial burden. *Health Affairs,* 20(2), 322-331. doi: 10.1377/hlthaff.2010.0584

13 Hamel, L., Norton, M., Pollitz, K., Levitt, L., Claxton, G., & Brodie, M. (2016, January 5). *The burden of medical debt: Results from the Kaiser Family Foundation/New York Times Medical Bills Survey. Section 4: Patients as consumers.* Retrieved from The Henry J. Kaiser Family Foundation website: http://kff.org/report-section/the-burden-of-medical-debt-section-4-patients-as-consumers

14 Collins, S. R., Gunja, M., Doty, M. M., & Beutel, S. (2015). *How high is America's health care cost burden? Findings from the Commonwealth Fund Health Care Affordability Tracking Survey, July-August 2015.* Washington, DC: The Commonwealth Fund. Retrieved from http://www.commonwealthfund.org/~/media/files/publications/issue-brief/2015/nov/1844_collins_how_high_is-americas_hlt_care_cost_burden_tb_v1.pdf

15 Singer A. J., Thode, H. C., Viccellio, P., & Pines, J. M. (2011). The association between length of emergency department boarding and mortality. *Academic Emergency Medicine,* 18(12), 1324-1329. doi:10.1111/j.1553-2712.2011.01236.x

16 Sun B. C., Hsia, R. Y., Weiss, R. E., Zingmond, D., Liang, L. J., Han, W. . . . Asch, S. M. (2013). Effect of emergency department crowding on outcomes of admitted patients. *Annals of Emergency Medicine,* 61(6), 605-611. doi:10.1016/j.annemergmed.2012.10.026

17 Liu, C., Srebotnjak, T., & Hsia, R. Y. (2014). California emergency department closures are associated with increased inpatient mortality at nearby hospitals. *Health Affairs,* 33(8), 1323-1329. doi: 10.1377/hlthaff.2013.1203

18 Emergency Medical Treatment and Labor Act of 1986, Pub. L. 42 U.S.C. § 1395dd.

19 U.S. Department of Health and Human Services, Centers for Medicare and Medicaid Services (2003). 42 CFR Parts 413, 482, and 489: Medicare program; Clarifying policies related to the responsibilities of Medicare-participating hospitals in treating individuals with emergency medical conditions. *Federal Register,* 68(174). Retrieved from https://www.gpo.gov/fdsys/pkg/FR-2003-09-09/pdf/03-22594.pdf

20 Petterson, S. M., Liaw, W. R., Phillips, R. L., Rabin, D. L., Meyers, D. S., & Bazemore, A. W. (2012). Projecting US primary care physician workforce

needs: 2010-2025. *Annals of Family Medicine,* 10(6), 503-509. doi:10.1370/afm.1431
21 U.S. Department of Health and Human Services, Health Resources and Services Administration Bureau of Health Professions, National Center for Health Workforce Analysis. (2013). *Projecting the supply and demand for primary care practitioners through 2020.* Rockville, MD: U.S. Department of Health and Human Services. Retrieved from http://bhpr.hrsa.gov/healthworkforce/supplydemand/usworkforce/primarycare/projectingprimarycare.pdf
22 Weiss, A. P., Chang, G., Rauch, S. L, Smallwood, J. A., Schechter, M., Kosowsky, J., . . . Orav, E. J. (2012). Patient- and practice-related determinants of emergency department length of stay for patients with psychiatric illness. *Annals of Emergency Medicine,* 60(2), 162-171.e5. doi: 10.1016/j.annemergmed.2012.01.037
23 Cheung, P. T., Wiler, J. L., Lowe, R. A., & Ginde, A. A. (2012). National study of barriers to timely primary care and emergency department utilization among Medicaid beneficiaries. *Annals of Emergency Medicine,* 60(1), 4-10e2. doi:10.1016/j.annemergmed.2012.01.035
24 Geissler, K. H., Lubin, B., & Marzilli Ericson, K. M. (2016). Access is not enough: Characteristics of physicians who treat Medicaid patients. *Medical Care,* 54(4), 350-358. doi:10.1097/MLR.0000000000000488
25 Decker, S. L. (2012). In 2011 nearly one-third of physicians said that they would not accept new Medicaid patients, but rising fees may help. *Health Affairs,* 31(8), 1673-1679. doi:10.1377/hlthaff.2012.0294
26 Capp, R., Kelley, L., Ellis, P., Carmona, J., Lofton, A., Cobbs-Lomax, D., & D'Onofrio, G. (2016). Reasons for frequent emergency department use by Medicaid enrollees: A qualitative study. *Academic Emergency Medicine,* 23(4), 476-481. doi:10.1111/acem.12952
27 Capp, R., Rooks, S. P., Wiler, J. L., Zane, R. D., & Ginde, A. A. (2014). National study of health insurance type and reasons for emergency department use. *Journal of General Internal Medicine,* 29(4), 621-627. doi: 10.1007/sl 1606-013-2734-4
28 Jiang, H. J., Boutwell, A. E., Maxwell, J., Bourgoin, A., Regenstein, M., & Andres, E. (2016). Understanding patient, provider, and system factors related to Medicaid readmissions. *The Joint Commission Journal on Quality and Patient Safety,* 42(3), 115-121.
29 Bernardi, B, & Wright, G. (2012, June 28). *Press release: ENA applauds Supreme Court decision upholding healthcare reform law.* Retrieved from the Emergency Nurses Association website: https://www.ena.org/about/media/PressReleases/2012/Pages/HealthCareLaw.aspx
30 The Henry J. Kaiser Family Foundation. (2015). *Hospital emergency room visits per 1,000 population by ownership type.* Retrieved from http://kff.org/other/state-indicator/emergency-room-visits-by-ownership/#graph
31 Pitts, S. R., Pines, J. M., Handrigan, M. T., & Kellermann, A. L. (2012).

National trends in emergency department occupancy, 2001 to 2008: Effect of inpatient admissions versus emergency department practice intensity. *Annals of Emergency Medicine,* 60(6), 679-686. doi:10.1016/j.annemergmed.2012.05.014

32 Tang, N., Stein, J., Hsia, R. Y., Maselli, J. H., & Gonzales, R. (2010). Trends and characteristics of U.S. emergency department visits, 1997-2007. *Journal of the American Medical Association,* 304(6), 664-670. doi:10.1001/jama.2010.1112.

33 Pukurdpol, P., Wiler, J. L., Hsia, R. Y., & Ginde, A. A. (2014). Association of Medicare and Medicaid insurance with increasing primary care-treatable emergency department visits in the United States. *Academic Emergency Medicine,* 21(10), 1135-1142. doi:10.1111/acem. 12490

34 U.S. Department of Health and Human Services, Centers for Disease Control and Prevention. (2014). *National Hospital Ambulatory Medical Care Survey: 2011 emergency department summary tables.* Retrieved from http://www.cdc.gov/nchs/data/ahcd/nhamcs_emergency/2011_ed_web_tables.pdf

35 U.S. Department of Health and Human Services, Centers for Disease Control and Prevention, National Center for Health Statistics. (2016). *Emergency department visits.* Retrieved from http://www.cdc.gov/nchs/fastats/emergency-department.htm

36 Kreider, A. R., French, B., Aysola, J., Saloner, B., Noonan, K. G., & Rubin, D. M. (2016). Quality of health insurance coverage and access to care for children in low-income families. *JAMA Pediatrics,* 170(1), 43-51. doi: 10.1001 /jamapediatrics.2015.3028

37 Baicker, K., Taubman, S. L., Allen, H. L., Bernstein, M., Gruber, J. H., Newhouse, J. P., . . . Finkelestein, A. N. (2013). The Oregon experiment — effects of Medicaid on clinical outcomes. *New England Journal of Medicine,* 368(18), 1713-1722. doi:10.1056/NEJMsa1212321

38 Taubman, S. L., Allen, H. L., Wright, B. J., Baicker, K., & Finkelstein, A. N. (2014). Medicaid increases emergency-department use: Evidence from Oregon's Health Insurance Experiment. *Science,* 343(6168), 263-268. doi: 10.1126/science. 1246183

39 DeLeire, T., Dague, L., Leininger, L., Voskuil, K., & Friedsam, D. (2013). Wisconsin experience indicates that expanding public insurance to low-income childless adults has health care impacts. *Health Affairs,* 32(6), 1037-1045. doi: 10.1377/hlthaff.2012.1026

40 Marketing General Incorporated. (2015). 2015 *ACEP poll Affordable Care Act research results.* Retrieved from https://www.heartland.Org/sites/default/files/2015acepacapollreportfinal1.pdf

41 Lo, N., Roby, D. H., Padilla, J., Chen, X, Salce, E. N., Pourat, N., & Kominski, G. F. (2014). *Increased service use following Medicaid expansion is mostly temporary: Evidence from California's Low Income Health Program.* Retrieved from the UCLA Center for Health Policy

Research website: http://healthpolicy.ucla.edu/publications/Documents/PDF/2014/Demand_PB_FINAL_10-8-14.pdf
42 Claxton, G., Rae, M., & Panchal, N. (2015, March 11). *Consumer assets and patient cost sharing*. Retrieved from The Fienry J. Kaiser Family Foundation website: http://kff.org/health-costs/issue-brief/consumer-assets-and-patient-cost-sharing/
43 Oberlander, J. (2014). Between liberal aspirations and market forces: Obamacare's precarious balancing act. *Journal of Law, Medicine, & Ethics,* 42(4), 431^441. doi:10.1111/jlme. 12166
44 Wharam, J. F., Zhang, F., Landon, B. E., LeCates, R., Soumerai, S., & Ross-Degnan, D. (2016). Colorectal cancer screening in a nationwide high-deductible health plan before and after the Affordable Care Act. *Medical Care,*54(5), 466^73. doi:10.1097/MLR.0000000000000521
45 Dusetzina, S. B., Winn, A. N., Abel, G. A., Huskamp, FI. A., & Keating, N. L. (2014). Cost sharing and adherence to tyrosine kinase inhibitors for patients with chronic myeloid leukemia. *Journal of Clinical Oncology,* 32(4), 306-311.
46 Hamel, L., Norton, M., Pollitz, K., Levitt, L., Claxton, G., & Brodie, M. (2016, January 5). *The burden of medical debt: Results from the Kaiser Family Foundation/New York Times Medical Bills Survey* (Section 3: Consequences of medical bill problems). Retrieved from The Henry J. Kaiser Family Foundation website: http://kff.org/report-section/the-burden-of-medical-debt-section-3-consequences-of-medical-bill-problems/
47 Hunter, W. G., Zhang, C. Z., Hesson, A., Davis, J. K., Kirby, C., Williamson, L. D., Barnett, J. A., Ubel, P. A. (2016). What strategies do physicians and patients discuss to reduce out-of-pocket costs? Analysis of the cost-saving strategies in 1755 outpatient clinic visits. *Medical Decision Making,* 30, 1-11. doi:10.1177/0272989X15626384
48 Zocchi, M. S., McClelland, M. S., & Pines, J. M. (2015). Increasing throughput: Results from a 42-hospital collaborative to improve emergency department flow. *The Joint Commission Journal on Quality and Patient Safety,* 41(12), 532-541.
49 Gindi, R. M., Black, L. I., & Cohen, R. A. (2016). Reasons for emergency room use among U. S. adults aged 18-64: National Health Interview Study, 2013 and 2014. *National Health Statistics Reports,* 90, 1-15. Retrieved from http://www.cdc.gov/nchs/data/nhsr/nhsr090.pdf
50 Kippenbrock, T., Lo, W-J., Odell, E., & Buron, B. (2015). The Southern states: NPs made an impact in rural and healthcare shortage areas. *Journal of the American Association of Nurse Practitioners* 27, 707-713.
51 Institute of Medicine Committee on the Robert Wood Johnson Foundation Initiative on the Future of Nursing, at the Institute of Medicine. (2011). *The future of nursing: Leading change, advancing health.* Washington, D.C.: National Academies Press, Part II, Chapter 3. Retrieved from http://www.ncbi.nlm.nih.gov/books/NBK209871/
52 Kim, T., Mortensen, C., & Eldridge, B. (2015). Linking uninsured patients

treated in the emergency department to primary care shows some promise in Maryland. *Health Affairs,* 34(5), 796-804. doi: 10.1377/hlthaff. 2014.1102

53 Pourat, N., Davis, A. C., Chen, X., Vrungos, S., & Kominski, G. F. (2015). In California, primary care continuity was associated with reduced emergency department use and fewer hospitalizations. *Health Affairs,* 34(7), 1113-1120.

54 Hines, A., Fraze, T., & Stocks, C. (2011). Emergency department visits in rural and non-rural community hospitals, 2008. *Healthcare Cost and Utilization Project (HCUP) Statistical Briefs #116.* Rockville, MD: Agency for Healthcare Policy and Research. Retrieved from http://www.hcup-us.ahrq.gov/reports/statbriefs/sbl 16.pdf

55 APRN Consensus Work Group & National Council of State Boards of Nursing APRN Advisory Committee. (2008). *Consensus model for APRN regulation: Licensure, accreditation, certification & education.* Chicago, IL: National Council of the State Boards of Nursing. Retrieved from https://www.ncsbn.org/Consensus_Model_for_APRN_Regulation_July_2008.pdf

56 Cubanski, J., & Neuman, T. (2015). *What's in store for Medicare's Part B premiums and deductible in 2016, and why?* Retrieved from The Henry J. Kaiser Family Foundation: http://kff.org/medicare/issue-brief/whats-in-store-for-medicares-part-b-premiums-and-deductible-in-2016-and-why/

57 The Henry J. Kaiser Family Foundation. (2016). *Total number of Medicare beneficiaries.* Retrieved from http://kff.org/medicare/state-indicator/total-medicare-beneficiaries/

58 The Henry J. Kaiser Family Foundation. (2012). *Seniors' knowledge and experience with Medicare's open enrollment period and choosing a plan: Key findings from the Kaiser Family Foundation 2012 National Survey of Seniors.* Retrieved from The Henry J. Kaiser Family Foundation website: http://kff.org/medicare/issue-brief/seniors-knowledge-and-experience-with-medicares-open/

59 Jacobsen, G., Swoope, C., & Neuman, T. (2015). *Income and assets of Medicare beneficiaries, 2014-2030.* Retrieved from The Henry J. Kaiser Family Foundation website: http://kff.org/medicare/issue-brief/income-and-assets-of-medicare-beneficiaries-2014-2030/

60 U.S. Senate. (2015). *Health insurance industry consolidation: What do we know from the past, is it relevant in light of the ACA, and what should we ask*: Hearings before the Committee on the Judiciary, Senate, 114th Cong. 1 (Testimony of Leemore S. Dafny). Retrieved from: http://www.judiciary.senate.gov/imo/media/doc/09-22-15%20Dafny%20Testimony%20Updated.pdf.

61 UnitedHealth Group. (2015, January 21). *UnitedHealth Group reports 2014 results, highlighted by strength in growth markets.* [Press release]. Retrieved from http://www.unitedhealthgroup.eom/~/media/2B5EEC6F00F446AC9051674E259BA80B.ashx

Authors

Authored by
Justin Winger, PhD, MA, BA
Reviewed by the Position Statement Committee
E. Marie Wilson, MPA, RN, Chair
Katie Bush, MA, RN, CEN, SANE-A
Melanie Crowley, MSN, RN, CEN
Kathy Dolan, MSHA, RN, CEN, CPHRM
Ellen Encapera, RN, CEN
Elizabeth Stone, MSN, RN, CPEN
ENA 2016 Board of Directors Liaison
Sally Snow, BSN, RN, CPEN, FAEN
ENA Staff Liaisons
Dale Wallerich, MBA, BSN, RN

Developed: 2016.
Approved by the ENA Board of Directors: 1988.
Revised and Approved by the ENA Board of Directors: 1990.
Revised and Approved by the ENA Board of Directors: September 1992.
Revised and Approved by the ENA Board of Directors: September 1994.
Revised and Approved by the ENA Board of Directors: May 1996.
Revised and Approved by the ENA Board of Directors: July 1998.
Revised and Approved by the ENA Board of Directors: September 2000.
Revised and Approved by the ENA Board of Directors: September 2002.
Revised and Approved by the ENA Board of Directors: February 2006.
Revised and Approved by the ENA Board of Directors: December 2010.
Revised and Approved by the ENA Board of Directors: July 2016.

Position Statement of the Emergency Nurses Association

Telephone Triage

Since the 1970's there has been an almost 400% increase in ED visits while the US population has increased by approximately 10% per decade.[3] Telephone triage, telephone advice counseling (Sabin) or telehealth nursing, as it is sometimes called today, became a popular method used by managed care and other private physician and health maintenance organization (HMO) groups in the 1970's to provide an entry into the healthcare system for an increasingly large number of patients.[1,2]

Today these formal commercial telephone triage programs function with specific physician-approved policies, protocols, staff education, patient documentation requirements, and quality improvement programs in order to function safely.[2,4,5] The chief advantage of telephone triage systems to the patient is timely access to a healthcare professional.[6] Successful systems of telephone triage have also been reported to make a positive difference in the appropriate use of the emergency department, patient satisfaction, and nurse/provider satisfaction.[7,8] By reducing unnecessary visits to a physician's office or an emergency department, the use of telephone triage may save time, patient costs and emotional trauma.[4,9] Although the goal of telephone triage is to provide the right level of care with the right provider at the right location at the right time there are challenges with the system.[6]

Identified concerns include: nurses, in spite of these protocols and decision-tree algorithms, may employ their own clinical judgment;[10] legal liability issues may put not only the nurse, but the physician and facility at risk of a lawsuit;[2] the inability to review the medical record or past medical history of the caller;[10] language barriers;[10] incomplete documentation issues;[10] lack of patient compliance and evaluating the appropriateness of decision-making algorithms.[6] When nurses were surveyed, they cited challenges assessing patients without visual cues and the demands of being the gatekeeper for large numbers of patients without a corresponding supply of available services.[11]

The Netherlands recently implemented a large scale, country-wide research intervention using the same five-level urgency markers for both physical and telephone triage in a primary care setting. Compliance to triage was good; safety was acceptable, however, as in other cases, further research is recommended to validate tool performance, compliance, decision-making and continued competence.[1,5,6,9]

ENA Position

It is the position of the Emergency Nurses Association that:

1 Emergency nurses do not give advice or clinical management recommendations over the telephone.
2 Formal commercial telephone triage nurses require specialized education; follow pre-established and physician-approved policies and protocols, complete patient documentation, and participate in quality improvement programs for safe and quality patient care.
3 Further research is recommended to determine if commercial telephone triage programs improve the use of available health services within the community.

Background

In 2010, the American College of Emergency Physicians (ACEP) and the Emergency Nurses Association (ENA) Joint Five-Level Triage Task Force approved a joint position statement stating "the quality of patient care benefits from implementing a standardized emergency department triage scale and acuity categorization process."[12] They went on to support the use of a reliable, valid five level triage scale such as the Emergency Severity Index (ESI)." Telephone triage is not addressed as a function of that process.

The Emergency Nursing Scope and Standards of Practice, Standard Ia Triage, approved and endorsed by the both the ENA and American Nurses Association (ANA), states, "the emergency registered nurse triages each health care consumer utilizing age, developmentally appropriate and culturally sensitive practices to care, prioritize and optimize health care consumer flow, expediting those health care consumers who require immediate care."[13, pg21] Telephone triage is not included within the scope of emergency nursing practice.

Giving advice over the phone outside of a formal telephone triage system can put the nurse, physician, and facility at risk.[2]

In a policy statement approved in 2013, ACEP recommends that "emergency department personnel not attempt medical assessment or management by telephone."[14] They further explain that callers with a mental health or limb- or life-threatening emergency are an exception and recommended they be instructed to access emergency medical services. As for patients recently discharged from the ED, ACEP recommends they be managed according to pre-determined protocols.[14] Emergency nurses are advised not to give advice or clinical management recommendations over the telephone.[10] However, if patients call with questions regarding ED discharge instructions and the chart is readily available, follow facility policy if clarifying instructions and notify the concerned patient to return to the emergency department, since the nurse may be liable for miscommunication.10 Instruct patients to dial 911 in cases of a mental health, life or limb threatening emergency after determining if they need assistance to make the call. And as always, observe common courtesy and handle these matters in a respectful, caring manner.

Resources

Briggs, J.K. (2012) *Telephone Triage Protocols for Nurses (4th Edition).*

Philadelphia, PA: Wolters Kluwer/Lippincott Williams & Wilkins.

References

1 Sabin, M. Telephone Triage Improves Demand Management Effectiveness. *Health Finance Management.* 1998;52(8):49-51. Retrieved from http://www.ncbi.nlm.nih.gov/pubmed/10182276

2 American College of Physicians-American Society of Internal Medicine: Telephone Triage. Philadelphia: American College of Physicians-American Society of Internal Medicine; 2000: White Paper. (Available from American College of Physicians-American Society of Internal Medicine, 190 N. Independence Mall West, Philadelphia, PA 19106.

3 Pines, J, Abualenain, J, Scott, J, Shesser, R. ed, *Emergency Care and the Pubic's Health,* Wiley Blackwell, 2014.

4 Dent, R.L. (2010). The effect of telephone nurse triage on the appropriate use of the emergency department. *Nursing Clinics of North America.* 45(1): 65-69.

5 Van Ierland, Y., van Veen, M., Huibers, L., Giesen, P. and Moll, H.A. (2011). Validity of telephone and physical triage in emergency care: The Netherlands Triage System. *Family Practice.* 28:334-341.

6 National Capital Poison Center. Retrieved from http://www.poison.org/about-us

7 Blank, L., Coster, J., O'Cathain, A., Knowles, E., Tosh, J., Turner, J., and Nicholl, J. (2012) The appropriateness of, and compliance with, telephone triage decisions: a systematic review and narrative synthesis. *Journal of Advanced Nursing.* 68(12): 2610-2621.

8 Bunn, F., Byrne, G., & Kendall, S. The effects of telephone consultation and triage on healthcare use and patient satisfaction: a systematic review. *The British Journal of General Practice.* 2005: 55(521): 956-961.

9 Hertz, A.& Schmitt, B. Decreasing ER Utilization with Nurse Telephone Triage and Establishing a National Network of Medical Call Centers. *American Academy of Pediatrics.* July 2011. Retrieved from http://www2.aap.org/sections/telecare/Decreasing%20ER%20Utilization%20with%20Nurse%20Telephone%20Tri.pdf

10 Huibers, L., Keizer, E., Geisen, P., Grol, R. and Wesing, M. (2012). Nurse telephone triage: good quality associated with appropriate decisions. *Family Practice.* 29:547-552.

11 Austin, S. Are you liable for telephone advice? *Nursing.* 2008;38:6-7. Retrieved from http://journals.lww.eom/nursing/fulltext/2008/09001/are_you_liable_for_telephone_advice_.2.aspx

12 Purc-Stephenson, R.J. and Thrasher, C. (2010). Nurses' experiences with telephone triage and advice: A meta-ethnography. *Journal of Advanced Nursing.* 66(3): 482-494

13 American College of Physicians (ACEP) and Emergency Nurses Association (ENA) joint position statement on Standardized ED Triage Scale and Acuity Categorization. ENA. July 2010. Retrieved from

https://www.ena.org/SiteCollectionDocuments/Position%20Statements/STANDARDIZEDEDTRIAGESCALEANDACUITYCATEGORIZATION.pdf
14 Emergency Nurses Association. (2011). Emergency Nursing Scope and Standards of Practice. 1st edition. Des Plaines, IL.
15 ACEP Policy Statement *"Providing Telephone Advice from the Emergency Department."* Retrieved from http://www.acep.org/Clinical—Practice-Management/Providing-Telephone-Advice-from-the-Emergency-Department/

Authors

Authored and Reviewed by the Position Statement Committee
Diane Gurney, MS, RN, CEN, FAEN, Chair
Katie Bush, MA, RN, CEN, SANE-A
Melanie Crowley, MSN, RN, CEN
Gordon Gillespie, PhD, DNP, RN, CEN, CPEN, CNE, PHCNS-BC, FAEN
Steven Jewell, BSN, RN
Robin Walsh, MS, BSN, RN
E. Marie Wilson, MPA, RN

ENA 2015 Board of Directors Liaison
Sally Snow, BSN, RN, CPEN, FAEN

ENA Staff Liaisons
Dale Wallerich, MBA, BSN, RN

Developed: 2015.
Approved by the ENA Board of Directors: April 1991.
Revised and Approved by the ENA Board of Directors: September 1992.
Revised and Approved by the ENA Board of Directors: September 1994.
Revised and Approved by the ENA Board of Directors: September 1996.
Revised and Approved by the ENA Board of Directors: September 1998.
Revised and Approved by the ENA Board of Directors: December 2001.
Revised and Approved by the ENA Board of Directors: July 2010.
Revised and Approved by the ENA Board of Directors: December, 2015.

This position statement, including the information and recommendations set forth herein, reflects ENA's current position with respect to the subject matter discussed herein based on current knowledge at the time of publication, is only current as of the publication date, and is subject to change without notice as new information and advances emerge. The positions, information and recommendations discussed herein are not codified into law or regulations. Variations in practice and a practitioner's best nursing judgment may warrant an approach that differs from the recommendations herein. ENA does not approve or endorse any specific sources of information referenced. ENA assumes no liability for any injury and/or damage to persons or property arising from the use of the information in this position statement.

APPENDIX C

Special Populations

Appendix C: Telephone Triage of Low Literacy Populations

These guidelines were designed to address the informational needs of low literacy populations as well as college educated callers. Thus, the home treatment instructions and disease descriptions are written at the fifth- to eighth-grade literacy level. This step facilitates communications by 'preprocessing the information, translating it into lay language at the most basic literacy level." This accomplishes two important functions: 1) Patients can quickly process the information, and 2) the nurse is spared those tasks, while she/he is performing the arduous intellectual task of critical thinking.

As a teaching and assessment tool, these protocols are designed to be user friendly. The true "end user" is the patient. For the caller with low literacy skills, questions and instructions must be clear, detailed and specific. Since the nurse often does not know when she/he is speaking to someone with low literacy skills, it is best to write instructions to the broadest possible literacy level—that of the fifth-grade reading level.

According to some experts, "23 million American adults may not be able to comprehend what health professionals are talking about." Communication is a complex process. While the low literacy client's listening comprehension may be better than reading comprehension, low literacy clients have special communication barriers. Common barriers to communication include Patient overcompliance, anxiety, and masking.

Over-compliance is a common coping mechanism of low literacy clients. They tend to agree to whatever is asked of them, perhaps out of embarrassment. It is best to explore the situation further when clients seem overcompliant.

A second barrier is patient anxiety. Patients may have difficulty processing information when they are worried or anxious about not understanding. We can help reduce anxiety by establishing trust and showing warmth, and writing protocols in language, which is easily understandable.

A third barrier to comprehension is "masking." "Masking" occurs when the client is very concrete or misunderstands the meaning of a word, which has many meanings. We can help to overcome this barrier by realizing that sometimes low literacy clients are very concrete or literal. We can ask the caller to repeat back our instructions to clarify their understanding.

In order to achieve strong patient understanding and reliable compliance, we must link already known information with new ideas—creating a frame of reference. There are two ways to do this: One is to make a point as vivid as possible and to teach the smallest amount of information to do the job.

Methods to make information vivid include

1. Writing at fourth or fifth grade reading level—avoid multisyllable words.
2. Using detailed, concrete, specific information.
3. Using a conversational style—short, precise, natural sounding sentences.
4. Using terminology consistently.

Teach the smallest amount possible to do the job. Organize information into chunks: "Advance organizers," tells the patient what you are about to tell them. Like explaining the "facts of life," don't overwhelm the listener with too much information or details. Think about what the client needs to know to "survive"—what, when, how and which complications to watch for. Finally, telling the caller "w'hy" they are doing a certain treatment w'ill help to get caller "buy in" and facilitate compliance. Examples of these can be found in the Supplemental Information Sections:

1. Signs/symptoms/cause
2. Possible complications
3. Prevention
4. Treatment goal (why) and activities

REFERENCES

Daugird, A. J,, & Spencer, D. C. (1989). Characteristics of patients who highly utilize telephone medical care in a private practice. *The Journal of Family Practice, 27,* 420-421.

Finley, R. (1995). *Polypharmacy and the elderly.* Presented at the Contemporary Forums Conference, Telephone Triage: Essential for Expert Practice, Dublin, CA.

Fletcher, K. (1995). *Polypharmacy in the elderly.* Presented at the Contemporary Forums Conference, Telephone Triage: Essential for Expert Practice, Dublin, CA.

Guy, D. H. (1995). Telephone care for elders. *Journal of Gerontological Nursing. 12,* 27-34.

Nobles-Knight, D. (1995). *Polypharmacy in the elderly.* Lecture presented at the Contemporary Forums Conference, Telephone Triage: Essential for Expert Practice, Dublin, CA.

Osgood, N.). (1985). *Suicide in the elderly.* Richmond, VA Aspen.

Wheeler, S. Q. (1993). *Telephone triage: Theory, practice and protocol development.* Albany, NY: Delmar.

APPENDIX D

Miscellaneous Supplemental Information

APPENDIX D: Miscellaneous Supplemental Information

BIOTERRORISM INFORMATION

PLEASE NOTE: It is advisable to establish a policy related to bioterrorism calls. Calls that arouse suspicions must be treated as emergent or urgent. Nurses should *always contact 911 first* to arrange for paramedic transport. In cases where there is suspicion of biochemical exposure, contact or transfer the call to 911 and Hazardous Materials teams to manage the call. Generally speaking, EMDs are more expert and have better access to resources than nurses do.

The telephone triage nurse may unwittingly be thrust into the role of first responder to initial or ongoing outbreaks of bioterrorism-related illness. The term "first responder" refers to the nurse's role in *identifying* suspicious-sounding symptoms. The nurse should use this information any time there are unusual symptom presentations or patterns. Assess all suspicious symptoms described by callers who may have, *unknowingly,* been exposed to biological or chemical weapons.

The list below was developed by the CDC and further adapted and modified for telephone triage nurse use. The Global pattern of biological or chemical terrorism is as follows:

- Symptoms: Sudden onset
- Patients: In large numbers
- Patients Not normally affected (i.e., young, previously healthy adults and children)
- Patient presentation Acutely ill
- Patient presentation: Rapid disease progression, i.e., from upper respiratory symptoms and bronchitis to life-threatening pneumonia and systemic infections

BIOTERRORISM RED FLAGS

Review' the Red Flags below frequently and remain alert for the following patterns, which may be indicators of bioterrorist events:

- Large numbers of ill persons calling with similar disease or syndrome
- Large numbers of unexplained disease, syndromes, or deaths
- Unusual increases in illness in a population (e.g., an increase in influenza-like illness that might be anthrax in disguise or an increase in poxlike illness that might be smallpox)
- Atypical geographic or seasonal distribution of a disease (e.g.. Tularemia in a nonendemic area, influenza in the summer)
- Atypical patient distribution (e.g., several adults with unexplained rash, previously healthy populations)
- 111 persons presenting near the same time (unusual surges in call volumes)
- Reports of death or illness among animals, which may be unexplained or attributed to a bioterrorist agent, that precedes or accompanies illness or death in humans
- Unusual disease presentation (e.g., pulmonary versus cutaneous anthrax)
- Unexplained increase in incidence in endemic disease (e.g.. Tularemia, plague)
- Simultaneous clusters of similar illness in noncontiguous areas (neither adjacent nor bordering), domestic or foreign disease transmitted through aerosols, food, or water suggestive of sabotage

In the case of confirmed bioterrorism diagnoses, EDs must inform the State Health Department, CDC, and FBI. For the latest information, refer to CDC Web site at www.bt.cdc.gov

Herbal Supplements Associated with Illnesses and Injuries

FREQUENTLY ASKED QUESTIONS

Who Should Not Use Supplements?

- Before starting a dietary supplement, check with your doctor. This is extremely important for people who
  —Are pregnant or breastfeeding.
  —Have chronic illness like HIV, heart problems, high blood pressure, diabetes.
  —Are over the age of 50 or under the age of 18.
  —Are taking any prescription or over-the-counter medicines. Certain supplements can raise blood levels of certain drugs to dangerous levels.
- For example, garlic and the supplement ginkgo biloba both thin the blood, which can be dangerous for people taking prescription medicines that also thin the blood.

Who Can Help Me Make Decisions?

- In addition to medical doctors, other health care professionals, such as registered pharmacists, registered dietitians and nutritionists, also can be sources of information about dietary supplements.

How Can I Tell if a Product Is Fraudulent?

- Fraudulent products are products that don't do what they say they can or don't contain what they say they contain. They waste consumers' money, and they may cause physical harm. You can tell which ones are fraudulent products by the types of claims made on labels and in advertising. Some possible signs of fraud are
  —Words like "secret cure,""breakthrough," "magical," "miracle cure," and "new discovery." If the product were a cure for a serious disease, it would be widely reported in the media and used by health care professionals.
  —Medical sounding words such as "detoxify," "purify," and "energize" to describe the way the product works. These claims are vague and hard to measure. So, they make it easier for the product makers to claim success, even though nothing has actually been accomplished.
  —Claims that the product can cure a lot of different diseases. No product can do that.
  —Claims that a product is backed by scientific studies that have no list of references (medical studies). In some cases, the references are incomplete, the citations cannot be traced, or if they are traceable, the studies are out-of-date, irrelevant, or poorly developed.
  —Claims that the supplement has only benefits—and no side effects. A product strong enough to help people will be strong enough to cause side effects.
  —Claims that the medical profession, drug companies, and the government are stopping information about it.
- Though it may be hard, consumers also can protect themselves from economic fraud. Economic fraud is the act of using inferior, cheaper ingredients and then passing it off as the real thing but at a lower cost. Avoid products sold for considerably less money than competing brands. If it's too cheap, the product is probably not what it's supposed to be.

How Can I Know if a Product Is High Quality?

- Poor manufacturing practices are not unique to dietary supplements, but the growing market for supplements in a less restrictive regulatory environment creates the potential for supplements to be prone to quality-control problems. For example, the FDA has identified several problems where some manufacturers were buying herbs, plants, and other ingredients without first adequately testing them to determine whether the product they ordered was actually what they received or whether the ingredients were free from contaminants. To help protect themselves, consumers should note the following:

—Look for ingredients in products with the U.S. Pharmacopoeia notation, which indicates the manufacturer followed standards established by the U.S. Pharmacopoeia.

—Realize that the label term "natural" doesn't guarantee that a product is safe. "Think of poisonous mushrooms," says one expert, "They're natural."

—Consider the name of the manufacturer or distributor. Supplements made by a nationally known food and drug manufacturer, for example, have likely been made under tight controls because these companies already have in place manufacturing standards for their other products.

—Write to the supplement manufacturer for more information. Ask the company about the conditions under which its products were made.

What Should I Do if I Have Side Effects?

- Consumers who use dietary supplements should always read product labels, follow' directions, and heed all warnings. Supplement users who suffer a serious harmful effect or illness that they think is related to supplement use should call a doctor or other health care provider. He or she in turn can report it to FDA MedWatch by calling 1 -800-FDA-1088 or going to http :/Avww.· fda.gov/medwatch/report/hcp.htm on the MedWatch Web site. Patients' names are kept confidential.
- Consumers also may call the toll-free MedWatch number or go to http :/Avww. fda.gov/medwatch/report/consumer/c onsurner.htm on the MedWatch Web site to report an adverse reaction. To file a report, consumers will be asked to provide

—Name, address, and telephone number of the person who became ill.

—Name and address of the doctor or hospital providing medical treatment.

—Description of the problem.

—Name of the product and store where it was bought.

- Consumers also should report the problem to the manufacturer or distributor listed on the product's label and to the store where the product was bought.

How Do I Get More Information?

The list of herbal supplements below is based on the 1998 list issued by the Food and Drug Administration Web site. For the most up-to-date information, visit http //www.fda.gov.

HERBAL INGREDIENTS

- Chaparral (a traditional American Indian medicine). Possible health hazards Liver disease, possibly irreversible.
- Comfrey. Possible health hazards: Obstruction of blood flow to liver, possibly leading to death.
- Slimming/dieter's teas. Possible health hazards Nausea, diarrhea, vomiting, stomach cramps, chronic constipation, fainting, possibly death (See Dieter's Brews Make Tea Time a Dangerous Affair in the July-August 1997 *FDA Consumer).*
- Ephedra (also known as Ma huang, Chinese Ephedra, and epitonin). Possible health hazards Ranges from high blood pressure, irregular heartbeat, nerve damage, injury, insomnia, tremors, and headaches to seizures, heart attack, stroke, and death.
- Germander. Possible health hazards: Liver disease, possibly leading to death.
- Lobelia (also known as Indian tobacco). Possible health hazards Ranges from breathing problems at low doses to sweating, rapid heartbeat, low blood pressure, and possibly coma and death at higher doses.
- Magnolia-Stephania preparation. Possible health hazards: Kidney disease, possibly leading to permanent kidney failure.
- Willow bark. Possible health hazards: Reye syndrome, a potentially fatal disease associated with aspirin intake in children with chickenpox or flu symptoms; allergic reaction in adults. (Willow bark is marketed as an aspirin-free product, although it actually contains an ingredient that converts to the same active ingredient in aspirin.)
- Wormwood. Possible health hazards Neurological symptoms, characterized by numbness of legs and arms, loss of intellect, delirium, and paralysis.

VITAMINS AND ESSENTIAL MINERALS

- Vitamin A (in doses of 25,000 or more International Units a day). Possible health hazards: Birth defects, bone abnormalities, and severe liver disease.
- Vitamin B_6 (in doses above 100 mg a day). Possible health hazards Balance difficulties, nerve injury causing changes in touch sensation.

- Niacin (in slow-released doses of 500 mg or more a day or immediate-release doses of 750 mg or more a day). Possible health hazards: Range from stomach pain, vomiting, bloating, nausea, cramping, and diarrhea to liver disease, muscle disease, eye damage, and heart injury.
- Selenium (in doses of about 800 meg to 1000 meg a day). Possible health hazards: Tissue damage.

OTHER SUPPLEMENTS

- Germanium (a nonessential mineral). Possible health hazards Kidney damage, possibly death.
- L-tryptophan (an amino acid). Possible health hazards: Eosinophil ia myalgia syndrome, a potentially fetal blood disorder that can cause high fever, muscle and joint pain, weakness, skin rash, and swelling of the arms and legs.

FEDERAL AGENCIES

Food and Drug Administration

Food Information Line
1-888-723-3366
(202)205-4314 in the Washington, D.C., area
FDA Web site http://www.cfsan.fda.gov/dms/supplmnt.html. Accessed 8/2008.

HEALTH PROFESSIONAL ORGANIZATIONS

You're Free to Reproduce the Information on the FDA Web Site

Unless otherwise noted, the contents of the FDA Web site ('http://www.fda.govL, both text and graphics, are *not* copyrighted. They are in the public domain and may be republished, reprinted, and otherwise used freely by anyone without the need to obtain permission from FDA. Credit to the U. S. Food and Drug Administration as the source is appreciated but not required. The *FDA also appreciate being informed about use of materials.* Contact FDA, HFI-40, Rockville, MD 20857 or E-mail: webmail@oc.fda.

APPENDIX E

Telephone Triage Standards and Performance Standards

APPENDIX E

TELEPHONE TRIAGE STANDARDS MANUAL

OVERVIEW OF TELEPHONE TRIAGE STANDARDS

A major goal of the Telephone Triage service is to optimize safe, timely access for patients and reduce decision error by the following means:

- Hire high quality RNs.
- Provide excellent training.
- Provide excellent protocols and documentation forms.
- Provide adequate staff (60 calls/8hr/RN).
- Provide feedback mechanism where possible.
- Provide for rotation of phone work and frequent breaks where possible.
- Support the reasonable, prudent approach where possible.

Secondarily, a goal for Telephone Triage services is to include the client population as part of the solution. Clients will not use services that they know nothing about. Therefore, it is reasonable to support the pretriage of calls through the mechanism of a patient brochure, which fosters patient independence and provides for a partnership which supports appropriate, timely access.

Overall management of the service is the responsibility of the program coordinator under the direction of the director of Ambulatory Care Services with the direction and support of upper management. Medical staff and associated departments will collaborate quarterly through Steering Committee meetings.

LINE MANAGEMENT

- The telephone triage program coordinator (PC) is a practitioner with appropriate clinical and managerial experience and/or the potential for it. The PC is selected by Ambulatory Care Administration to assume responsibility for the effective functioning of staff, including collaborating with clinic managers on their development and evaluation. The PC is responsible for the efficient functioning of telephone triage and the quality of telephone triage provided in this setting.
- The clinic manager assigns a shift coordinator to oversee the 8 (10 or 12) hr shift in order to facilitate service communication, coordination, and delivery of patient care.
- Nursing standards will be reviewed and updated annually by the Steering Committee. After approval from nursing and medical administration, these standards will outline additional nursing functions and responsibilities within telephone triage.

MEDICAL ADMINISTRATION

- The chiefs of the various medical, surgical, and special services shall be available to the PC, clinic managers, and shift coordinators for the purpose of resolving conflicts and/or providing medical direction in the case of unavailability of a primary care physician.
- The director of Ambulatory Care Services shall be available to the PC and clinic managers regarding nurse-physician communications, adequacy of direction provided to the nursing staff, and general working relationships.

STEERING COMMITTEE

This committee is an ad hoc group consisting of representatives from Poison Control, Medicine, Emergency Department, Education and Professional Development, Marketing Ambulatory Care Administration, and Nursing Staff and Management. This committee meets quarterly to discuss matters related to the Telephone Triage Program. The Director of Ambulatory Care Services selects members.

HOURS OF OPERATION

Telephone Triage is a telephone management system, which provides adult triage during clinic hours and after hours (all day, year round).

USE OF TELEPHONE TRIAGE SERVICES

Criteria

- All callers are considered clients for Telephone Triage services, whether they are experiencing acute, or potentially acute illness or injury in single or multiple body systems, or are seeking education, information, counseling, advocacy or referral.
- Telephone recordings will be available in three languages, notifying clients that they are on hold and will be helped soon. Callers will be advised to call 911 for life-threatening emergencies and to call Poison Control for poisoning information and assistance.
- Other client populations served include
  —Clients seeking medical advice and education for home treatment.
  —Clients seeking health-related information including hospital approved written reference materials, community resources, and hotlines.

—Clients seeking referrals, i.e., physician, pharmacist, community resource, support groups, hotlines, hospital services, and in-house self-care and self-help programs.

—Clients seeking emotional support and counseling.

—Clients seeking information and support as health consumer or self-advocate (patients' rights, second opinions, living wills, etc.)

Limitations

- Telephone Triage is not designed as a message-answering service for physicians.
- Telephone Triage will not fill prescriptions at client request.
- AIDS related questions would be referred directly to the AIDS hotline.
- Drug-related questions will be referred directly to the pharmacist.
- Poison related questions will be transferred directly to Poison Control.
- Crisis level calls will be managed per the appropriate crisis intervention protocol.

Demand for Information/Service Beyond Capacity (Call Volume)

- The capacity of Telephone Triage is 60 calls per 8 hr per practitioner (7 calls/hr). When call volume is in excess of budgeted daily call volume, it is the responsibility of the shift coordinator to notify the clinic manager for staffing consideration.
- Nursing staff (shift coordinator) will collaborate as needed with clinic manager to validate call acuity, volume, and peak volume times, including

—"Flu season"

—Weekends, Holidays

—Peak hours

—Disaster

Call Duration (Talk Time)

- General guidelines. Client and problem acuity and need for emotional/informational support determines the amount of time spent on each call.
- Average duration of call. The *average duration* of call is 8.5 min. Generally, this time period allows for safe, effective interactions for all populations, including elderly, high risk, low income, and multicultural populations.
- Timely disposition. All available resources will be used to facilitate timely disposition of all calls, i.e., crisis intervention, referral, informational, educational, and counseling.
- Chronic callers. Chronic callers shall be noted by shift coordinators and referred to Department of Social Services or Public Health Nurses as necessary.

Disposition

- Information. All disposition information will be documented.
- Disposition (When, where, and by whom client will be seen/treated). Clients will be classified according to one or more of the following criteria:

—Emergent ("Immediate"—0 min—1 hr)

—Urgent (I hr—8 hr)

—Acute (8—24 hours)

—Nonacute/Appt (24+ hr)

—Advice

GOVERNING RULES OF AREA

General Safety

- Traffic/visitor control. Telephone Triage is not to be used by hospital personnel as a thoroughfare. Traffic is limited to physicians and staff conducting the business of client service.
- Students. The management staff of Telephone Triage will adhere to the Department of Nursing Policy regarding institutional affiliation as well as specific role of nursing students as described in Addendum B.

Confidentiality and HIPAA

- Client information. All client information is highly confidential and is protected by the Health Insurance Portability and Accountability Act of 1996 (HIPAA) and Hospital Patient Bill of Rights.
- Discussion of client information in areas of public traffic is a violation of hospital policy and is considered a major disciplinary offense.
- Client records are to be in the hands of the appropriate employee at all times. Clients requesting to see own records may do so in the presence of medial record staff.
- Media request for information. Telephone Triage staff may not give out information by phone to any media representative unless prior arrangements have been made with administration (See Hospital Policy on Confidentiality).
- Duplication of client records. No client record may be copied except that which is for transfer or educational activity (See Hospital Policy on Client Records).
- Regulations governing AIDS testing Knows and adheres to current AIDS confidentiality laws.

STAFFING

Quantity

- Staffing. Telephone Triage is staffed with sufficient number of professional personnel to provide established minutes of nursing care to an average daily call volume as outlined in the annual budget. Staffing will always provide for no less than 75% regular service staff.
- Acuity levels. Changing acuity levels and/or increased call volume demanding increased nursing coverage shall be met via intervention of the shift coordinator and/or PC. Additional staff is provided via (1) approved overtime by full-time employees (double shifts), (2) additional hours by part-time employees, and (3) use of per diem ambulator)' care float personnel. Appropriate records of staff utilization are maintained by the service.
- The program manager/clinic manager in cooperation with the shift coordinator makes staffing adjustments.
- Regular scheduling. The clinic manager defines and has responsibility for adhering to the Telephone Triage staffing pattern. This pattern is based on staffing parameters outlined above as well as Personnel Policy regarding staffing.
- Clinic manager is responsible for scheduling nursing staff to provide adequate Telephone Triage services to clients and adhering to policy that all clients have access to an RN staff member (See Addendum A, Scheduling Policies).
- Management coverage. The clinic manager will designate a responsible person to manage in their absence.
- Assignments and protocols will be addressed as outlined in Delivery of Care Methodology of these policies.

Delivery of Care Methodology

- The method of patient care delivery of Telephone Triage is consistent with the goals and philosophy of the Ambulatory Care Health Services.
- See Addendum C for "Delivery of Care Methodology" on Telephone Triage.

Preparation

- Selection

  —The program/clinic manager in collaboration with the director of Ambulatory Care Services will hire staff for Telephone Triage service. Staff selection will be based on current vacancies, educational and experiential background, and the interview process.

  —See Addendum D.

- Orientation

  —All Telephone Triage staff will participate in hospital and service orientation programs, which are structured, formalized, and individualized.

  —See Addendum D.

- Basic preparation/internship

  —All staff will have an additional period of review at the end of the 3-wk orientation period based on Telephone Triage standards, nursing responsibilities for the specific client population, and identified learning needs of the new staff member.

  —Orientation schedule is as follows:

  c Week 1,2,3: Meet weekly with the preceptor to set goals for the next week,

  o Weeks 4,8, and 12 Meet with preceptor, clinic manager, and AHN and Education and Professional Development person to set goals for the following month.

  o Month 6 and 9: Meet with above people for written evaluation and goals.

- Continuing education

  —All staff will participate in continuing education related to the Telephone Triage service. These educational activities will be based on routine and new responsibilities of nursing staff, patient care review activities.

  —Staff will be expected to attend all mandatory events dealing with the following issues:

  c CPR and Emergency Measures

  o Safety (general, electrical, fire, and disaster)

  o Infection control review

  c AIDS update

  c General hazardous materials

  —Educational records will be maintained within the Telephone Triage service. It is the responsibility of each staff member to maintain her/his own record. This record will be updated quarterly. Participation in continuing education is an essential component of the employee appraisal process and Telephone Triage quality improvement plans.

- Maintaining/assuring competency

  —All staff will be expected to participate in periodic evaluation to determine learning needs. This will include surveys, questionnaires, and unsolicited suggestions for continuing education programs.

  —Staff will also be expected to participate in competency evaluations, which will be conducted as joint activity by Clinical Educations, Clinical Specialist, and Telephone Triage management team. Annual testing will be conducted to validate cognitive and skill knowledge base relative to the work and client population.

—Finally, staff will be expected to participate in ongoing quality improvement activities for the ongoing purpose of assuring compliance to Telephone Triage standards, identifying learning needs and identify ing/resoling staff/unit/patient-care problems.

RESPONSIBILITIES—ADVICE NURSES

- Demonstrates knowledge of and use of nursing process in carrying out Telephone Triage services to include triage, crises intervention, and client education.
- Demonstrates knowledge of and use of physical/psychosocial assessment skills as specified in protocols.
- Acts as public relations representative for the hospital.
- Markets hospital services and programs, as appropriate.
- Identifies need for protocol and forms update and revisions as necessary. Submits suggestions to PC.

Organization Chart Narrative

Telephone Triage is a patient service that facilitates appropriate and timely access, while enhancing system cost effectiveness.

The success of Telephone Triage depends on quality service. It is therefore recommended that a steering committee meet on a regular basis to guide this project, but maintain a direct reporting system to one department to ensure program effectiveness.

The organizational charts reflect the optional reporting system, but they both include a Steering Committee made up of the following departments: Nursing, ED, Marketing, Administration, and Medicine.

TELEPHONE ORGANIZATION CHART

DIRECTOR, AMULATORY CARE SERVICES

I

TELEPHONE TRIAGE
STEERING COMMITTEE

I

TELEPHONE TRIAGE
PROJECT COORDINATOR

I

CLINIC MANAGERS

I

SHIFT COORDINATOR

l

TELEPHONE TRIAGE NURSES

Job Description

Position Title Program Coordinator, Telephone Triage
Reports to Director of Ambulatory Care Services
Summary The *program coordinator* is a first line manager designated as the leader for Telephone Triage service, its patient population, and assigned staff He/she has responsibility and accountability for all Telephone Triage activities, service operation, and staff function.

SPECIAL CHARACTERISTICS

- The program coordinator is a skilled communicator who is experienced in maintaining communication mechanisms among professional staff, outside agencies, patients, and family.
- The program coordinator demonstrates leadership skills to include delegation, organization, and problem Identification/solving skills.
- Functions as a role model in his/her clinical specialty.

DUTIES AND RESPONSIBILITIES

The program coordinator will

- Demonstrate competency in clinical knowledge of Telephone Triage, judgment, and technical skills. Provide clinical direction to staff Evaluate the level of care provided by the nursing staff.
- Demonstrate awareness of hospital and departmental policies, participate in their development as appropriate, and use these as a basis for decision making for both clinical and management issues.
- Demonstrate awareness of and adherence to safety and legal requirements established at the hospital and department level w'ith emphasis on those pertinent to the Telephone Triage service.
- Participate in budgetary planning and implementation for the department.
- Serve on committees, task forces, and work groups on a voluntary and appointed basis at the department and hospital level. Participate actively, and complete follow-up activities in a consistent manner.
- Participate in the development of criteria-based job descriptions as directed. Write performance standards for employees of Telephone Triage service.
- Actively develop standards for the Telephone Triage service to define service function, staff performance, and patient care activities.
- Actively participate in licensing and accreditation process.
- Plan and implement service-based quality improvement activities. Share results for integration at the department level.
- Participate in personnel functions to include (1) annual and ongoing performance appraisal on employees; (2) engage in annual licensure validation for employees; (3) recruit, interview, select and hire nursing employees. Endeavor to maintain stable staff and minimize staff turnover.
- Independently and in conjunction with others, plan and participate in the clinical and leadership development of employees in the Telephone Triage service. Maintain accurate records and evaluate effectiveness of activities.
- Assess self-learning needs. Seeks ways to meet those needs and to maintain current competency and respond to new clinical and management demands.
- Remain aware of current nursing research and implement relevant findings as appropriate.

QUALIFICATIONS

- Current State License
- BSN required
- Prior proven experience and medical surgical nursing (minimum 3-5 yr)
- Prior proven experience and expertise in management
- Excellent verbal and written communication skills
- Strong pediatric and OB/GYN background preferred
- Telephone Triage experience or formal training
- Demonstrates computer literacy
- Meets requirements of employee physical

Job Description

Position Title: Telephone Triage Nurse

Reports to: Clinic Manager

JOB SUMMARY

The telephone triage nurse is a health care professional that assumes responsibility and accountability for a group of clients for a designated time frame. The triage nurse provides Telephone Triage services to clients via therapeutic use of self, protocols, the environment/instrumentation, and other telephone triage and crises intervention team members.

- Demonstrates knowledge of and use of nursing process in carrying out Telephone Triage.
- Demonstrates knowledge of and use of physical/ psychosocial assessment skills as specified in key questions and protocols.
- Acts as public relations representative for facility services and programs, as appropriate.
- Acts as an information broker and referral agent, using approved references and referrals.
- Identifies need for protocol and forms update and revisions as necessary. Submits suggestions to manager.

SPECIAL CHARACTERISTICS

- Demonstrates an awareness of own responsibility and accountability for professional practice.
- Demonstrates strong communication skills. Uses lines of authority appropriately. Delegates tasks and duties appropriately when directing and coordinating health care team members, client care, and department activities.
- Demonstrates effective problem identification and resolution skills as a method of sound decision making.

DUTIES/RESPONSIBILITIES:

The telephone triage nurse will

- Demonstrate a sound knowledge base and decision making for a diverse client population with a w'ide range of problems and acuity.
- Perform effectively in crisis intervention, follow established protocols, remaining calm, informing appropriate persons, and documenting events.
- Perform assessment/data collection in an ongoing and systematic manner, focusing on physiological, psychological, educations, resource referral, and cognitive status.
- Document in timely, accurate, comprehensive and concise manner.
- Formulate sound working diagnosis.
- Select protocols appropriately.
- Instruct patients in an articulate, skillful, consistent and professional manner.
- Base client care on expressed needs and available resources of time, personnel, and equipment.
- Evaluate effectiveness of client self-care as appropriate.
- Identify client/significant other learning needs and implement appropriate measures to meet these.
- Demonstrate awareness and sensitivity to rights of client, as identified within the institution.
- Demonstrate awareness of legal issues in all aspects of Telephone Triage service function. Strive to manage situations to reduce legal risks.
- Seek validation of knowledge base, skill level, and decision making as necessary. Assertively seek guidance in areas of question. Participate in continuing education to meet own professional development.
- Participate in peer review, and Telephone Triage service and department quality improvement activities as well as standards development.
- Be aware of safety issues as identified by the institution.
- Participate actively as preceptor for staff development activities for Telephone Triage service personnel.
- Participate in nursing research activities as requested.
- Remain flexible in staffing patterns and resolution of staffing conflicts; perform related duties as required.

TELEPHONE TRIAGE NURSE—JOB QUALIFICATIONS

All attempts will be made to employ staff with previous medical/surgical experience compatible with the Telephone Triage population of clients and surrounding community. If this is not possible, applicant learning ability, motivation, or leadership potential will be carefully considered at the time of the interview'. The ideal candidate will be a trained, mature, and experienced RN with good judgment.

Personal Qualifications

- Ability to make good medical decisions under conditions of uncertainty and urgency
- Ability to set priorities
- Good judgment
- Excellent written and spoken communications skill
- Excellent interpersonal skills

In addition, applicants with the following life/work experience are preferred:

- Applicants who are parents or possess pediatric experience
- Applicants who possess OB/GYN experience. Generally, applicants will have
  - —A minimum of 5 yrs recent experience in medical/surgical nursing or clinic setting
  - —Recent experience in Critical Care or Emergency Department desirable
- Triage experience (walk-in or telephone)—Preferred
- Case management skill—Preferred
- Bilingual (preferred)—Spanish
- Current BLS certification
- Demonstrates good judgment and problem solving skills
- Demonstrates a caring manner with clients
- Works well independently
- Functions well under pressure
- Works effectively with
  - —Culturally diverse populations
  - —Educationally diverse and illiterate populations
  - —Non-English speaking populations
  - —High-risk populations
- Able to serve as resource/liaison for clients, clerical staff, physicians, nurses, telephone triage nurses, medical assistants,____________________________ ED staff,____________________________ poison control, and clinic administrators.

Applicants lacking the above experience are required to take refresher courses as part of the conditions of employment

Sample Performance Standards

Title RN Performance Standards for the Telephone Triage function

Clinic:____

Purpose: To define the daily expectation of this employee category

CONTENT

Nursing Process

Assessment

- Performs client assessment for all callers to Telephone Triage services
- Documents required data on triage form (per triage form directives and guidelines) or electronic medical record (EMR) (per EMR guidelines)
- Obtains specific data (physical, psychosocial, and cultural) from patient and family, significant others, other health care providers and medical record(s) as appropriate
- Assesses and interprets client symptoms
- Able to assess clients within an average of 7-10 min, as appropriate, using the appropriate guidelines and protocol(s)
- Documents working diagnosis and states to client
- Performs follow-up assessment, as appropriate, 1-24 hr after initial call

Plan

- Selects and implements the appropriate protocol(s) (plan of care) utilizing assessment information
- Implements protocol directives (per protocol directives and guidelines)
- Modifies and/or individualizes plan as appropriate and documents all modifications to protocol plan
- Establishes priorities for care based on
  —Presenting symptoms/chief complaint
  —Appointment availability
- Includes patient/family/significant others in the development of nursing care
- Collaborates with other health disciplines as necessary (Pharmacy, Poison Control, 911, Suicide Prevention, Community Resources and others)

Intervention

- Appropriately implements crisis intervention for life-threatening symptoms.
- Advises (and/or schedules) same day and future appointments appropriately
- Initiates referrals with appropriate agencies
- Provides advice from protocols or approved texts
- Offers counseling and emotional support as appropriate

Evaluation/Teaching for Client Self-Evaluation

- Evaluates the effectiveness of advice as appropriate by
  —For advice only clients: Follow up call(s) as appropriate
  —For appointment clients Chart (EMR) review within 1 wk
- Evaluates client's ability and resources available to effectively carry out self-care measures at home. Determines availability of home treatment materials (OTC meds, thermometer, specific diet, etc.).
- Demonstrates ability to quickl and effectively assess client's learning needs and carry out teaching/advice segment for basic protocols. 15.
- Evaluates client response to protocols in areas specified in protocol and documents as appropriate.
- Judges the effectiveness of current protocol(s) on patient.
- Judges the effectiveness of comfort measures including all nonprescription medications taken within 2-8 hr as appropriate.
- Evaluates client's response to physical and psychological self-care procedures as appropriate
- Evaluates client's/significant other's (SO) ability to carry out self-care, home treatment, and teaching.

Modifies teaching as appropriate.

- Evaluates protocol advice effectiveness as appropriate related to
  —OTC and approved prescription medications
  —First aid measures/home treatment
  —Client advocacy
  —Referral

EDUCATION

Patient, Family, Significant Others

- Maintains adequate amount of client brochures as w>ell as other patient education literature.

Ensures that each caller is aware of client brochure.

- Identifies needed education literature that is needed for clinic managers.
- Refers/schedules patient, family and significant others to appropriate educational classes within the hospital/community, based on identified learning needs.
- Documents actions taken.

- Demonstrates cultural sensitivity in regard to client's learning needs and literacy level. Observes principles of cultural sensitivity when carrying out teaching related to all protocols.
- Uses "layman's language" in communicating with client.
- Acts as patient advocate as appropriate
  —Demonstrates working knowledge and endeavors to meet client needs in the following items:
  oHIPAA
  8 Patient's Bill of Rights
  ⁰ Informed consent
  o Second medical opinions
  —Client Dissatisfaction. Refers dissatisfied clients to_________________________
  —Referrals. Makes appropriate and timely referrals to appropriate self help and support groups, community agencies, and in-house programs and meetings.

Staff and Students

- Functions as a preceptor for new staff as part of orientation programs.
- Acts as a resource for
  —Nursing staff
  —Medical staff
  —Clerical staff
- Provides learning opportunities for students/staff based on identified needs within legal guidelines.
- Evaluates competency level of staff in relation to the learning objectives.

Self-Growth and Development

- Assesses own knowledge, skill, and junction on an ongoing basis. Seeks on-going high practice level. Verifies knowledge and practice constantly. Sets high standards of practice and constantly seeks to fulfill them.
- Participates in formal credentialing mechanism annually. Pursues identified follow-up activities assertively in a timely manner.
- Maintains own records of professional practice. Documents strengths and weaknesses and evidence of professional practice.
- Participates in self-evaluation at performance appraisal by completing evaluation tool, providing documentation of practice, and mutually setting goals for achievement with PC.
- Participates in quarterly coaching and counseling sessions with PC to review accomplishments and short-term goal development.
- Participates in peer review' at performance appraisal time.
- Demonstrates w'illingness to critique own daily practice for errors.
- Documents errors from problem sheets or occurrence reports, and pursues corrective action.
- Demonstrates willingness to critique the practice of coworkers and report inappropriate actions on a timely basis.
- Attends minimum of three in-services per year (given by other staff).
- Reports back on all outside conferences within period of next staff' meeting or six weeks, whichever is appropriate.
- Attends all annual mandatory educational and licensure sessions.
- Engages in daily, informal teaching of other staff members. Documents these activities on own practice record. Communicates general needs to PC for planning purposes.

Practice Management

Orientation:

- Actively participates in staff orientation by
  —Accepting coach/mentor position as requested
  —Using *Service Orientation Manual* as designed
  —Maintaining Orientation Evaluation Tool
  —Giving weekly feedback to clinic manager re orientee performance and progress
  —Participating in orientation evaluation conference

Licensure:

- Maintains current licensure and provides assistant head nurse with copies of
  —RN license
  —State/national certificates
  —Hospital required certifications

Shift Coordinator:

- Each shift will have a shift coordinator assigned by the clinic manager. There will be a back up assigned incase of illness.
- In summary, this role includes but is not limited to
  —Assignments of duties and breaks
  —Coordination of emergency situations as necessary
  —Maintaining contact with the (nurse supervisor) regarding unit problems and staffing
  —Supervision and direction of new staff members
  —Handling of complaints from clients, physicians, and staff, as well as interdepartmental problems

—Preparation and submission of daily log

—Completion of "shift report" for submission to clinic manager; facilitation of nursing office report at end of shift.

—Planning, coordination, and presentation of educational programs in collaboration with PC

—Charge responsibilities (as noted in site-specific manual)

Goal Setting/Attainment:

- Actively commits self to goal accomplishment. Reviews goals as a staff member weekly and participates in quarterly goal summary with clinic manager and staff. Contributes suggestions for new goals.
- Actively volunteers or accepts assignment for projects to achieve Telephone Triage Department goals.

Communications/Meetings (as per site specific standards)

- Documentation. Documents appropriately, using approved terminology and abbreviations. Follows guidelines for use of triage form.
- Bulletin board update. Utilizes bulletin board as communication support.
- Shift report. Gives shift report to shift coordinator as appropriate.
- Communications. Demonstrates effective verbal communication skills in following areas:

  —Telephone

  —Concise report
- Medical consultation. Calls primary MD (after hours-ED/MD on Call) in a timely and appropriate manner to

  —Report client incidents

  —Report abnormal lab work that is likely to require immediate intervention

  —Report changes in client's condition relative to deteriorating vital signs or negative response to home treatment
- Effectively elicits information relative to client needs, comfort and concerns.
- Report. Adheres to report activities by timely and regular attendance as outlined in Delivery of Care Methodology.
- Staff meetings. Attends 75% of service staff meetings; reads minutes when not able to attend; reads posted agenda before meeting; actively participates in discussions of problem identification and resolution.
- Emergency department. Calls ED as appropriate to notify of impending arrival of emergent and urgent level acuity clients.
- Crisis intervention. Communicates effectively and appropriately with members of Crisis Intervention Team (911, Poison Control, Drug Crisis, etc).

Technical Computer Skills

- Is computer literate
- Able to type 50 wpm.
- Competently operates required software programs and EMR.

Safety

- Demonstrates appropriate use of occurrence reports with

  —All unusual calls (homicide, suicide, rape, drug-related, child/spousal/elder abuse)

  —Medication errors

  —All lawsuit threats

Emergency Situations:

- Demonstrates effective response to the following service/client crisis situations as outlined in the telephone advice protocols:

  —Symptoms of shock

  —Symptoms of cardiac arrest

  —Symptoms of respiratory crisis

  —Trauma related symptoms

  —Symptoms of hemorrhage

  —Neurologic complications (seizures, unconsciousness)

  —Symptoms of severe emotional disturbance

  —Symptoms of drug-related problems

  —Documents essential data and disposition for all crisis level calls

Quality Improvement

Poiicy/Procedures/Protocois

- Complies with current applicable standards
- Actively participates in protocol development and review process
- Participates on task forces/quality teams/clinical practice groups as needed and/or requested by clinic manager
- Maintains competency for protocols and support materials contained in protocol book

Knowledge Base

- Is aware of location of, possesses working knowledge of, and ability to use following manuals/references on the unit

  —Telephone Triage protocols in hard copy and electronic versions

—Standards Manual

—Quality Improvement Manual

—Infection Control Manual

—Hazardous Substance Program Manual

—Occupational Injury and Illness Prevention Program Manual

—Emergency Preparedness Manual

- Accesses and utilizes the following reference manuals/ Telephone Triage reference books including, but not l imited to

—Formulary or Drug Reference

—Merck Manual

—Telephone Triage Approved Reference Library

—Communicable Diseases in Man

- Demonstrates ability to locate and use other reference manuals and books on the nursing unit:

—County Phone Book

—Directory of Human Services

—Hospital library

- Demonstrates working knowledge of the following agencies and departments:

—Public health

—Home care

—Hospice management

- Demonstrates ability to interpret lab values and report abnormalities to the physicians.
- Demonstrates the ability to provide Telephone Triage services for clients requiring the following interventions

—Crisis intervention (medical and emotional)

—Telephone Triage (assessment and advice for medical problems)

—Physician referral

—Health education

—Community resource referral (self-help and support groups)

—Hospital programs and services referral

—Hotline referral

o Parental stress

o AIDS

o Sexual assault

o Poison control

—Advocacy, health consumerism

- Demonstrates working knowledge of the following major classification of medications as well as current knowledge of new medications and pharmacological trends. Uses drug references as needed.

—Analgesics

—Anti-inflammatory drugs

—Anesthetics

—Antiasthmatic drugs

—Antibiotics

—Anticonvulsants

—Antifungal drugs

—Antiviral drugs

—Cardiovascular drugs cardiac glycosides, calcium channel blockers, Ace inhibitors, antidysrhythmics, antihypertensive, diuretics, vasodilators, anticoagulants, thrombolytics, antihyperlipidemics

—I mmunosuppressants, immunomodulators

—Chemotherapy

—Contraceptive medications and devices

—Hormone replacement therapy

—Psychotropic drugs

—Steroids

- Demonstrates ability to modify protocol advice after clearly considering implications of appropriateness for client, relationship to current therapy, and integration with nursing standards.

Standards

- Standards/protocol development. Actively identifies new areas for standards/protocol development and communicates these to PC.
- Protocol update/review. Reviews and critiques current protocols and standards for areas of obsolescence or ineffectiveness; participates in annual review[1].
- Continuous quality improvement. Participates in CQI sessions.
- Analysis of present problems. Uses past experiences and results to analyze present problem situations for effective decision making. Demonstrates ability to transfer information from one situation to another.
- Minor problem solving. Assertively attempts to solve minor problems of care, relationships, equipment, supplies, environment prior to PC intervention; documents actions and communicates actions to PC.

Delegalion/Coordinalion

- Carries out shift coordinator role when assigned that duty.
- Participates in Delivery of Care Methodology defined in service structure (Addendum C—Delivery of Care Methodology) with regard to

—Assignment mechanism of clients and unit duties

—Use of nonprofessional personnel

- Actively supervises other members of his/her assignment team via verbal interaction to validate call volume, acuity, and problems.
- Functions as dependable team member, assisting when requested and volunteering when need is obvious. Perceived by other team members as a helpful team member.
- Accepts assignment willingly or discusses concerns appropriately with shift coordinator, keeping continuity and quality of care uppermost in mind.
- Delegates assigned "follow-up clients" to responsible team member in report when going off duty.
- Demonstrates priority setting ability and organizational skills by

—Completing assignment in allotted time

—Maintaining clean and orderly work area

—Minimal use of overtime and obtaining approval ahead of time when possible

—Taking scheduled breaks and dinner times

—Integrating care conferences and in services into work schedule

—Preparing for and attending meetings

—Utilizing clerk for clerical tasks and phone calls

—Timely notification of physician as to client's condition

—Appropriate use of the PC and shift coordinator for problem resolution

Working Relationships/Behaviors

Working Relationships

- Cultivates and maintains effective working relationships with professional staff, coworkers, physicians, and members of Crisis Intervention Team.
- Cultivates and develops working relationships characterized by mutual support, open communication, trust, and respect.
- Separates personal biases and private life from work setting.
- Participates as desired in planning and conducting service social activities (approved by PC in advance) to celebrate personal events for the purpose of maintaining staff morale. Takes into considerations hospital policy governing appropriate and safe social activities.
- Reports irreconcilable differences among coworkers to PC for intervention and possible assignment considerations.
- Gives criticism to others in a private, constructive manner.
- Accepts criticism in a positive manner.
- Demonstrates ability to appropriately challenge questionable protocol treatment and advice.
- Demonstrates appropriate use of colleagues (clinical specialists, medical librarian, physicians, other RNs, dietitian, social worker, pharmacist, hospice, and home health care nurse). Effectively collaborates and coordinates with these resources in planning and delivering service.
- Demonstrates ability to work effectively with the following Crisis Intervention agencies:

—Medical Dispatchers (911)

—Suicide Prevention

—Sexual Assault

—Poison Control

- Demonstrates collaboration and coordination skills in planning and giving telephone advice.

Behaviors

- Is punctual in reporting to work and required meeting.
- Maintains good attendance record. Uses sick time sparingly; adheres to call-in policy defined by Telephone Triage.
- Adheres to facility dress code.
- Maintains positive public relations image with clients/visitors at all times by phone, in rooms, on elevator, and in public places.
- Responds to client request with promptness, empathy, and genuine interest as perceived by clients and coworkers.
- Participates in Telephone Triage annual needs assessment to identify new topics for continuing education.
- Volunteers to teach minimum of two 20-min in services per year to service staff on selected Telephone Triage topics.

Staffing/Flexibilily

- Time schedules. Checks and records posted time schedules on a weekly basis to remain up to date with changes.
- Schedule changes. Demonstrates flexibility in requesting and time changes.
- Floating. Floats to other areas as requested following policy on temporary reassignment.
- Staffing adjustments. Works with shift coordinator in conjunction with PC when staffing assistance is required. Works with shift coordinator to adjust assignments and set priorities to complete assignments.

TELEPHONE TRIAGE ADDENDA

ADDENDUM A

Staffing and Scheduling Policies

MODEL-STAFFING PATTERN FOR TELEPHONE TRIAGE

Weekdays

- Day Shift (trained Telephone Triage RNs)
  —Preferred Staff___________________
  —Minimum Staff___________________
- Evening Shift (trained Telephone Triage RNs)
  —Preferred Staff___________________
  —Minimum Staff___________________
- Night Shift (trained telephone triage RNs)
  —Preferred Staff___________________
  —Minimum Staff___________________

Weekends and Holidays

- Day Shift (trained telephone triage RNs)
  —Preferred Staff___________________
  —Minimum Staff___________________
- Evening Shift (trained Telephone Triage RNs)
  —Preferred Staff___________________
  —Minimum Staff___________________
- Night Shift (trained Telephone Triage RNs)
  —Preferred Staff___________________
  —Minimum Staff___________________

Scheduling is the responsibility of the PC. Time schedules will be written for 6-wk time periods. The draft will be

- Written in the first week of the month (schedule posted)
- Approved in the second week of the month (schedule posted)
- Posted in the third week of the month (schedule posted)

All staff may be scheduled on a rotating basis.

- A request form is used for staff requests for special time on or off. Every effort is made to honor reasonable requests. Request must be submitted in writing at least 6 wk in advance.
- Vacations will be handled as outlined in department policy.
- Staff may trade shifts only after receiving approval from management and completing change request form.

ADDENDUM B
Nursing Students' Observations of Telephone Triage

Students from various university settings often affiliate with the Department of Nursing. Nursing students will be limited in responsibilities to observation only when working within the Telephone Triage system. Nursing instructors will be responsible for establishing orientation dates for themselves and the student groups.

ADDENDUM C
Delivery of Care Methodology for Telephone Triage

METHOD

The method of client care delivery for Telephone Triage is compatible with current goals and philosophy of ambulator)- nursing.

- Call volume. Nurses are assigned to provide Telephone Triage for all incoming calls not to exceed more than 10/hr. Nurses are to perform with consistency and maintain patient continuity.
- Level of urgency. All nurses are assigned to answer all levels of calls from routine to crisis level.
- Staffing. Nurses will deliver care over an 8-, 10-, or 12-hr period.
- Supervision. The RN is responsible for supervision of all other staff that works with Telephone Triage area when management is not available.
- The nurse will always perform the initial assessment on all new callers.
- Telephone Triage means earn ing out all aspects of the nursing process for those tasks that cannot be delegated to nonprofessional staff including:

  —Assessment (data collection and analysis)

  —Problem identification ("working diagnosis" or "impression")

  —Formulation of a client plan of action and disposition

  —Instruction for client self-evaluation of effectiveness of nursing intervention(s) or home treatment

  —Closure and disclaimer

  —Use of appropriate Protocols

  —Medication/treatment advice

  —Documentation

  —Interaction with physician, family, client. Crisis Intervention Team

  —Carrying out teaching from prescribed Protocols and approved books

  —Counseling for emotional or psychological stress

  —Regular shifts are traditionally 8 hr long

ASSIGNMENTS

- Assignments are made by the Clinic Manager.

  —Assignments are based on

  o Client acuity

  ⁰ Staff availability

  ⁰ Staff learning needs, interest, variety

  ⁰ Continuity of client care

  o Limiting the call volume to the maximum projected number of 60 calls per nurse per 8-hr shift

  o Seasonal increases in call volume (i.e., "flu season")

  o Weekly increases in call volume (weekends, holidays)

  ⁰ Predictable patterns of peak call volume (peak times)

  —Assignments may be changed during or after report as deemed necessary by the Shift Coordinator

Report

- Shift report will be written on a shift report form and given orally to the oncoming staff. Routine report will cover:

  —The current status of call volume and acuity

  —Review of current problem calls

  —Review of needed "follow-up" calls. All relevant calls will be reviewed as follows:

  ⁰ Name

  ⁰ Phone number

  ⁰ Age

  ⁰ Symptoms

  ⁰ "Working diagnosis"

  ° Plan

  ⁰ Disposition

  o Immediate needs relevant to next 8 hours

  ⁰ Significant changes in plan for nursing care

  ⁰ Significant emotional, communications, psychological, educational needs or problems

- All staff will give report, remain attentive to client status, and take notes as appropriate.
- Immediately after report, all oncoming staff RNs will make verbal contact with off going staff to validate report information, clarify any questions, and update any changes.
- Immediately following this routine, the oncoming staff will begin answering calls.

ADDENDUM D
Staffing Policies

The following policies are designed to augment current and future staffing policies established by the Nursing and Personnel Departments. They are found in the *Standards Manuals of the Telephone Triage Service* and are shared with new staff. Reviews and updates are preformed on an annual basis.

ORIENTATION

- All new staff in the Telephone Triage service shall receive the general hospital. Department of Nursing, and Ambulatory Services orientation before independent assignment within the Telephone Triage service.
- In Addition, each staff member will receive an additional orientation to the nursing standards and responsibilities of the Telephone Triage service. This orientation period will have written objectives, and structured content. It will consist of a 1-day formal class. This class will consist of a Telephone Triage "core program" and protocol and standards review. During the 4-wk orientation period, calls will be supervised.
- The above Telephone Triage service orientation may be extended as appropriate if the PC feels that the additional time will result in safe, effective, knowledgeable staff members.
- During the additional orientation, educational content may be modified according to the employee's self-evaluation and demonstrated learning needs.

HIRING

- Staff may be recruited from outside the hospital or in-house. The PC will interview all staff after their resume is reviewed for education and nursing experience. All interviewees will be given a tour of the Telephone Triage service. The PC will review the appropriate job description and performance standards with the applicant as well as the Standards Manual. Specific issues discussed will be nursing responsibilities, scheduling, and participative style of unit management.
- All attempts will be made to employ staff with previous medical/surgical experience compatible with the Telephone Triage population of clients and surrounding community. If this is not possible, applicant learning ability, motivation or leadership potential will be carefully considered at the time of the interview.
- Generally, applicants will have
  —At least 3-yr recent experience in medical/surgical nursing or
  —At least 1- to 3- yr recent experience in Critical Care or Emergency Department or in addition, applicants with the following life/work experience are preferred:
  - o Applicants who are parents or possess pediatric experience
  - o Applicants who possess OB/GYN experience

Applicants lacking the above experience are required to take refresher courses as part of the conditions of employment.

- Generally, contingent staff will not be utilized unless extreme staffing shortages exist.
- Part-time staff hired for Telephone Triage will be expected to participate in the general and service orientation schedule on a full-time basis before beginning their part-time schedule.
- Staff members transferring into the Telephone Triage service will be expected to go through the Telephone Triage orientation.
- Regular part-time status is limited to 4 shifts per 2-wk period in order for telephone advice nurse staff to maintain nursing skills, contribute to telephone Triage projects, and keep abreast of communication and changes in the Department and within the Telephone Triage service.

STAFF PREPARATION AND RESPONSIBILITY

- New staff are expected to meet minimum requirements for continued employment by the end of the probationary (3 mo) period to include (but not limited to) the following:
  —Demonstrated clinical competency in basic Telephone Triage assessment and communication skills, plan of action, intervention, and evaluation of education (application of nursing process).
  —Communication skills with peers, physicians, supervisory staff, clients/families. Crisis Intervention Team, pharmacologist.
  —Appropriate documentation according to hospital/department requirements (standards).
  —Demonstrated knowledge of Telephone Triage policy, procedure, and all written standards.
  —Minimum crisis level intervention competency (mock call practicums, Appendix D).

- Staff will perform self-evaluation methods during orientation to identify learning needs; staff will collaborate with PC to need educational deeds by taking advantage of Telephone Triage service continuing education.
- Staff will participate in review of calls at monthly staff meetings. This responsibility is assigned to meet specific learning needs, refine techniques, increase sophistication of work habits, and enhance overall knowledge.

Role-Playing Practicum

Using the scripts, the protocols, a copy of the documentation form and the QA score sheet, three participants take turns role-playing nurse, patient, and evaluator.

- In the nurse role, that participant will use the protocol and documentation form, while interviewing the caller.
- In the patient/caller role, that participant will use the mock call scripts to present the symptoms. "Patients" should neither volunteer too much information initially, nor make it unduly difficult for the nurse to collect information. If information is not included in the script, it is acceptable to "make it up" during the interview process.
- In the evaluator role, that participant should assess whether the nurse is collecting the information listed on the QA score sheet. Listen for key questions and evaluate the documentation as well. Each item collected counts for 2 points. Each item that is volunteered by the patient also counts for 2 points. Items that don't apply (such as questions regarding breastfeeding/pregnancy, inappropriate for males) still count as 2 points. A perfect score is 100 points. A passing score is 70. Failure to obtain the caller's age, be helpful, or ask open-ended questions initially will result in a loss of 10 points for those three reasons. That is because these criteria are so critically important in the history-taking process.
- Each "call" should take no longer that 15 minutes initially, and time efficiency should improve with practice.
- Participants should each take a turn as patient, nurse, or evaluator.
- Feel free to make up your own "mock calls" for ongoing training.
- Ideally, it would be best if the patient calls the nurse from another room, thereby making the call more realistic.

QA AUDIT

ROLE *(*7,10, 15 16)*	Call 1	Call 2	Call 3	Call 4
Helpful Manner: Warm, Friendly, "Business-like"				
Inquisitive, Investigative, timely decisionmaking				
Teaching: Uses Effective, Lay Language				
Crisis Management: Proficiently management of life-threatening & emergent calls. Proficient Warm Transfers				
COMMUNICATION *(*11 Communication)*				
Call Management is Confident, Timely, Professional				
Performs Preliminary Assessment prior to Selecting Guideline & before using "Smart Phrases"				
Consistently inquires about & documents ***repeat Calls***				
Inquires & Rules out Symptoms of Sepsis & Dehydration				
States Impression (Working Diagnosis) in Lay Terms				
States Disposition (When, Where, Why) As Appropriate				
Verbalizes Precautions				
Provides Informed Consent: Understanding & Agreement				
ASSESSMENT *(* 1 Systematic Data Collection)*				
SAVED + 1 or more Assessment Tools				
1. Severe, Strange, Suspicious Symptoms				
2. Age				
3. Veracity				
4. Emotional Distress				
5. Red Flag Symptoms & Populations				
6. SCHOLAR (6-8 items)	#			
7. RAMP (4-5 items)	#			
8. ADL (6-8 items)	#			
9. A DEMERIT (6-8 items)	#			
DECISION MAKING & DISPOSITION *(*2 Data Analysis)*				
Selects Appropriate Guideline				
Uses Guideline Correctly				
Uses Master Guideline Appropriately				
Able to Estimate Symptom Urgency (5-Tier Triage)				
DOCUMENTATION *(*11 Communication)*				
Guideline Title				
Impression with acuity level				
Disposition using 5-Tier Triage Method				
Documents in "real time"				
CONTINUITY: *(*4 Continuity, Coordination)*				
Provides for safe, timely, 5-Tier Triage Dispositions				
SCORE:				

Score 1 point per question, except Assessment tools. NA- 1 for Not Applicable. O for errors.
Total Possible Score: 25-29 . Acceptable Score: 25
**Related 2011 AAACN Standards noted in parentheses*
Related Measures to Avoid Root causes of Error (Joint Commision)

WALL CHART

SAVED: RED FLAG POPULATIONS

Severe/Strange/Suspicious Symptoms:

Severe pain, bleeding, trauma, etc.

Age

Sexually active adolescents (male or female)
All women of childbearing age
All frail elderly

Veracity

Second-party calls
Low literacy
Language barrier
In Elderly: Suspected substance abuse: Incoherent or slurred speech in patient/caretaker
In Elderly: Caretaker unfamiliar w patient

Emotional Status (Caretaker and/or Child)

Hysteria or denial; inappropriate affect in caretaker
Parent or caretaker with history of abuse (physical or sexual), psychiatric problems, or substance abuse

Debilitation

In general, debilitation refers to chronic illness. Chronic illnesses may include but are not limited to the following:

All Populations
AIDS
Asthma
Diabetes
Sickle Cell

Immunocompromised
Lack of adequate immunizations
Chemotherapy
HIV
Splenectomy
Steroid therapy/chronic
Transplants
Nephrotic Syndrome

Adult/Frail Elderly
Cardiac Problems
COPD
Dementia

Distance

Parent/caretaker calling from remote location over 1 hr from hospital.

In emergent situation: Unable to arrive by car within 1 hr because of traffic or lack of available car. Must take public transportation that is sporadic or nonexistent after certain hours at night.

SCHOLAR: PROBLEM HISTORY

Symptoms and associated symptoms
Is it an isolated symptom or a complex of symptoms?
Course of symptoms: Is it better ? Worse? The same?
Characteristics (aids in precise description)
Quantitative (scale of 10)
Qualitative (sharp, dull, pounding)
History of complaint in past
What was done? By whom?
When!' Results?
Onset of symptoms
When started? How long present?
Sudden or gradual? (Sudden = Higher acuity)
Location of symptoms
Strive for precision.
Radiation? (Localized = Higher acuity)
Aggravating factors: What makes it worse?
Relieving factors: What makes it better?

PAMPER: PATIENT HISTORY

Pregnancy/breastfeeding?
Ask all women between ages of 12-50:
"Is there any chance you might be pregnant?
"Have you used birth control consistently and correctly?
Allergies
Food, chemical, drugs, insect bites, cosmetics?
Medications
Current OTC, Rx, and BCP, recreational drugs, alcohol
Previous chronic illness
Recurrent illness, multiple surgeries, family history
Emotional state
Psychiatric history, current reaction to illness
Recent injury, illness, ingestion
Recent accident or child/elder/spouse abuse/neglect
Exposure to communicable disease
Possible ingestion

STRESS BUSTER PROGRAM

Stress Reduction

Hackman and Oldham's Job Characteristics Model

Stress reduction and job satisfaction can be increased by developing the following job characteristics. The more skill variety, task identity and significance, autonomy and feedback that managers can build into the task of telephone triage, the higher will be job satisfaction and stress reduction.

1. Skill variety—the degree to which the job requires a variety of different activities so the worker can use a number of different skills and talents
2. Task identity—the degree to which the job requires completion of a whole and identifiable piece of work
3. Task significance—the degree to which the job has a substantial impact on the lives or work of other people
4. Autonomy—the degree to which the job provides substantial freedom, independence, and discretion to the individual in scheduling the work, and in determining the procedures to be used in carrying it out
5. Feedback—the degree to which carrying out the work activities required by the job results in the individual obtaining direct and clear information about the effectiveness of his or her performance

Why is Telephone Triage So Stressful?

"Telephone Triage is ... high stakes activity ... making decisions under conditions of uncertainty and urgency ... like work of air traffic controller, fire captain, emergency medical dispatcher" (Patel 1995).

1. High-volume systems
2. Lack of training/knowledge
3. Sensory deprivation
4. Lack of acknowledgment/status
5. Angry callers
6. High-stress work
7. Uncertainty: Lack of feedback about outcome and QA

Job satisfaction can be increased by managing the volume, knowledge deficits, sensory deprivation, lack of status, caller hostility, and uncertainty to any degree that is reasonably possible.

"STRESS BUSTER" PROGRAM

The cumulative effect of several stressors can result in burnout and high levels of stress. Conversely, certain activities and remedies can also have a cumulative effect of stress reduction. Create a workspace and mental attitude that is rich in stress reduction triggers as illustrated below:

The External Environment

1. Clear your desk: Uncluttered, pleasant workspaces are restful and calming. Clutter is visually tiring.
2. Personalize your workspace: Pictures of places and people and/or things (plants, stones, icons, and goldfish) can calm and center you between calls.

   Visual vacations Posters of scenes you won't tire of, like vacation spots or nature.
3. Workstation Ergonomic/head set/light/air/quiet/ sense of repose/openable window looking onto nature.
4. Dim, warm light Pink light bulbs, neither too bright nor too low; nonglare screen on your computer.
5. Paint your office soft green or blue.
6. Sound and music resources: Most relaxing: Classical, light jazz, new age, or nature sounds (ocean, rain, birds).

   Music can actually trigger relaxation response.

   Low-level volume just above level of awareness.
7. Aroma therapy: A few drops of lavender, rosemary, or mint oil on warm light bulb.

The Internal Environment

Stress is inevitable. We cannot remake the world, but according to most experts and spiritual leaders, we can change our attitudes. Anything that "stills the mind" can help.

1. Clear your mind: Like clearing your desk, clearing your mind helps reduce stress.

   Take allotted breaks.

   Use your breaks to clear your mind and emotions, NOT as "catch up" time on work.

   Leave your workstation completely. Take a brisk walk outdoors.

   Take a mental vacation—Read a short story, magazine, poetry, inspirational readings.

   Meditate/mindfulness.

   Emphasize your desire to serve.
2. Workstation exercises: Create a short exercise to mentally "clear your mind between calls."

   Breathe Diaphragmatic breathing: Count as you breathe in, or recite an affirmation. Breathe deeply and smile.

Shoulder: Shoulder lifts and rolls.

Back: Stand, bend forward and shake out neck and shoulders.

Arms/hands: Lace fingers together, lift, palms to ceiling, and stretch.

3. Mental preparation: Decide who you would be, then develop a repertoire or package of consumer friendly, but effective responses (Nordstrom's/ED/car talk). Be ready for the inevitable "difficult call": Mentally rehearse or write down statements to use to handle certain predictable difficult situation. After difficult calls: Debrief as needed.
4. Develop tools of communication as a way to manage stress. Practice communication techniques to reduce stress by diffusing anger, setting limits, or managing conflicts. Share your experience and expertise through "war stories," tales of difficult but successfully managed calls.
5. Create and implement a realistic exercise program: The best antidotes to stress are moderate exercise three times a week, three balanced meals daily, and good friends.
6. Monitor and adjust: Are you at risk for burn out? Danger signs include: prolonged fatigue, insomnia, lack of appetite, loss of libido, inability to concentrate, or feeling your life is out of control.

COMPETENCY TESTING

Generally speaking, three domains of skill comprise most jobs: Interpersonal, clinical/technical, and critical thinking skills. Of these three, in telephone triage the most important domains are interpersonal and critical thinking skills. In addition, telehealth competency integrates the several domains of nursing practice and expertise adapted from the work of Pat Benner, the author of ***From Novice to Expert***. These domains and roles include helper/teacher/coach, diagnostic/crisis management, and coordination.

It is also important to differentiate between competency and performance reviews. Competency assessment evaluates the ongoing skills, knowledge, abilities, and behaviors needed to carry out job functions. Its primary purpose is to assure that the "right person" is doing the "right job" ongoing. In addition, competency changes as the employee develops, addressing the dynamic nature of a job.

Performance reviews assure that employees are fulfilling contractual agreements of the job and organizational policies and procedures. It is based on organizational policies, practice standards, and the job description. It may be used to evaluate whether an employee will advance or receive more compensation for work performed. Examples include such things as attendance, policy compliance, and professional ethics.

Competency testing may be verified by the following methods:

- Exemplars
- Self-assessment
- Posttests
- Return demonstrations
- Mock calls
- Observation
- Peer reviews

The following competency parameters may be evaluated utilizing any one of the previous listed methods. One simple way for managers to evaluate staff during orientation is to review five random calls, using an audio recording, documentation form and the Q&A score sheet. Evaluate at 3-mo intervals in the first year. Evaluate annually thereafter.

DOMAIN: INTERPERSONAL SKILLS

Helper—Enabler, Support, Facilitator

- Serves as patient advocate.
- Excellent listening skills. Is fully present and accessible to client.
- Articulate. Communicates well. Uses voice to give comfort.
- Projects a helpful, responsive, and welcoming manner.
- Demonstrates ability to form instant rapport with client.
- Concrete in data collection and teaching.
- Uses confrontation appropriately.
- Facilitates informed consent by stating disclaimer.
- Demonstrates cultural sensitivity.
- Demonstrates good conflict management skills.
- Demonstrates respect for the individual.

DOMAIN: EDUCATOR/COACH SKILLS

Teaching/Coaching

- Maximizes client participation
- Demonstrates a collaborative approach
- Encourages ownership of problems and solutions
- Uses a client-centered approach; collaborates with clients
- Uses timing appropriately
- Elicits clients' perception of the problem
- Provides appropriate information or referral for clients
- Modifies referrals and information to ensure they are current and useful

DOMAIN: CRITICAL THINKING

Diagnostician/Monitoring

- Uses nursing process
- Performs systematic patient assessment utilizing SCHOLAR, PAMPER, and ADL
- Detects, anticipates, and documents significant symptoms and changes in client condition
- Demonstrates appropriate suspiciousness
- Utilizes intuitive approach
- Correctly identifies Red Herrings
- Utilizes Rules of Thumb appropriately
- Uses appropriate interview techniques (open-ended, leading questions, and pertinent negatives)
- Selects the appropriate protocol(s)
- Uses protocols consistently, appropriately, and judiciously
- Overrides protocols appropriately
- Documents deviations to protocols as appropriate
- Elicits and addresses the caller's hidden agendas
- Provides adequate information for monitoring of treatment and illness

- Correctly identified Red Flag Populations and symptoms:
  —Severe, subtle, or suspicious symptoms
  —"Big Five" symptoms: Abdomen, chest, respiratory, dizziness/fainting, flu symptoms
  —High-risk age groups and age-based conditions
  —Veracity: Communication barriers
  —Emotional distress/stress
  —Debilitation/distance

DOMAIN: CRISIS INTERVENTION

« Manages rapidly changing situation with dispatch and composure

- Grasps problems readily and prioritizes appropriately

® Demonstrates effective, sophisticated psychological skill

® Interfaces well and appropriately with other crisis team members

DOMAIN: CLINICAL/TECHNICAL

Organizational Skills

° Organized

® Works well with minimal direction

- Confident in own decision making
- Seeks collaboration when appropriate and necessary
- Willing to acknowledge and address limitations
- Develops a plan for personal/professional growth and development

e Functions well as a team member

® Coordinates well with coworkers and other team members

® Sets priorities well

» Meets multiple patients' needs well

- Coordination: Determines the time, place, steps necessary for appropriate referral

Technical Skills

- Proficient use of equipment (telephone, headset, computer)

® Able to schedule appointments

® Proficiently uses documentation form (complete, accurate, timely)

® Proficiently uses protocols

® Call length commensurate with call complexity, patient's needs

Communication Skills

® Excellent communication skills: written and verbal

® Communicates completely, accurately in timely fashion

® Maintains patient confidentiality

o Identifies and appropriately addresses caller concerns

® Effectively defuses angry/demanding callers

® Interacts effectively with colleagues

® Confirms caller understanding/intent to comply with plan of care

® Invites caller to call back if necessary

® Appropriately accesses community resources

Avoids Common Errors of Practice/ Communications

® Leading questions

® Medical jargon

® Failure to collect adequate data

® Failure to allow adequate "talk time"

® Failure to talk directly with the patient

- Second guessing the caller

® Premature acceptance of patient self-diagnosis

® Minimizing problem seriousness/risk

0 Ignoring patient concerns

® Fails to err on the side of caution

o Stereotyping patients or symptoms

® Jumping to conclusions or premature closure

® Overreacting and underreacting

PERFORMANCE REVIEW

© Maintains current nursing licensure

° Complies with all relevant nurse practice acts

® Complies with all policies and procedures regarding licensure and retraining

- Knowledgeable of, and applies organizational policies

® Participates in relevant CE to maintain/enhance clinical knowledge base

- Demonstrates excellent customer-service attitude

® Demonstrates ability to respond to constructive criticism

0 Seeks continued professional growth

SUGGESTED READING

Robbins, S. P. (1991). *Organizational Behavior: Concepts, Controversies, and Applications.*, Englewood Cliffs, NJ: Prentice Hall, pp. 205-207.

Community Needs Assessment

Describe your community in relation to the following characteristics:

- Average age
  - —Elderly
  - —Young families
  - —Young adults (college population)
  - —Other____________
- Environmental dangers
  - —Nuclear waste/accidents
  - —Coal mining
  - —High crime rate
  - —Toxic waste dumps
  - —Other______________
- Type of community/population
  - —Suburb
  - —Inner city
  - —Rural
  - —Small town
  - —Military
  - —Veteran
  - —Other_____________
- Socioeconomic resources
  - —Working poor
  - —Middle income
  - —Upper income
  - —Other______________
- Literacy level
  - —8th grade
  - —12th grade
  - —College level
  - —Graduate
- Addiction
  - —Alcohol/drug abuse
  - —Other_________
- Endemic diseases
  - —High-risk mothers/babies
  - —Sickle cell disease
  - —AIDS
  - —Other___________
- Cultural/religious factors and resources
  - —Religious practices (diet, gender-based attitudes)
  - —Religious prohibitions
  - —Other____________
- Consumer awareness (patient rights, health options, informed consent, etc.)
  - —Low
  - —Medium
  - —High
- Languages spoken (other than English)

  ____

  ____

  ____
- Self-help, self-care resources
  - —Few support groups, hotlines
  - —Several support groups and hotlines
  - —Many support groups and hotlines
  - —Other

Patient Brochure

Please take the opportunity to customize this brochure for your individual practice.

TELEPHONE ADVICE SERVICES

We now offer telephone advice services 24 hours a day, 365 days a year. Call the advice nurse if you have symptoms, questions, need advice about any health problem, information about counseling, and referrals to community resources. They have had special training to help you. If your symptoms are not serious, you may not need an appointment; the advice nurse will tell you how to treat the problem at home. We can help you decide whether the problem needs an appointment right away or whether your symptoms can be safely treated at home.

Thank you in advance for taking the time to read this brochure. Please keep and use this list of important phone numbers. Attach it to the wall close to your telephone. Please tell others about this service. This pamphlet is available in English, Spanish, Vietnamese, and Cambodian at all clinics. You can get more pamphlets by calling:

HOW TO HELP THE ADVICE NURSE TO HELP YOU

There are many ways you can help the advice nurse. First, unless it is an emergency, please call the advice nurse *before* you come in. Also, if you can't keep your appointment, please call the clinic and let us know, so we can give that appointment to someone else. You can also help the advice nurse by providing a current address and phone number, so the nurse can call you back later. Also, let the nurse know if you do not have the medicine we advise or the home-treatment materials needed to follow the advice given.

WHAT TO TELL THE ADVICE NURSE

The advice nurse will want to talk directly with the sick person if that person is old enough and well enough to give good information. The information you give us helps us decide whether the symptoms are serious and whether an appointment is necessary. Please be ready to answer the following questions, if at all possible:

When did the symptom(s) start?

Is it getting worse?

If there is pain? Where is it?

Have you had this symptom before?

What makes it better?

What makes it worse?

How have you treated it?

Are you taking any medicines?

Are you pregnant or breastfeeding?

Do you have any allergies?

Have you had any recent injury, surgery, infection, illness?

Has there been any possible ingestion of toxic material or poisons?

Do you have any chronic disease?

HELP BY PHONE FOR EMERGENCIES

Problems like suicide or poisoning need quick help from hotlines like Suicide Prevention or Poison Control. The hotlines listed here are free and will give you fast help by telephone, 24 hr a day to all callers:

HOTLINES

- Poison Control (24 Hour/day)
- Suicide Prevention
- Parental Stress
- ® Spousal Abuse/Crisis Care
- "Warm Line" for Kids

HELP BY PHONE FOR CHRONIC EMOTIONAL OR PHYSICAL PROBLEMS

You can get help by phone for chronic emotional and physical problems, such as depression, AIDS, or drug and alcohol abuse. Learn about the groups listed in this brochure. Use them, and tell others about them.

- AIDS
- Drug/Alcohol Help Line
- Alcoholics Anonymous, AlAnon, Alateen
- Emotional Problems
- Seniors
- Teens

IMPORTANT PHONE NUMBERS

Clinic Hours/Days: Phone No.:

PRESCRIPTION REFILLS 24-HOUR NUMBER (Please call at least a week before your medication runs out):

MEDICATION QUESTIONS: Pharmacist

TRANSPORTATION:

MEDICARE INFORMATION:

MEDICAL INFORMATION:

LAB TEST RESULTS

Glossary of Terminology

ALGORITHM: A step-by-step procedure for solving a problem or accomplishing some end, esp. by computer. *[Merriam-Webster's Dictionary,* (1994). (10th ed.) Springfield, MA.]

DECISION-MAKING EXPERT SYSTEM: An expert system which allows an unqualified person to make a decision that is beyond his/her level of training and experience." [Widman, L.E., (1995). "Expert Systems in Medicine" Internet Home Page.]

DECISION SUPPORT EXPERT SYSTEM: An expert system that reminds an experienced decision maker of options or issues to consider that she/he once knew but may have forgotten. (Widman, L.E., 1995, "Expert Systems in Medicine" Internet Home Page.)

DIAGNOSIS: The art or act of identifying a disease from its signs and symptoms. [*Merriam-Webster's Dictionary,* (1994). (10th ed.) Springfield, MA.]

EMPIRICAL: Capable of being verified or disproved by observation or experiment. *[Merriam-Webster's Dictionary,* (1994). (10th ed.) Springfield, MA.]

FUZZY LOGIC: Everything is a matter of degree—nothing is absolute. Fuzzy logic mimics the workings of the human brain.

GUIDELINE: An indication or outline of policy or conduct. [Merriam-Webster's Dictionary, 1994. (10th ed.) Springfield, MA.]

A single statement or a set of statements which relate to a specific condition or patient problem, covering both medical and nursing care, supported by scientific evidence, not tradition or intuition. [Dracup (1996, February) Putting the Clinical Practice Guidelines to work, *Nursing* 96, p 41-45.)

HEURISTIC: Rule of thumb. (Patel 1997) (See below)

NEURAL NETWORK: Nonlinear, dynamica system. Can recall or recognize a stored pattern. Trained by showing examples. Intuition.

NURSING DIAGNOSIS: A concise phrase or term summarizing a cluster of empirical indicators. [Roy C. (1982) Theoretical framework for classification of nursing diagnosis in Kim and Moritz, Classification of nursing diagnosis; Proceedings of the third and fourth national conferences. New York, McGraw Hill.]

NURSING PROCESS: Organized, systematic, deliberate approach to the practice of nursing. [Yura and Walsh (1978). The Nursing Process: Assessing, Planning, Implementing and Evaluating. New York: Appleton-Century-Crofts.]

Dynamic and adaptable to any practice setting, components maybe used sequentially or concurrently. [Christensen and Kenney, (1990). *The Nursing Process: Application of Conceptual Models.* (3rd ed.) St Louis, MO: Mosby).

PROCEDURE: A set of how-to action steps, based on scientific knowledge and published data, focused on a specific treatment. [Dracup (1996, February) Putting the Clinical Practice Guidelines to work, *Nursing 96,* p 41-45.)

PROTOCOL: A detailed plan of a scientific or medical experiment, treatment or procedure. [Merriam-Webster's Dictionary (1994). (10th ed), Springfield, MA.]

RED FLAG: A warning signal; something that attracts attention. [Merriam-Webster's Dictionary (1994). (10th ed.) Springfield, MA.)

RULE OF THUMB: A method or procedure based on experience and common sense. A general principle regarded as roughly correct but not intended to be scientifically accurate. [Merriam-Webster's Dictionary, (1994). (10th ed.) Springfield, MA.]

TELEPHONE TRIAGE: The safe, effective, appropriate disposition of health-related problems by phone. May include assessment, advice, triage, information dispensing, referral, counseling, and crisis intervention. [Wheeler, S. Q. (1993). *Telephone Triage: Theory, Practice and Protocol Development.* San Anselmo, CA: TeleTriage Systems (www.teletriage.com).]

WORKING (DIAGNOSIS): Adequate to permit work to be done, assumed or adopted to permit or facilitate further work or activity. [Merriam-Webster's Dictionary, (1994). (10th ed.) Springfield, MA.]

Protocol-Specific References

Abdomen Problem

Briggs, J. K. (2007). *Telephone Triage Protocols for Nurses.* New York: Wolters Kluwer.

Brunicardi, F. C., Andersen, D. K., Billiar, T. R., et al. (Eds.). (2005). *Schwartz's Principles of Surgery* (8th ed.). New York: McGraw-Hill Companies, Inc.

Goldman, L., and Ausiello, D. (Eds.). (2007). *Cecil Medicine* (23rd ed.). Philadelphia: Elsevier Inc.

Karmath, B,, Holden, M.D., Hussain, N. et al. (2004, April). Chest pain: Differentiating cardiac from non-cardiac causes. *Hospital Physician,* 24-28.

Lafferty, S,, and Baird, M. (2001). *Telenurse: Telephone Triage Protocols.* Albany, NY: Delmar Thomson Learning.

Long, V., and McMullen, P.C. (2003). *Telephone Triage for Obstetrics and Gynecology.* New York: Lippincott Williams and Wilkins.

Marx, J. A., Hockberger, R. S., Wall, R. M., et al. (Eds.). (2006). *Rosen's Emergency Medicine: Concepts and Clinical Practice* (6th ed.). Philadelphia: Mosby Elsevier.

Porter, R. D,, Kaplan, J. D,, Homeier, B. P., et al. (Eds.). (2006). *The Merck Manual of Diagnosis and Therapy* (18th ed.). Whitehouse Station, NJ: Merck and Co., Inc.

Teichman,). M. (2004). Clinical Practice. Acute Renal Colic from Ureteral Calculus. *New England Journal of Medicine, 350,* 684-693.

Abuse

American Medical Association. (1992). Violence: A Compendium from JAMA, American Medical News and Specialty Journals of the AMA. *JAMA.* Chicago: American Medical Association.

Briggs, J. K. (2007). *Telephone Triage Protocols for Nurses.* New York: Wolters Kluwer.

Cowell, N. A., and Burgess, A. W. (Eds.). (1996). *Understanding Violence against Women.* Washington, DC: National Academy Press.

Jezierski, M. (1999). Family violence screening: Opportunities in prehospital settings. *Journal of Emergency Nursing,* 25(3), 201-205.

Lee, D., and Anderson, L. F. (1995). *Improving Your Community Clinic's Response to Domestic Violence.* Sacramento, CA: California Department of Health Services.

Lipscomb, G. H., et al. (1992). Male victims of sexual assault. *Journal of the American Medical Association, 267(22),* 3064-3066.

Markus, K. (1999, April 19). Reporting signs of abuse. *Nurse Week,* 13.

Reece, R. M. (1994). *Child Abuse: Medical Diagnosis and Management.* Philadelphia: Lea and Febiger.

Shea, C.A., Mahoney, M., and Lacey, J. K. M. (1997). Breaking through the barriers to domestic violence intervention. *American Journal of Nursing,* 97(6), 26-33.

West, C. M. (1999). *Partner Violence in Military Families.* Durham, NH: University of New Hampshire, Family Research Laboratory.

Winfrey, M. E., and Smith, A. R. (1999). The suspiciousness factor: Critical care nursing and forensics. *Critical Care Nursing,* 22(1), 1-7.

Back Problem

Briggs, J. K. (2007). *Telephone Triage Protocols for Nurses.* New York: Wolters Kluwer.

Goldman, L., and Ausiello, D. (Eds.). (2007). *Cecil Medicine* (23rd ed.). Philadelphia: Elsevier Inc.

Karmath, B., Holden, M.D., Hussain, N. et al. (2004, April). Chest pain: Differentiating cardiac from non-cardiac causes. *Hospital Physician,* 24-28.

Lafferty, S., and Baird, M. (2001). *Telenurse: Telephone Triage Protocols.* Albany, NY: Delmar Thomson Learning.

Marx, J. A., Hockberger, R. S., Wall, R. M., et al. (Eds.). (2006). *Rosens Emergency Medicine: Concepts and Clinical Practice* (6th ed.). Philadelphia: Mosby Elsevier.

Bowel Problem

Briggs, J. K. (2007). *Telephone Triage Protocols for Nurses.* New York: Wolters Kluwer.

Goldman, L., and Ausiello, D. (Eds.). (2007). *Cecil Medicine* (23rd ed.). Philadelphia: Elsevier Inc.

Lafferty, S., and Baird, M. (2001). *Telenurse: Telephone Triage Protocols.* Albany, NY: Delmar Thomson Learning.

Marx, J. A., Hockberger, R. S., Wall, R. M., et al. (Eds.). (2006). *Rosen's Emergency Medicine: Concepts and Clinical Practice* (6th ed.). Philadelphia: Mosby Elsevier.

Porter, R. D., Kaplan, J. D., Homeier, B. P., et al. (Eds.). (2006). *The Merck Manual of Diagnosis and Therapy* (18th ed.). Whitehouse Station, NJ: Merck and Co., Inc.

General References

- Baumeister & Tierney (2011) Will Power
- Donabedian (2003) An Introduction to Quality Assurance in Health Care
- Donabedian A. Quality assurance. Structure, process and outcome. Nursing Standard (Royal College Of Nursing (Great Britain). 1992;7(11 Suppl).
- Gawande (2009) The Checklist Manifesto
- Institute of Medicine. To Err is Human: Building a Safer Health System. . In: Institute of Medicine Committee on the Quality of Health Care in America, editor. Washington DC: Institute of Medicine; 1999.
- Kahneman (2011) Thinking Fast and Slow
- Joint Commission. Sentinel Event Data: Root Causes by Event Type 2004-2Q 2012. In: Commission TJ, editor. Washington, DC: The Joint Commission, Office of Quality Monitoring; 2012.
- Johns Hopkins Research, 5/4/16. BMJ http://www.hopkinsmedicine.org/news/media/releases/study_suggests_medical_errors_now_third_leading_cause_of_death_in_the_us
- Lephrohon, J. & Patel, V. (1995). Decision Strategies In Emergency Telephone Triage. Medical Decision-Making. 15 (3): 240 -253.
- Mahlmeister, L, & Van Mullen, C. (2000). The Process Of Triage In Perinatal Settings: Clinical And Legal Issues. J Perinatal Neonatal Nurse 2000 Mar; 13(4): 13-30
- Perrin EC, Goodman HC. Telephone management of acute pediatric illnesses. The New England Journal of Medicine 1978;298(3): 130-5 , Washington,
- Wachter (2015) The Digital Doctor: Hope, Hype and Harm Medicine's Computer Age
- Wheeler, et al. (2015) Safety of Clinical & Non-Clinical Decision Makers in Telephone Triage. Journal of Telemedicine & Telecare, Sep;21(6):305-22.
- Wheeler, S. Q. (2009). Telephone Triage Guidelines For Adult Populations with Women's Health, TeleTriage Systems Publishers, San Anselmo, CA
- Wheeler, S.Q. (2017) Telephone Triage: Essentials for Expert Practice. Preceptor Workbook. TeleTriage Systems Publishers(teletriage.com)

Safety References

- Huibers L, Smits M, Renaud V, Giesen P, Wensing M. Safety of telephone triage in out-of-hours care: a systematic review. Scandinavian Journal of Primary Health Care. 2011 Dec;29(4): 198-209.
- Wheeler SQ. Telephone triage protocols for adult populations. New York City: McGraw Hill Publishers; 2009.
- The Lancet. Nurse-telephone triage. The Lancet. 2001;357(9253):323.

- Perrin EC, Goodman HC. Telephone management of acute pediatric illnesses. The New England Journal of Medicine 1978;298(3): 130-5.
- Blank L, Coster J, O'Cathain A, Knowles E, Tosh J, Turner J, et al. The appropriateness of, and compliance with telephone triage decisions: a systemic review and narrative synthesis.. Journal of Advanced Nursing 2012;68(12):2610-21.
- Bunn F, Byrne G, Kendall S. Telephone consultation and triage: effects on health care use and patient satisfaction (Review). The Cochrane Library. 2009;1:1-36.
- Carrasqueiro S, Oliveira M, Encamacao P. Evaluation of Telephone Triage and Advice Services: a Systematic Review on Methods, Metrics and Results. Fairfax, VA: IOS Press; 2011 [cited.
- Donabedian A. Quality assurance. Structure, process and outcome. Nursing Standard (Royal College Of Nursing (Great Britain). 1992;7(11 Suppl).
- Flannery M, Moses G, Cykert S, Ogden P, Keyserling T, Elnicki M, et al. Telephone management training in internal medicine residencies: a national survey of program directors. Academic Medicine 1995;70(12): 1138-41.
- Brown JL. Pediatric telephone medicine: principles, triage, and advice. Philadelphia: Lippincott Williams & Wilkins; 1994.
- Katz H, Telephone Manual of Paediatric Care, Wiley, 1982
- Schmitt B. Pediatric Telephone Advice. Boston, MA: Little Brown & Co; 1980.
- Wheeler, S & Windt, J. Telephone Triage: Theory, Practice and Protocol Development, Delmar Publishers, Albany, NY. 1993
- Leprohon J, Patel V. Decision-making Strategies for Telephone Triage in Emergency Medical Services. Medical Decision Making. 1995;15:240-53.
- Reisman AB, Brown KE. Preventing communication errors in telephone medicine: A case based approach. Journal of general internal medicine. 2005 Oct;20:959-63.
- Mahlmeister, 2012, Affordable Care Act and Telephone Triage, Online CE Course available through TeleTriage Systems, In press TeleTriage Systems,
- Smith, 2005, Telephone Triage Risk Management, Online CE Course available through TeleTriage Systems teletriage.com
- lDahlberg CP. State probes whether Kaiser call centers endanger patients. The Kaiser Papers, A Public Service Page Sacramento, CA: Sacramento Bee; 2009.
- Greatbatch D, Hanlon G, Goode J, O'Caithain A, Strangleman T, Luff D. Telephone triage expert systems and clinical expertise. Sociology of Health & Illness. 2005;27(6):802-30.
- Rutenberg C, Greenberg L. The Art and Science of Telephone Triage. Consulting TT, editor. Hot Springs, Arkansas: Telephone Triage Consulting; 2012.

- Deakin CD, Alasaad M, King P, Thompson F. Is ambulance telephone triage using advanced medical priority dispatch protocols able to identify patients with acute stroke correctly? Emergency Medicine Journal. 2009 Jun;26(6):442-5. (NOTED IN TABLE 3 Decision Maker Frame work)
- Institute of Medicine. To Err is Human: Building a Safer Health System. . In: Institute of Medicine Committee on the Quality of Health Care in America, editor. Washington DC: Institute of Medicine; 1999.
- Norman GR, Eva KW. Diagnostic error and clinical reasoning. Medical Education 2010;44:94-100.
- The Joint Commission. Sentinel Event Data: Root Causes by Event Type 2004-2Q 2012. In: Commission TJ, editor. Washington, DC: The Joint Commission, Office of Quality Monitoring; 2012.
- Deakin CD, Sherwood DM, Smith A, Cassidy M. Does telephone triage of emergency (999) calls using Advanced Medical Priority Dispatch (AMPDS) with Department of Health (DH) call prioritisation effectively identify patients with an acute coronary syndrome? An audit of 42,657 emergency calls to Hampshire Ambulance Service NHS Trust. Emergency medicine journal: EMJ. 2006 Mar;23(3):232-5.
- Kempe A, Bunik M, Ellis J. How safe is triage by an after-hours telephone call center? . Pediatrics 2006;118:457-63.
- Kempe A, Luberti A, Belman S, Hertz A, Sherman H, Amin D, et al. Outcomes Associated With Pediatric After-Hours Care by Call Centers: A Multicenter Study. Ambulatory Pediatrics. 2003;3:211-7.
- Lee TJ, BaraffLJ, Guzy J, Johnson D, Woo H. Does telephone triage delay significant medical treatment? Archives of Pediatrics and Adolescent Medicine. 2003;157:635-41., 32
- Andrews J, Armstrong K, Fraser J. Professional telephone advice to parents with sick children: time for quality control! Journal of paediatrics and child health. 2002;38:23-6.
- Katz H, Kaltsounis D, Halloran L, Mondor M. Patient safety and telephone medicine: some lessons from closed claim case review. Journal of general internal medicine. 2008;23:517-22.
- Killip S, Ireson CL, Love MM, Fleming ST, Katirai W, Sandford K. Patient Safety in After-hours Telephone Medicine. Family Medicine. 2007;39:404-9.
- Foumy M, Lucas AS, Belle L, Debaty G, Casez P, Bouvaist H, et al. Inappropriate dispatcher decision for emergency medical service users with acute myocardial infarction. The American journal of emergency medicine. 2011 Jan;29(l):37-42.
- Hildebrandt DE, Westfall JM, Femald DH, Pace WD. Harm resulting from inappropriate telephone triage in primary care.. The Journal of the American Board of Family Medicine. 2006;19(5):437-42.

- Hildebrandt DE, Westfall JM, Smith PC. After hours telephone triage affects patient safety. Journal of Family Practice. 2003;52(3):222-7.
- Klasner A, King W, Crews T, Monroe K. Accuracy and response time when clerks are used for telephone triage. Clinical Pediatrics. 2006;45:267-9.
- Derkx HP, Rethans J-JE, Muijtjens AM, Maiburg BH, Winkens R, van Rooij HG, et al. Quality of clinical aspects of call handling at Dutch out of hours centres: cross
- North F, Odunukan O, Varkey P. The value of telephone triage for patients with appendicitis. Journal of Telemedicine and Telecare. 2011;17:417-20.
- Emesäter A, Engstrom M, Holmstrom I, Winblad U. Incident reporting in nurse-led national telephone triage in Sweden: the reported errors reveal a pattern that needs to be broken. Journal of Telemedicine and Telecare. 2010 Jul;16(5):243-7.
- Emesäter A, Winblad U, Engstrom M, Holmstrom IK. Malpractice claims regarding calls to Swedish telephone advice nursing: what went wrong and why? Journal of Telemedicine and Telecare. 2012 Aug 24.
- Hirsh DA, Simon HK, Massey R, Thornton L, Simon JE. The host hospital 24-hour underreferral rate: an automated measure of call-center safety. Pediatrics. 2007;119:1139-44.
- Giesen P, Ferwerda R, Tijssen R, Mokkink H, Drijver R, van den Bosch W, et al. Safety of telephone triage in general practitioner cooperatives: do triage nurses correctly estimate urgency? Quality and Safety in Health Care. 2007;16:181-4.
- Huibers L, Giesen P, Smits M, Mokkink H, Grola R, Wensing M. Nurse telephone triage in Dutch out-of-hours primary care: the relation between history taking and urgency estimation. European Journal of Emergency Medicine 2012;19:309-15.
- Marklund B, Ström M, Månsson J, Borgquist L, Baigi A, Fridlund B. Computer-supported telephone nurse triage: an evaluation of medical quality and costs. Journal of Nursing Management 2007;15:180-7.
- Hannan TJ, Celia C. Are doctors the structural weakness in the e-health building? Internal Medicine Journal 2013;43:1155-64.

Task Force Biographies

TASK FORCE LEADER

Sheila Quilter Wheeler, RN, MS, has practiced nursing for over 30 years, primarily in the critical care, ED, and clinic settings. She is an accomplished writer, educator, and researcher. Since 1984, Ms Wheeler has pioneered the field of telephone triage. Ms Wheeler is the author of *Telephone Triage: Theory, Practice, and Protocol Development,* has written for the *Journal of Emergency Nursing;* and lectures nationally. She is the founder of the annual national conference "Telephone Triage: Essentials for Expert Practice." In addition to an MA in film, Ms Wheeler holds an MS degree in community health nursing from the University of California, San Francisco.

2009 Contributing Authors/Medical Reviewers

Expert Reviewers

Elsa Tsutaoka, MD, has practiced family medicine in the San Francisco area since 1998. She has a primary care practice in an urban underserved area in San Francisco. Dr. Tsutaoka also serves as assistant clinical professor in the Department of Family and Community Medicine, University of California at San Francisco. She also works in Urgent Care in various locations in the San Francisco bay area, from urban to suburban settings, and has a practice as a student health center physician at City College of San Francisco.

Dr. Tsutaoka's interests include chronic disease care, community involvement, and self-management. She also works in Urgent Care and Student Health Centers. She graduated from UC, San Diego.

Cindy Lamendola, MSN, ANP, is an adult nurse practitioner and clinical research coordinator at the Stanford University in Stanford, California. Ms. Lamendola has a specialized practice in cardiovascular nursing. She currently researches and practices in the areas of insulin resistance, Type 2 diabetes, and cardiovascular disease.

Ms. Lamendola has an extensive background in cardiac rehabilitation and risk factor management. She has lectured nationally and published articles on insulin resistance and CVD risk factors. She is a founding member and past president of the Preventive Cardiovascular Nurses Association and a fellow of the American Heart Association.

Adult/Geriatric Physician Medical Reviewers

Russ J. Kino, MD, is currently director of emergency services at St. John's Hospital and Health Center, Santa Monica, California. He is also assistant clinical professor of medicine at UCLA Medical Center in Los Angeles as well as director of ER on Call, a telephone triage program at St. John's. Dr. Kino has broad experience in emergency medicine both in the United States and in Western Australia, where he did internship and residency rotations at the Royal Perth Hospital. Awards for achievement include the Jack Bercove Memorial Prize in general practice, best scientific paper, National Conference of the Australian College for Emergency Medicine, and Buchanan Prize for top score in National Examination for Fellow of Australian College for Emergency Medicine. Dr. Kino has given numerous presentations on a wide range of topics internationally. His research articles have appeared in peer-reviewed publications.

Edwin Cary Pigman, MD, has served as the medical director of World Access Group, an international travel and medical assistance service organization. Dr. Pigman is assistant professor of Emergency Medicine at George Washington University Medical Center, Washington, DC, and has received awards for excellence in teaching and research. In addition to numerous presentations, Dr. Pigman is a frequent contributor to the *American Journal of Emergency Medicine, Annals of Emergency Medicine,* and others. Dr. Pigman graduated from the Ohio University College of Medicine and received a B. of S. from Edgecliff College of Xavier University, Cincinnati, Ohio.

Pediatric Physician Medical Reviewer

Robert H. Pantell, MD, is chief of the General Pediatrics Division and professor of pediatrics at the University of California, San Francisco. Past positions include chief of adolescent medicine and associate professor of pediatrics, family medicine, and biometry at Medical University of South Carolina; assistant coordinator of ambulatory pediatrics at Stanford University Medical Center; and pediatrician at a community health program in rural Idaho. Since 1974, Dr. Pantell has received numerous awards for his writing and research. He is winner of the American Medical Writers Association award, Robert Wood Johnson Foundation grant, David and Lucille Packard grant, Agency for Health Care Policy and Research grant award, and many others. Dr. Pantell has served as contributor and author for numerous articles and books and is a frequent presenter at regional and national forums. The major focuses of his creative activities are Doctor-Patient Communications, Common Clinical Problems, Health Care Provider Behavior and Modification by Education. Dr. Pantell received his MD from Boston University in 1969, completed his pediatrics residency at North Carolina Memorial Hospital in Chapel Hill in 1972, and a fellowship as a Robert Wood Johnson clinical scholar at Stanford University in 1977.

Adult/Geriatric Nurse Task Force Members

Jeff Howell, RN, CEN, has practiced emergency and trauma nursing for 10 years. He has practiced in New York City and San Francisco. He currently resides and practices in Sonoma County, California. He has also worked as an MICN, paramedic clinical preceptor, telephone triage RN, drug/AIDS counselor at San Francisco General Hospital, and emergency flight transport nurse in the Bahamas. Mr. Howell is currently at work on his MA at San Francisco State University.

Jean Berg Meddaugh, RN, began working for the East Valley Clinic in 1968 when she converted a small room in the Alexian Brothers Hospital into a satellite clinic for the Santa Clara Valley Medical Center. Over the years, she has managed the clinic, which has expanded to become an important community resource, committed to providing care to seniors and the medically underserved on the east side of San Jose. In 1993, Ms. Meddaugh coordinated the development of an Urgent Care Center that offers pediatric and adult medical services seven days a week.

Bertha A. Ruiz, DNSc, RN, GNP, CS, has been a nurse for 15 years, primarily in the areas of medical-surgical nursing and as a gerontological nurse practitioner. Her research and written work has focused on patient health care outcomes and cost effectiveness of nursing interventions. Dr. Ruiz's current research project addresses hip fracture recovery in older persons. She has been active locally, statewide, and nationally on issues regarding education of ethnic populations, specifically those of Latinos. Dr. Ruiz is the founder and immediate past president of the San Francisco Bay Area Chapter of the National Association of Hispanic Nurses and a key member of the California Nursing Coalition for the Emerging Majority. She holds a DNSc degree from the University of California, San Francisco. Dr. Ruiz has held various nursing positions in Oregon, Idaho, Utah, and California.

Adult/OB/GYN Nurse Task Force Members

Laura Wachter Alexander, RN, BSN, IBCLC, has a broad background in nursing as a clinical instructor and patient educator. Ms. Alexander currently works as a lactation consultant and prenatal instructor to California Pacific Medical Center, San Francisco. In the past she has worked for the National Center for Education in Maternal and Child Health, Washington, DC. Ms. Alexander graduated from Northern Illinois University School of Nursing and has practiced nursing since 1979.

Stacy Bischoff, RN, NP, has practiced for more than 19 yr as a women's health care nurse practitioner. She has practiced most recently with Women's Medical Associates, a private OB/GYN practice in Greenbrae, California. Ms. Bischoff has worked extensively for the last 10 years in the areas of family planning and planned parenthood, specializing in infertility, patient education, and adoption counseling. Most recently, Ms. Bischoff has worked in integrative medicine and women's health. Ms. Bisehoff received her diploma from Norton Medical Infirmary and nurse practitioner training at Harbor-UCLA Medical Center.

Joan Marks, BSN, NP, has been in a private OB/GYN practice for the last 20 yr in Marin County with Richard H. Printz, MD. Women's health is her primary interest. Ms. Marks received her Nurse Practitioner Certificate from University of California at San Francisco in 1977. She is a graduate of the University of Colorado School of Nursing, 1969.

Suellen Miller, RN, CNM, MHA, PhD, is currently a postdoctoral research fellow at the Institute for Health Policy Studies at the University of California, San Francisco, School of Medicine. Dr. Miller has practiced as a certified nurse-midwife since 1977. She has worked with international organizations as a researcher, educator, and technical advisor in the Philippines, West Indies, and Thailand. Dr. Miller has authored numerous articles and books and is a regular presenter on women's issues. Dr. Miller received her PhD at UCSF, MHA at Antioch University West, San Francisco, and nurse-midwifery at Meharry Medical School in Nashville, Tennessee.

Pediatric Nurse Task Force Members

Jeff Howell, RN, CEN (See Adult/Geriatric Nurse Task Force Members.).

Elizabeth San Luis, MSN, PNP, has practiced nursing since 1972, primarily in the areas of intensive care, dialysis, and pediatrics. Currently Ms. San Luis practices at the Ambulatory Care Center at the University of California Medical Center, where she services low-income, high-risk pediatric patients. Ms. San Luis developed the Clinic for Children of Teen Parents to provide primary care. She provides breastfeeding consultation to patients and providers. Ms. San Luis also provides primary care in a unique family-oriented clinic for children with HIV or AIDS. Ms. San Luis received a MS and a degree as a pediatric nurse practitioner at the University of California, San Francisco.

Susan Valeriote, RN, CPNP, MS, has worked as a pediatric nurse practitioner since 1984. Ms. Valeriote worked for seven years in the Pulmonary Center at Children's Hospital in Oakland, caring for a predominantly Medi-Cal population—single young mothers of minority, lower socioeconomic status with children. As a pediatric nurse practitioner, she was responsible for all telephone triage at the center. Her publications include a tracheotomy care booklet and teaching videos for tracheotomy care and bronchodilator therapy. Most recently she was a clinical professor at the University of California, San Francisco, in the Pediatric Nurse Practitioner program. She holds a BS in nursing from USF, a BSB from Santa Clara University, and an MS from UCSF.

Expert Reviewers

Patricia A. Crane, MSN, RNC, NP, has practiced nursing for 25 yr. Ms. Crane attended the University of Texas Health Science Center at Dallas' Women's Health Care

Nurse Practitioner program and obtained her MSN degree from the University of California, San Francisco, in 1991. As an educator and practitioner, Ms. Crane has provided reproductive health care in a variety of settings and coordinated and lectured in the education program Associate Women's Health Care Nurse Practitioner program for 5 years. As a forensic nurse consultant, she has spoken at national and international conferences on medical-legal issues, specifically interpersonal violence and the cultural practice of female genital mutilation.

Eve R. Meyer, MSW, MSHA, has been executive director of San Francisco Suicide Prevention for 12 yr. She has specialized in training staff members of small community organizations to be part of the larger mental health system. Prior to working in Suicide Prevention, she was marketing director for a group of for-profit health care facilities. She worked at California Pacific Medical in marketing, and for SMP Health Care Architects in system design. She received a masters in social work at the University of Chicago and an MSHA at the University of Michigan.

Adrienne Plasse, MPH, CNM, has been a certified nurse-midwife since 1978, when she graduated from Johns Hopkins School of Public Health's Nurse-Midwifery program. She has worked primarily in underserved communities, Planned Parenthood, and in Central America. She has served in faculty positions at Case Western Reserve University, The Frontier School of Midwifery in Kentucky, and currently at the University of California, San Francisco, in both the School of Medicine and the Nurse-Midwifery Education Program. Ms. Plasse has extensive and current experience in protocol design for OB/GYN, NP, and CNM practice. At present, she works in a community-based women's health clinic and attends births at Marin General Hospital, in Marin County, California.

Donna M. Vincent, RN, BSN, MA, has practiced nursing for 28 yr. She began her career in the neonatal intensive care unit of a large academic center and then went on to develop and teach a perinatal outreach education program for the Robert Wood Johnson Foundation Rural Infant Care Project. Ms. Vincent acted as the director of the Perinatal Advisory Council for Los Angeles communities, which published guidelines for perinatal and neonatal care. She has served as director of four major telephone triage programs across the United States, including those at Boston Children's Hospital at Harvard and Stanford Medical Centers. Ms. Vincent has published numerous articles in the areas of perinatal/neonatal care and telehealth and has presented lectures at several natural conferences.

Lindsay Wheeler, DC, has been a practitioner of chiropractic since 1982. She has a private practice in Berkeley, California. She lectures frequently on back injury prevention and rehabilitation. She has published numerous articles in chiropractic journals. She has a longstanding interest in self-care and education in the treatment of back pain.

AFTERWORD

"We don't look for patterns of our recurrent mistakes or devise and refine potential solutions for them. But we could, and that is the ultimate point". Gawande, 2009

Any mistake or failure in the diagnostic process can lead to a diagnosis that is wrong, missed or delayed. Inpatient diagnostic errors tend to be more lethal, however more diagnostic errors occur in ambulatory settings Gröszkruger,

It has been my life's work to devise solutions for patterns of error in practice and systems. In 1993,1 authored the fust "how to" training manual in telephone triage. Two years later, I led a Task Force of 25+ expert nurses, nurse practitioners and physicians to complete the fust three-volume set of age-specific, 5-Level Triage adult and pediatric guidelines. Our goal was to create a decision support tool that met the needs of clinicians.

Twenty Years Later

Evidence-based practice Since 1995, research and standards have validated the guideline structure, process and system (training, guidelines, documentation, standards). For example,

- Research on patient safety and error (Institute of Medicine) has emphasized the use of a system-based approach. The guidelines are one part of a system.
- The Joint Commission has pointed out root causes of error (inadequacies of assessment, communications, cognitive error, informed consent, and continuity) -- which these guidelines and system reduce through improved nursing process, force functions and checklists.
- Clinical Call center standards have emerged (URAC), as have practice standards (American Academy of Ambulatory Care Nursing) - both supported by the structure and process of the guideline and system.
- The guidelines improve communications through refined and clarified triage nomenclature developed by American College of Emergency Physicians.
- Finally, Emergency Medicine Standards have been published that emphasize the use of pattern recognition, context and identification of high-risk populations.

In the light of these developments, I felt the guidelines needed to be revised and updated, because these differences constitute significant change.

Health Information Technology Also during the same 20-year period technology literally exploded — Internet, Healthcare Informational Technology, the electronic medical record (EMR) and electronic guidelines known as Computerized Decision Support Systems (CDSS). In 2011, the global telemedicine market was $11.6 billion in 2011 and is expected to triple to $27.3 billion in 2016, according to a BCC report ('http://www.bccresearch.com/pressroom/hlc/global-telemedicine-market-reach-$27.3-billion-2016). Professionally, however, the field lagged behind technology.

"All learned occupations have a definition ofprofessionalism, a code of conduct. It is where they spell out their ideals and duties. They all have at least three

common elements: expectation of selflessness; of skill; and of trustworthiness. Aviators have a fourth expectation — discipline". (Gawande, 2010)

Malpractice in Telephone Triage Since 1995,1 have served as an expert witness related to telephone triage malpractice — reviewing and analyzing between 30-35 cases. In the majority of cases, malpractice was related to recurrent patterns of error — inadequate assessments, incomplete documentation, poor communication, and cognitive bias and as well as inadequate systems.

Many malpractice cases are related to *Delay in Care.* Telephone triage is a risk-prone clinical subspecialty due to challenges of assessing the symptoms of invisible patients. The propensity for cognitive bias is worsened due to ambiguity, decision fatigue and a time-driven work atmosphere that stresses efficiency over proficiency.

By virtue of its difficulty, telephone triage — of all clinical specialties — requires a high degree of professionalism. Early on in the guideline development process, I was informed that patient patterns of distress are predictable (for example, potential for sepsis and dehydration in pediatric populations). The information leads us to develop guidelines to *routinely* investigate and try to rule out these patterns. Our goal was to develop tools that would anticipate problems, resulting in timely referrals. However, over that 20-year span, 1 found that in 30-40% of malpractice cases on which 1 consulted the outcome were sepsis *-problems that other guidelines had failed to anticipate and address.*

Research: Current Decision Maker Safety In 2015 1 performed a narrative review of the literature (2002-2012), to evaluate the status of Decision maker Safety in telephone triage. Despite the small number of substantive studies I found an adequate number upon which to base the review. Not surprisingly, we found nurses to be as proficient and safer than physicians; nurses appear to be the best match of clinician to the task of telephone triage. This prospective conclusion may be due to:

- more *complete* systems
- use of pattern recognition and context in decision-making
- right strategy: estimation of symptom urgency rather than differential diagnosis

It is important to note that after decades of practicing *telephone medicine,* physicians still have no formal telephone triage system, and their documentation is inconsistent. It appears that physicians are largely unfamiliar how nurses perform the task — urgency estimation, pattern recognition, context, the nursing process (for telephone triage). Yet, since the mid-90's, physicians have developed electronic guidelines (CDSS) that nurses are required to use.

Despite the introduction of physician-developed CDSS — presumably designed to make the process safer - mistriage and delays in care persist. In my opinion, nurses best utilized as guideline developers, and physicians as reviewers.

Current CDSS Approach to Decision Making

Differential Diagnosis vs Urgency Estimation To date, no independent research has demonstrated the validity and reliability of a given CDSS (Marklund, Randell). In fact, researchers have found that savvy nurses resist using software as intended, instead developing "workaround approaches" (Greatbatch, Holmstrom).

Many current CDSS developers use algorithms. It may be overly deterministic — aimed at a differential diagnosis. Whereas, medical diagnoses are based on face-to-face encounters and one or more of the following processes http://omerad.msu.edu/ebm/Diagnosis/Diagnosis2.html With the exception of pattern recognition (modified for phone encounters) these diagnostic approaches appear to break down in telephone triage for the reasons described in Box 1.

BOX 1: Medical Diagnostic Processes

***Diagnosis** may be defined as the "'process of using the history, physical examination, laboratory, imaging studies, and other tests to identify the disease responsible for the patient's complaint. Diagnoses help clinicians make informed decision about treatment and prognosis. Physicians use several types of reasoning during the diagnostic process:*

- ***Pattern-recognition** — "instant recognition " of a disease commonly used for diagnosis of common conditions such as urinary tract infection or sinusitis.*
- ***Algorithmic** — using flowcharts and algorithms, this approach is useful for conditions where patient information is discrete and accurate, such as diagnosis of anemia or an abnormal liver function test. Decision trees of individual symptoms are dependent upon automated reasoning, with little or no pattern elicitation, or working hypothesis. Automated reasoning is deterministic (diagnostic; establish a cause) it requires accurate, complete information.*
- ***Exhaustive** — gathering every possible piece of data. Used for unusual presentations where other modes of decision-making have failed and after patients have already received a basic evaluation. However, it is generally inefficient in the primary care setting for an initial evaluation.*
- ***Hypothetic deductive** — generating and rejecting hypotheses as more data are collected, involves proposing a differential diagnosis, asking a question, using the answer to refine the differential diagnosis, asking another question, again refining the differential, and so on ".*

ADAPTED AND MODIFIED FROM
http.V/omerad. msu. edu/ebm/Diagnosis/Diagnosis2. html

Telephone triage is time-limited, and is not face-to-face. Unlike office or ED visits, there is no immediate access to lab results, x-rays or other resources. The best approach appears to be to use a solid operating procedure - the nursing process — including thorough assessments, pattern recognition, and urgency estimation.

The algorithmic approach (currently employed in CDSS) appears to be the wrong match of tool to task because it requires accurate information and uses "automated reasoning". In addition, the exhaustive, or hypothetico-deductive approaches are both extremely time-consuming and impractical. Thus, pattern recognition with urgency estimation appear to be the best match of tools to task.

However, in order for pattern recognition to be effective, clinicians must follow the nursing process, perform comprehensive assessments, communicate effectively, provide informed consent, ensure continuity and avoid cognitive bias. These elements are built into the design for the guidelines and system we have developed. We integrated standards and components in order to achieve safety and quality.

They differ from other guidelines in several ways. Some electronic software appear to function like *decision-making* systems (CDMS) and are devoid of clinical training programs or professional standards. These guidelines are *decision support* tools and include an integrated form for documentation as well as standards with optional training. The structure and processes supporting guidelines are robust, reliable and used consistently - in other words, a strong system and professional discipline.

Design Standards for Guidelines

In 2011 the Institute of Medicine recommended that developers set forth design standards for the assumptions, analytic methods, and rationales used in any guideline development. In Clinical Practice Guidelines We Can Trust (2011), IOM sets forth seven criteria required for appraising Guidelines (p 213, Appendix C). While such design standards apply to all telephone triage guidelines, no developer has produced evidence that their guidelines meet such standards. Our goal has always been to meet and surpass these standards, and to make the guidelines as evidence-based as possible.

These guidelines are based on evidence (Goodman & Perrin, 1978; Patel, 1995) related to a clinical pattern recognition strategy (by nurses and nurse practitioners) in telephone triage. They are also derived from categories and descriptions established by ACEP. Finally, they are based on a 5-Tier Triage approach supported by ENA. They were specifically designed to meet and/or exceed the following IOM criteria:

Validity - if guidelines are followed, it will lead to expected outcomes — one of 5 Level dispositions

Reliability/reproducibility - given the same data and using the guidelines, another set of nurses would produce the same results or expected outcomes — safe, timely 5-Tier dispositions

Clinical applicability - explicitly states the populations to which they apply

Flexibility - identifies exceptions to their recommendations

Clarity & Transparency - unambiguous language, precisely defined terms, easy to follow mode of presentation

1) *Validity and Reliability/Reproducibility*

If followed, it will lead to expected outcomes. Reliable: given the same data, another set of nurses using these guidelines would produce the same outcomes. Validity and reproducibility are feasible only if qualified nurses — with adequate clinical training — operate them.

2) *Clinical applicability*

Guidelines were designed to explicitly address three distinct populations: Adults (Age 18+), School Age (Age 6-18), and Infant Child age groups (Birth to Six years) of all risk levels, socioeconomic status and literacy levels.

3) *Flexibility*

The Users Guide identifies exceptions to guideline recommendations, rules or provisions for situations, which do not fall into typical presentations. Some examples include:

- When dealing with high-risk patients, atypical symptoms or situations
- When in doubt about what is the right decision
- When the nurse wishes to upgrade or downgrade
- A robust Standardized Guideline, used as a "go to" or "fall back" guideline for situations where no specific guideline seems to apply.

4) *Clarity*

The authors of the protocols made every attempt to achieve the goal of clarity. As recommended by the Manchester Triage Group (2016), we worked tirelessly to create a product with unambiguous language, precisely defined terms, clear operating instructions and a consistent and user-friendly presentation.

We used 5th - 8th grade level language, so information could be *read directly* to the caller, rather than risk introducing error by having to "retranslate" it from medical jargon or college to 8th grade level.

We simplified the format to streamline the process and to direct the eye through the guideline. Table of Contents are Site-based for ease of locating the correct title.

Guideline dispositions are based on the 5-Tier Triage model, which provides complete instructions for when, where, and why patients should be seen for each of five levels of acuity. The guidelines have been 5-Level since 1995 — when first published in 1993.

5) *Transparency*

By their very nature, books are transparent. Similar to the classic Merck Manual reference, which describes a broad array of symptom patterns, these guidelines are also a reference book format. In addition, the User's Guide has full instructions. The reader can easily understand how the manuals operate.

Changes to 2017 Edition

Since 1995, several experts have reviewed and contributed content revisions to the fust editions of Infant-Child, School Age and Adult versions in 2003, 2005 and 2009 respectively. The structure and process are further bolstered by the aforementioned research and standards. We have reframed several key features of the Guidelines — Checklists (Gawande, Wachter), Force Functions (Wachter) and 5-Tier Triage (Emergency Severity Index, Manchester Triage Group). In the light of new research and standards, these updates can enhance safety and quality.

Built-In Standards to avoid Error

Telephone triage interactions represent "virtual visits", not unlike an ED visit. Early research emphasized thorough assessment, contextual and pattern recognition leading to decisions (Perrin, Patel). One method is the use of checklists — *a key feature of these guidelines.*

Checklists

In the 1995 versions of the guidelines, we developed four Assessment Checklists to use with the guidelines: SAVED, SCHOLAR, RAMP, and ADL. Those checklists remain intact with minor modifications and additions (DEMERIT and SEPSIS). The new approach is to rely heavily on these checklists.

Atul Gawande, MD, set out to improve safety in the surgical process by developing a checklist that would prevent clinicians from forgetting key steps. Dr. Gawande based his book on checklists used by very risk averse industries — the airline and the building industries. Pilots use the aviation industry checklist before taking off in order to prevent plane crashes. Building contractors consult detailed lists for constructing high-rise buildings - to prevent them from falling down. The World Health Organization noted that as numbers of surgeries increased worldwide, so were complications and deaths. WHO asked Gawande to develop a checklist to make surgery safer.

Gawande saw that two lists were necessary - a detailed list for critical steps to be taken (process); and a list of required communications (assessment). In 1993,1 developed checklists to improve communications by avoiding cursory assessments assess symptoms, using the nursing process to insure consistent communication, informed consent and (patient flow) continuity. All of these are consistently built into the process

- Assessment Checklists (SAVED, RAMP, SCHOLAR, ADL, ADEMERIT)
    - Identify high risk populations by age, chronic illness, communication problems, immunodeficiency and other risk factors
    - Identify and rule out certain high risk symptoms
    - Rule out sepsis and dehydration — more common in high-risk populations

(elderly, debilitated, disabled and pediatric populations).

Force Functions or Safety Features

Guidelines have built-in safety features to avoid errors related to:

- *Assessment to support adequate assessments related to symptoms, patient history, and identifying high risk symptoms and patients.*
- *Communication* to ensure clear, accurate instructions throughout the process. Promote improved oral, written, electronic communications, among staff, with physicians, patient or family.
- *Continuity* to strengthen and promote safe, timely access, correct sites for care, and continuity of care.
- *Human Error* to improve decision-making, reduce decision fatigue, distraction, complacency
- *Patient Rights* elements to ensure informed consent, participation in care, pain management

5-Tier Triage Approach to Dispositions

Telephone Triage Task Force worked tirelessly to simplify - in a reasonable, prudent way — what can be a mentally arduous and labor-intensive process - that of eliciting, recognizing and sorting symptoms (triage). This approach, now known as "5-Tier Triage" is a current trend (ENA). Early telephone triage research (Perrin, Lephrohon,1985) hypothesized that pattern recognition was the cognitive skill shown to aid decision making without the benefit of visualization or guidelines.

- *2015 ENA Policy Statement (see Appendix B) outlines a policy to develop a 5-level urgency approach for face-to-face triage **and** telephone triage. Our approach has been based on 5-Level Urgency Triage since 1995. It includes flexible time frames and sites for further evaluation that apply 24/7/365, rather than limited to Office Hours.*

Disposition Clarity and Transparency

A "body of knowledge" for triage requires agreed-upon triage terminology (Manchester Triage Group, 2015)

- nomenclature (Classifications: 5-Tier)
- definitions (Definitions for emergent, urgent, etc)
- teaching (Medical and legal tradition, Joint Commission, evidence-based)
- methodology (Nursing Process)
- audit (QA based on AAACN standards)

Our five-level approach builds upon nomenclature based upon ACEP and Manchester Triage Group standards, dividing symptom patterns into five categories of Urgency as follows:

Life Threatening

- Emergent
- Urgent
- Acute
- Non-Acute

Each level has a time frame and access sites to be further evaluated — as appropriate — depending upon the time and day of the week. Each urgency level is intended as a flexible *time frame and* a flexible *access venue* for the nurse to determine what is safe, timely and prudent. Nurses have a professional responsibility to use good judgment. A common rule of thumb to apply being "when in doubt, err on the side of caution, and bring patients in sooner rather than later".

Life threatening symptoms always require paramedic transport to ED within minutes. They must be kept NPO. Remain on the line with the caller. Whenever possible, institute a three-way conference call with both parties (patient and EMS services, Suicide Prevention, Rape Crisis or Poison center, for example) as directed by your policies.

Emergent level symptoms always require ED services. Some must be kept NPO. Some patients will require paramedic transport; some may be brought by car by a person who can safely bring them in within the appropriate time frame (0-1 hour). Always notify Labor and Delivery or Emergency Department of pending arrivals of any patient coming via car.

Urgent symptoms typically require evaluation within 1-8 hours (same-day appointment). Some may require evaluation within the hour and are instructed by guideline to "Come in now". Depending upon the time of day and day of the week, some patients may be directed, as appropriate, to Emergency Department, Urgent Care, or office settings for further evaluation.

Some patients in Urgent category may also require paramedic transport due to transportation problems. Some may require other reliable, timely transport as is practical, i.e. Uber, Lyft or Taxi etc. if there is no readily available car or if relatives are too anxious to drive them in. Always notify Labor and Delivery or Emergency Department of pending arrivals any patient arriving via car.

Acute Symptoms typically require evaluation within an 8-24 hour time frame, or a next day appointment. Depending upon the time of day and day of the week, some patients may be directed, as appropriate, to Emergency Department, Urgent Care, or office settings for further evaluation. Always notify Labor and Delivery Department, Emergency Department or Psychiatric Emergency of any pending arrivals of patient being transported via car.

Non-Acute Symptoms may require evaluation within a 24+ time frames or future appointment or advice only. Depending upon the time of day and day of the week (available access), these patients may be directed to Emergency Department, Urgent Care, or office settings for further evaluation, as appropriate.

CONTINUING EDUCATION OPTIONS

PLEASE NOTE: *The Preceptor Workbook (details below) is only available with one of the following CE training packages from teletriage.com in CE section:*

"The Update Package" for Telephone Triage: 18 CE Order online at teletriage.com *(CE is available to a single individual only) Provides an update to recent trends in safety, regulations and legal issues in telephone triage.*

- *Risk Management 1 In Telepractice (2005, 2014) (3 CE)*
- *Risk Management 2 In Telepractice (2005, 2014) (3 CE)*
- *Risk Management 3 in Telepractice (2014) (1 CE)*
- *Safety of Decision makers in Telephone Triage (2015) (6 CE)*
- *Protocol Competency (2012) (5 CE)* Includes one volume of Adult or Pediatric Guidelines
- *Audiolinks to* 10 case studies (2009)
- Preceptor Workbook Download 200 pages (Free)
- Standards Manual Download 80 pages (Free)

Guideline Competency: 5 CE Course may be ordered online at teletriage.com.

- A single volume of Adult, Infant-Child or School-Age Guidelines
- Audio links to 10 case studies (2009)
- Preceptor Workbook Download 200 pages (Free)
- Standards Manual Download 80 pages (Free)

PRECEPTOR WORKBOOK

Telephone Triage: Essentials for Expert Clinical Practice

Description: 200-page workbook with Answer Key serves as an update to the 1993 training manual. It focuses on the essential elements the Role, Risks, Rules of Thumb, Red Flags, Red Herrings, Right Assessment, Right Disposition, and the clinical decision-making process. It also emphasizes methods to reduce errors related to inadequacies in assessment, communication, continuity and human error. The goal of the training manual is to teach participants to get patients to the right place, at the right time, for the right reason.

This training program and tools, processes and strategies utilized in it (for Assessment, Documentation, and Decision Making) represent best practices grounded in an evidence- and standards- based, complete, comprehensive *system* (training program, standards, guidelines, documentation form).

Workbook with Exercises utilizes the methodologies of reading, workbook exercises, and analysis and critique and triage practicum with case studies. Includes 50 Adult and Pediatric written case studies, End of Chapter Exercises and Answer Key. Participants may practice triage skills with Adult and Pediatric written case studies, using a Master

(Generic) Guideline and QA score sheet. Participants will be able to coach less experienced nurses to an adequate level of competency in these areas:

- How to avoid five root causes of error related to telephone triage
- How to utilize Rules of Thumb, Red Flags to make better decisions
- How to utilize five assessment Check Lists and purpose of each
- Improved clinical decision-making process (nursing process), with an emphasis on assessment and communications
- Consistently select safe, timely dispositions from 5-Tier System using 50 Adult and Pediatric case studies

The content contained in this workbook is based on recent research and an article from the American Society of Risk Managers (Groszkruger, D. (2014) Diagnostic Error: Untapped Potential For Improving Patient Safety? Journal of Healthcare Risk Management, Vol 34, No 1, P 38-41), wherein the author stresses the current lack of knowledge about the extent of diagnostic error, and uncertainty about error characteristics and variations in definitions. He recommends remedies such as evidence-based guidelines, remedial education, organizational efforts to reduce human error, improved decision support systems, triggers to identify high risk populations, simulations, post mortem examinations, audits and patient involvement.

Table of Contents

Made in United States
North Haven, CT
10 November 2026

22095619R00200